INTUITIVE
EATING

INTUITIVE EATING

A Revolutionary Anti-Diet Approach

4TH EDITION

EVELYN TRIBOLE, MS, RDN, CEDRD-S
ELYSE RESCH, MS, RDN, CEDRD-S, FAND

ST. MARTIN'S
ESSENTIALS
NEW YORK

In the writing of this book we have changed the names and occupations of all of our personal clients so that their true identities will not, in any way, be revealed, in order to maintain their anonymity. In addition, we use the pronouns *we* and *us* when referring to our work with individual clients, rather than specifying each time which of us has worked with a particular client. It should be noted, however, that each of us has a private clientele; we do not see clients together as a team. When referring to an event in the private life of either of us, we do differentiate between us by putting in parentheses the initials of the one involved—hence (ET) refers to Evelyn Tribole and (ER) refers to Elyse Resch.

First published in the United States by St. Martin's Essentials, an imprint of St. Martin's Publishing Group

INTUITIVE EATING FOURTH EDITION. Copyright © 1995, 2003, 2012, 2020 by Evelyn Tribole, MS, RDN, CEDRD-S, and Elyse Resch, MS, RDN, CEDRD-S, FAND. All rights reserved. Printed in the United States of America. For information, address St. Martin's Publishing Group, 120 Broadway, New York, NY 10271.

www.stmartins.com

The Library of Congress Cataloging-in-Publication Data is available upon request.

ISBN 978-1-250-25519-8 (trade paperback)
ISBN 978-1-250-75828-6 (ebook)

Our books may be purchased in bulk for promotional, educational, or business use. Please contact your local bookseller or the Macmillan Corporate and Premium Sales Department at 1-800-221-7945, extension 5442, or by email at MacmillanSpecialMarkets@macmillan.com.

First Edition: 2020

10 9 8

We dedicate this book to our past and present clients and future
Intuitive Eaters, and to the health professionals doing this work:

May you have dignity, health, and happiness—regardless
of your body size or shape.
May you never doubt your inner wisdom or experiences.

Contents

Contents

Acknowledgments

We are grateful to many people, including, but not limited to the following:

David Hale Smith, Inkwell Management, LLC, our agent, for championing our work from the very beginning, and his associate, Naomi Eisenbeiss, for her swift attention to detail.

Jennifer Weis, former editor of St. Martin's Press, for her enthusiastic vision, and the editorial team for their guidance, especially Sallie Lotz, Assistant Editor, St. Martin's Publishing Group.

Tracy Tylka, PhD, for validating Intuitive Eating through her seminal research and creating the Intuitive Eating Assessment Scales.

Deb Burgard, PhD, FAED, for her critical and compassionate feedback.

The following researchers for sharing their tools and insight:
Kristin Neff, PhD, Lindo Bacon, PhD, Carl Lavie, MD, Catherine Cook-Cottone, PhD, Janet Polivy, PhD, and C. Peter Herman, PhD, Ellen Satter, MS, RDN, MSSW, Susie Ohrbach, Jane Hirschmann, PhD, and Carol Munter, Laurel Mellin, PhD, Rachel Calgero, PhD, Diane Neumark-Sztainer, PhD, MPH, RD, Traci Mann, PhD, Leann Birch, PhD, Cynthia Price, PhD, MA, LMT.

To the following communities for advocating Intuitive Eating:
Health at Every Size, Certified Intuitive Eating Counselors & Facilitators, the Intuitive Eating Online Community, the Instagram #IntuitiveEatingVillage, #IntuitiveEatingOfficial, and the EDRD Pro Community.

Arlene Drake, PhD, LMFT, my wife, for her constant and nurturing support, advice, and patience. (ER)

Daniel P. Brown, PhD, my meditation teacher, for his insight and guidance. (ET)

Ellen Ledley, LCSW, my therapist, for her wisdom and understanding. (ER)

Chrissy Roletter for her marketing vision to help spread the word on Intuitive Eating. (ET)

Karen Freeman, MS, RDN, CSSD, my dearest friend, for a lifetime of support, especially during this project. (ER)

Ryan Seay, PhD, and Lisa Du Breuil, LICSW, for their wise counsel. (ET)

Shazi Shabatian, MS, RDN (Associate) and the members of the professional group I supervise, for their input and encouragement. (ER)

Samantha Mullen for her reliable support with all Intuitive Eating projects and Greta Jarvis, MS, for helping with social media. (ET)

To our family and friends, whose unselfish understanding gave us the freedom to complete this book.

And lastly, to the outstanding Intuitive Eating professionals who are carrying on the torch of our work to generations to come.

Foreword

*This [the brain's] integrative function illuminates how reasoning,
once thought to be a "purely logical" mode of thinking, is in fact,
dependent on the nonrational processing of our bodies.*
—Daniel Siegel, M.D., *Mindsight*, 2010

Intuitive Eating was originally published in 1995. Over the years, hundreds of thousands of people have read this book. While reading it, they have had a sense, at a gut level, of "getting it." We've gotten many letters and emails saying "you're writing about me," or "how did you know I felt this way," or "finally someone gets it." Just as so many have "gotten it"—there are others who have asked what Intuitive Eating really means. Are we just driven by instinct? Do we just "know" what and how much and when to eat? In introducing this fourth edition, we'd like to take this opportunity to be as clear as we can in answering the question of what Intuitive Eating really is.

Knowing a bit about the human brain can help us to understand why we're born with all the wisdom we need to be Intuitive Eaters. It can also help us to see how we're able to live an Intuitive Eating life, even while being bombarded by the unending choices of natural and refined foods available to us every day—and the relentless diet messages that abound.

Humans are privileged to experience a dynamic interplay of instinct, emotion, and thought, which work together to orchestrate life, and are mediated by the brain. Psychiatrist and mindfulness expert Daniel Siegel, MD, calls this process "Mindsight." There are three regions of the brain responsible for this powerful integration.

The first region is called the reptilian brain, because when the early reptiles roamed the Earth, they acted and responded exclusively by instinct. They didn't rationalize or feel—they simply went for it. As life evolved, another level of brain function developed, called the limbic brain, which mammals also possess. Emotions and social behaviors originate here. In the limbic brain, feelings are layered upon the instincts of the reptilian brain. The instincts originating from the reptilian brain are sent to the limbic brain, which serves to expand awareness (Levine 1997). Eventually, the third key region of the brain, called the rational brain, or the neo-cortex, evolved. The rational brain integrates instincts and feelings from the other two brain regions. The rational brain does not control instincts—instead, it perceives the instinctual and feeling parts of our beings and reflects upon them. The rational brain creates thoughts and language.

Intuitive Eating embraces all three parts of the human brain. In infancy and toddlerhood, eating is mostly instinctual. As we grow older, thoughts and feelings often play a part in our decisions about eating. As we often tell our clients, our bodies are not just composed of the tongue and the stomach, but also the mind. We have often heard someone say, "I thought that as an Intuitive Eater, I could eat whatever I wanted. So now I eat whatever I want and as much as I want, whenever I feel like it!" This comment actually distorts the premise of Intuitive Eating. Yes, make peace with food, and eat what pleases your palate. Yes, give yourself the freedom to eat unconditionally, and eat as much as you need to satisfy your body. But eating whenever you feel like it, without regard to hunger and fullness, might not be a very satisfying experience and might also cause physical discomfort. Attunement with your body's satiety cues is an important part of this process.

As an Intuitive Eater, you will be honoring your brain, because it is part of your body. As you go through the principles of Intuitive Eating, you will be storing information in the memory "files" that you create and house in your brain. When you feel hungry, you will need to pull up several of these files while deciding what to eat. You will evaluate how hungry you feel and then think about what foods might satisfy your hunger and your taste buds. You might even go through a series of sensual imaginings of the taste and texture and temperature of different foods. You also may open the file to reflect on past eating experiences. You might ask yourself whether your present eating choice has worked out for you when you've eaten it in the past. Did it sustain you long enough? Did it make your blood sugar crash? Did you end up with indigestion? Or did you thoroughly enjoy the food and want to have it again? Your emotions may also come into play when you have the desire to eat. Might you be upset and craving food to comfort and soothe yourself? Or are you bored and thinking about eating as a distraction? Considering these possibilities might inform your decision of what to eat, or even whether to eat at all.

In the beginning of your journey to reclaim your Intuitive Eater, you will probably be hyperconscious of hunger, fullness, satisfaction, thoughts, and emotions. Your brain will need to be highly in tune with your tongue and your stomach. As you become more adept at recognizing your inner signals, you may find that your instincts and intuitive wisdom take a more prominent role in your eating experience. Intuitive Eating is truly about trusting that you will be able to access all of the information you need, by using all aspects of your brain—your reptilian instincts, your limbic connection with your emotions, and your rational thoughts.

Getting back to the roots of this book, it is hard for us to believe that it has been twenty-five years since *Intuitive Eating* was originally published. Although the time has flown by rapidly, the years have been packed with profound experiences. We have received innumerable phone calls, emails, social media messages, and letters from people in all parts of the country and around the world. These communications have brought us into the lives of people we could never have known without this book. We have heard stories about how *Intuitive Eating* has changed lives and healed relationships with food and body. We have talked with people who are in the beginning of their journey and are reaching out to us for more individualized intensive work—whether in person, by telephone, or virtually. We have also received thanks from those who have used the book as a springboard for their own personal healing and have succeeded in the process on their own.

We have been asked to refer people to nutrition therapists and other health professionals in other locales who are familiar with Intuitive Eating. In order to spread the word, we have trained more than one thousand professionals throughout the world to become Certified Intuitive Eating Counselors and Lay Facilitators. We have given talks at professional meetings, as well as to students and to the lay public, and have made television appearances and been interviewed on the radio and for podcasts. We have been quoted in articles in newspapers, magazines, and on the internet. In addition, professional colleagues have asked our permission to use *Intuitive Eating* as the basis of college lectures, workshops, and seminars of their own.

The impact of all of these experiences has been deeply meaningful for us. It has given us the opportunity to broaden the work that we had previously done in our offices, by telephone, or virtually, working with individuals, one on one. We have been able to extend the philosophy of *Intuitive Eating* to those whom we would have never been able to reach if not for the book.

It has touched our souls to be able to hear how *Intuitive Eating* has changed the lives of so many. One of the most frequent comments that we have heard from people concerns the despair they felt after years and years of failed dieting experiences and the new hope that blossomed after finding and reading *Intuitive Eating*. We have heard how some have cleared their minds of punitive and obsessive thoughts about their eating and body perception. This clearing has made room for positive thinking and determination to make serious life changes. Self-esteem has catapulted, as people have reported the empowerment they have felt by working with a process that honors the validity of one's inner voice. Through *Intuitive Eating*, they have learned to trust the wisdom that has always been within but has been blunted by years of self-doubt. Doubting their innate eating signals had extended to doubting their beliefs about many other aspects of their lives.

We have heard stories about people who have left abusive relationships, made peace with estranged loved ones, and made significant career changes once their struggle with food and body had been resolved. We have also heard about new romances that, for some, could not have been possible while they were occupied with body concerns and focused on the latest doomed diet attempt. *Intuitive Eating* has freed all of these people to go on with their lives, while leaving behind self-doubt and the despair that had resulted from their painful relationship with food. (It needs to be kept in consideration, however, that higher-weight people are likely to continue to face discrimination, even after they have become Intuitive Eaters.)

Intuitive Eating has also changed the lives of many of our professional colleagues. At every conference we attend, we hear comments from nutrition therapists and psychotherapists about how grateful they are to have this book to give to their patients. They tell us how it makes their lives easier, having it for use as a guidebook in their private practices, for classes they teach, and for seminars they give. We have also found, in our own professional lives, that having a book that we have written available for our patients to take home with them to use as a reference is an invaluable aid in our practices. We've been told that it helps some people feel that they can carry a part of us with them for support when they need it!

In this fourth edition, there are some new additions that we hope will reach a broader base of readers and will offer some new tools for everyone. First, we have added a section on baby-led weaning/solids to the chapter on raising an Intuitive Eater. Our goal is to help parents protect their children's inner wisdom about eating, with which they were born. We also want to give advice to parents about repairing a fractured relationship that they may have with their children around the eating experience. How wonderful it would be if all children were able to retain their inborn Intuitive Eating throughout their lives!

Second, we have expanded the chapter on the research validating the benefits of Intuitive Eating. When we originally cultivated the premise of Intuitive Eating, we reviewed evidence from hundreds of studies, which, in addition to our clinical experience, ultimately formed the basis of the ten Intuitive Eating principles. Although our original concept is evidenced-based (or, more accurately, evidenced-inspired), it's really not the same thing as saying, "studies show that Intuitive Eating works." Until recently, that is.

When we first wrote *Intuitive Eating*, we had no idea that our concept would generate many studies, which we find absolutely exciting! To date, there have been more than 125 studies on Intuitive Eating, with several that are currently underway. In this update, we discuss the exciting research on interoceptive awareness, which is the underpinning of Intuitive Eating. The basic definition of interoceptive awareness is our ability to perceive physical sensations that arise from within the body. This includes bodily states such as a full bladder or racing heart, and satiety and hunger cues. Every emotion has a unique felt sensation in the body, like a physical fingerprint. When we listen to our bodies via interoceptive awareness we have a treasure trove of information to get our biological and psychological needs met! In other words, our wants, needs, and emotions are very much tied to the direct experience of sensations in our here-and-now bodies. The Intuitive Eating principles work by either increasing interoceptive awareness, or by removing the obstacles to this "superpower." The obstacles usually arise from the mind in the form of rules, beliefs, and thoughts.

We have continued to direct our focus to satisfaction as a driving force in the Intuitive Eating process. You will see how seeking satisfaction in your eating will both profoundly inform all of the other principles in the book, as well as how the other principles will affect finding satisfaction. Updates have also been made throughout. Over the years, we have especially become sensitive to the impact that any mention of numbers has on our readers. Whether the numbers refer to weight, height, or serving sizes and recommendations, these numbers can trigger comparison and negative feelings. So, wherever possible, numbers have been removed. In addition to numbers, most statements regarding weight have been removed, as we believe that any focus on weight can only perpetuate the toxic weight stigma that exists in our culture. This problem is so pervasive that we added sections on diet culture and weight stigma so you can really understand how it impacts you, even if you are not consciously dieting!

Be sure to check out our new Intuitive Eating resources section, which provides information on resources (including our Intuitive Eating Online Community, *The Intuitive Eating Workbook,* and the *Intuitive Eating Workbook for Teens*)—to give you the tools and information to further support your Intuitive Eating journey.

We have also felt that it was very important to keep the appendix, entitled "Step-by-Step Guidelines," in this version of the book. This readily accessible outline will be a boon to old and new readers as you go through this journey. If it's your first time around with the book, you can choose to read the book in its entirety and then use the outline to remind you of the whole process. Readers already familiar with the Intuitive Eating process can use this section as a way to review the concept and as a handy shorthand method of checking in. Or, you might decide to read about one principle at a time and then use the part of the outline that refers to that principle to fortify your focus on each step. (And just a word about the order of the principles: some people may find that they're drawn to a particular principle and want to read about it out of order. There is no "right way" to absorb Intuitive Eating—just go with your gut, as you read the entire book.) Whatever you choose, we hope that the step-by-step guidelines will provide a helpful tool for you in your Intuitive Eating work.

Finally, we would like to express our gratitude to the many people we have had the honor to meet and work with over the years. You have been our teachers, even as we have counseled you on your healing path. You have inspired us to continue this work and bring out this fourth edition of *Intuitive Eating.* Thank you!

If you could cash in every diet like a frequent-flyer mileage program, most of us would have earned a trip to the moon and back. The global weight-loss industry market is expected to reach $278.95 billion by 2023, which could finance the trip for generations to come. Ironically, we seem to have more respect for our cars than for ourselves. If you took your car to an auto mechanic for regular tune-ups, and after time and money spent the car didn't work, you wouldn't blame yourself.* Yet in spite of the fact that up to 95 percent of all diets fail, you tend to blame yourself, not the diet! Isn't it ironic that with a massive failure rate for dieting we don't blame the *process* of dieting?

But what does failure really mean? It has traditionally referred to the fact that the majority of people who go on diets and lose weight gain it back, with many gaining even more weight. (Studies show that up to two-thirds of folks will regain more weight than they lost!) To focus on weight loss as the definition of failure fails to address the root issue: Why are people so focused on losing weight? Why is there a valuing of thinner over fatter bodies? Why do people value themselves based on the number on the scale? The failure of dieting is that it promotes weight stigma by not recognizing that people come in all sizes and shapes and that each individual is worthy just as they are. In this book, we want to provide you with information that may let you stop blaming yourself and your body. We'll present some new ideas that will help you value your individuality and everything that makes you your authentic self.

---

* This industry report includes: bariatric surgery, foods, fitness equipment and gyms, weight-loss products and programs. https://tinyurl.com/Global-stats

Initially, when we ventured into the world of private practice, we did not know each other. Yet separately, we had remarkably similar counseling experiences that caused us to rethink how we work. This led to a considerable change in how we practice and years later was the impetus for this book.

Although we practiced independently of each other, unknowingly each of us got started by making a vow to avoid the trap of working with "weight control." We didn't want to prescribe a process that was only set up to fail. But while we tried to avoid weight-loss counseling, physicians kept referring their patients to us. Typically, their blood pressure or cholesterol was high. Whatever their medical problems, weight loss was thought to be the key to treatment. Because we wanted to help these patients, we embarked on the weight-loss issue with a commitment to do it differently: Our patients would succeed. They would be among that small 5 percent success group. Clearly, our consciousness had not as yet been raised to even question the whole focus on weight that pervades much of society. Also, at that time there was not the body of research that we have today, which shows dismal failure rates and harm from dieting.

We created beautiful meal plans according to our patients' likes and dislikes, lifestyles, and specific needs. These plans were based on the widely accepted "exchange system," commonly used for diabetic meal planning and "weight control." We told them that this was not a diet, for even back then we knew that diets didn't work. We rationalized that these meal plans were not diets, because patients could choose among chicken, turkey, fish, or lean meat. They could have a bagel, a muffin, or toast. If they really wanted a cookie, they could have one (not five!). They could fill up with "free foods" galore, so that they never had to feel hungry. We told them that if they had a craving for a particular food, they could go ahead and eat it without guilt. But we also reinforced, gently yet firmly, that sticking to their personalized plans would help them achieve their goals. As the weeks went by, our clients were eager to please us and followed their meal plans. We weighed them each week (something we would never do now!), and, finally, their weight goals were met.

Unfortunately, however, some time later we started getting calls from some of these same people telling us how much they needed us again. Somehow, the weight had come back on again. Their calls were very apologetic. Somehow, they couldn't stick to the plan anymore. Maybe they needed someone to monitor them. Maybe they didn't have enough self-control. Maybe they just weren't any good at this, and they felt guilty and demoralized.

In spite of the "failure," our patients put all the blame on themselves. After all, they trusted us—we were the "great nutritionists" who had helped them lose weight. Therefore, *they* had done something wrong, not us. As time went on, it became clear that something was very wrong with this approach. All of our good intentions were only reinforcing some very negative, self-effacing notions that our patients had about themselves— that they didn't have self-control, they couldn't do it; therefore they were bad or wrong. This led to guilt, guilt, guilt.

By this time, we had both reached a turning point in the way we counseled. How could we ethically go on teaching people things that seemed logical and nutritionally sound, yet triggered such emotional upheaval? On the other hand, how could we neglect an area of treatment that could have such a profound effect on a patient's future health? (Or so we had been trained to think!)

As we struggled with these issues, we began to explore some of the popular literature, as well as scientific studies that suggested a 180-degree departure from dieting of any kind (even dietitian-approved). Some of the founding professionals who paved the way via a non-diet approach and influenced us included Jane R. Hirschmann, CSW; Carol H. Munter; Lela Zaphiropoulos, CSW; Susie Orbach, PhD; Janet Polivy, PhD; C. Peter Herman, PhD; and Leann L. Birch, PhD; among others. They proposed a way of eating that allowed for any and all food choices but did not address nutrition. Our initial reactions were highly skeptical, if not downright rejecting. How could we, as nutritionists (registered dietitians), trained to look at the connections between nutrition and health, sanction a way of eating that seemed to reject the very foundation of our knowledge?

The struggle continued. The "healthy" meal plans were keeping people attached to diet culture, with the intermittent despair that came with it, yet the "demand feeding" described in the popular psychology books in the late 1960s through the '80s seemed incomplete.

Eventually, we resolved the conflict by developing the Intuitive Eating process with ten principles. Special note to health professionals: We have come to realize that this conflict, or cognitive dissonance, is a common experience for health professionals, who have been trained in weight-centric health care—that a person's weight determines their health. There's a lot more to health than what you eat—your relationship with food, mental health, social determinants of health, to name a few. Besides, body weight is not a behavior. It becomes a journey of the great unlearning and it feels uncomfortable at first. Just know that you are not alone in this reckoning.

Our book became a bridge between the growing anti-diet movement and the health community. How do you reconcile forbidden food issues and still eat nutritiously, while not dieting? We will tell you how in this book.

If you are like most of our clients, you are weary of dieting and following rigid food plans yet terrified of eating. Most of our clients arrive in our offices uncomfortable in their bodies. *Intuitive Eating* provides a new way of eating that is ultimately struggle-free and healthy for your mind and body. It is a process that unleashes the shackles of dieting (which can only lead to deprivation, rebellion, and rebound weight gain). It means getting back to your roots—trusting your body and your signals. *Intuitive Eating* will not only change your relationship with food; it will change your life. In fact, many of the clients mentioned in this book came to us simply for the purpose of losing weight. Even though they may have mentioned physical discomfort in their bodies or emotional discomfort, believing that they were not good enough unless they lost weight, they eventually learned to find comfort and gratitude in the "here and now."

We do not judge people for their desire to lose weight—it's a consequence of diet culture, which is ubiquitous and problematic. It's a societal system of beliefs, messages, and behaviors that places value on a person's weight and appearance, rather than well-being, which unfortunately, has become common and normalized. Diet culture reifies thinness, equating it with health and moral virtue, while demonizing some foods and elevating others. It's difficult to go even a single day without hearing conversations, seeing ads, scrolling through social media that involve some aspect of shrinking bodies. Health professionals are not immune to diet culture, as some health care professionals put patients on calorie-restricted or entire food group–restricted diets, even though there is not a single study to date showing that it's sustainable or efficacious in the long run, or without harm. Sadly, research indicates that health professionals are one of the main perpetuators of weight stigma.

The problem is that any focus on weight loss will sabotage your ability to reconnect with your body's Intuitive Eating signals. When you focus on weight, it places your attention on external measures for eating—such as the portions of foods, the macros of food—rather than connecting you with your internal cues. (That's why we like to say that Intuitive Eating is an inside job.) Instead, focusing on your day-to-day progress—such as getting more satisfaction from your meals and staying more present in eating and life—will give you a sense of connection, which can lead to feelings of joy and well-being.

But before we go on, we want to mention a caveat. This book was written by two cis-gender white women with thin privilege who feel grateful for the many privileges each acknowledges. Neither of us has dealt with food insecurity or the weight stigma that is experienced by many who may be reading this book.

It will be important to work with a practitioner who is trained both in Intuitive Eating and in the specialty issue affecting you, including but not limited to: trauma, medical nutrition therapy, eating disorders, and mental illness. In addition, some people don't have access to the resources they need in order to learn this process, and that needs to be acknowledged. We acknowledge that we don't even know all the reasons that might prevent people from accessing these resources. Intuitive Eating is a privilege.

We wish that the suffering that so many experience in this world did not exist. We will keep working toward making this a better world—one in which Intuitive Eating can be accessible to all bodies. Intuitive Eating is one tool, and we are constantly learning and striving toward radical inclusivity.

Intuitive Eating is a compassionate, self-care eating framework that treats all bodies with dignity and respect.

We care deeply about the relationship you have with your body and the relationship that may form between us as the authors and you as the reader. We are humbly open to feedback on how we can do better.

We hope you find that Intuitive Eating will make a difference in your life; it has for our clients. In fact, when our clients learned that we were writing this book, they wanted to share some specific turning points with you:

- "Be sure to tell them that if they have a binge, it can actually turn out to be a great experience, because they'll learn so much about their thoughts and feelings, as a result of the binge."
- "Tell them that taking a time-out to see if they're hungry doesn't mean that they can't eat if they find they're not hungry. It's just a time-out to make sure that they're not eating on autopilot. If they want to eat anyway, they can!"
- "When I come to a session, I feel as if I'm going to the priest

for confession. That comes from all the times I used to go to the diet doctor, and I would have to tell him how I had sinned after he had weighed me. This isn't coming from you, but the inner Food Police."

• "I feel like I'm out of prison. I'm free and not thinking about food all the time anymore."

• "Sometimes I get angry, because food has lost its magic. Nothing tastes quite as good as it did when it was forbidden. I kept looking for the old thrill that food used to give me until I realized that my excitement in life wasn't going to come from my eating anymore."

• "With permission comes choice. And making choices based on what I want and not on what somebody else is telling me feels so empowering."

• "After giving up bingeing, I ended up feeling pretty low some of the time and even rageful at other times. I realized that the food was covering up my bad feelings. But it was also covering up my good feelings. I'd rather feel good and bad rather than not feel at all!"

• "When I saw how much I was using dieting and eating to cope with life, I realized that I had to change some of the stress in my life if I ever wanted to let go of food as a coping mechanism."

• "Sometimes I have hungry days, and sometimes I have full days. It's so nice to eat more sometimes and not feel guilty that I'm going against some plan."

• "I get so exhilarated when I see a food I used to restrict. Now I think—it's free, it's there, and it's mine!"

• "I'm so glad you're writing this book; it will help me explain what I'm doing. All I know is that it works!"

• "When I'm in the diet mentality, I can't think about the real problems in my life."

• "This is the best I've ever taken care of myself in my life."

Note: We recognize that gender is a spectrum, and in this version of Intuitive Eating we will be gender inclusive by using gender-neutral language and pronouns, unless we are referring to a specific person who has specified their pronoun.

Chapter 1

The Science Behind
Intuitive Eating

When we cultivated the premise of Intuitive Eating, we reviewed evidence from hundreds of studies, which, in addition to our clinical experience, ultimately formed the basis for the ten Intuitive Eating principles. Today, the research on Intuitive Eating itself is robust, with more than 125 published studies showing benefits—with the growing recognition that IE is an adaptive eating style, which influences positive psychological and physical well-being. We've decided to begin by highlighting some of the studies validating the process, benefits, and characteristics of Intuitive Eating, in order to give you a glimpse of the changes that may occur in your life when you rediscover your inner Intuitive Eater.

For a complete list of the studies, see the References: *Intuitive Eating Studies.*

MEDIA IGNITES PUBLIC AND SCIENTIFIC INTEREST

Although our book was originally published in 1995, the tipping point for both research and public interest in our work occurred ten years later, triggered by the publication of two different studies on Intuitive Eating, which sparked global media attention.

In 2005, a professor of health science at Brigham Young University, Steven Hawks, and his colleagues published one of the first studies exploring Intuitive Eating in college students (Hawks et al. 2005). It was a small study, in which women scoring high on an Intuitive Eating scale developed by Hawks and colleagues (2004) were shown to have lower fat levels in the blood and a reduction in the overall risk for heart disease, compared with participants who scored low. In other words, Intuitive

Eaters were associated with better health indicators. This study caught the attention of the media.

Very soon afterward, Dr. Hawks and I (ET) appeared on the *Today* show, discussing Intuitive Eating. Dr. Hawks did several more interviews, including CNN, MSNBC, and the *Washington Post*.

SCIENTIFICALLY DEFINING AND MEASURING INTUITIVE EATING

In 2006, Dr. Tracy Tylka of Ohio State University published a seminal study on nearly thirteen hundred college women, which validated three key features of Intuitive Eating (Tylka 2006):

1. Unconditional permission to eat when hungry and what food is desired.
2. Eating for physical rather than emotional reasons.
3. Reliance on internal hunger and satiety cues to determine when and how much to eat.

Tylka's research was a big undertaking, because in order to assess and validate the key components of Intuitive Eating, a series of four studies were conducted. In the first part of the study, Tylka created and validated the Intuitive Eating Scale (IES) to measure and identify Intuitive Eaters.

Next, the college women completed the Intuitive Eating Scale, along with a series of other tests, in order to evaluate the relationship between Intuitive Eating and several indicators reflecting mental health, body awareness, and eating disorder symptoms.

Women scoring high on the Intuitive Eating Scale were identified as Intuitive Eaters. Compared to women scoring low on this scale, Intuitive Eaters were found to have higher body satisfaction, without internalizing the thin ideal, which indicates that Intuitive Eaters are less likely to base their self-worth on being thin. Intuitive Eating Scale total scores were positively associated with self-esteem, satisfaction with life, optimism, and proactive coping.

In 2013, Tylka updated the Intuitive Eating Scale, with an even larger study of 1,405 women and 1,195 men. This study also validated a fourth characteristic of Intuitive Eaters—the Body-Food Choice Congruence, which reflects the Gentle Nutrition principle and how food feels in your body (Tylka and Kroon Van Diest 2013). Of note, this was the first time that the scale was validated for men.

Notably, Hawks and Tylka independently developed and validated different tools to assess Intuitive Eating characteristics. Hawks's Intuitive Eating Scale (2004a) has four components:

1. Intrinsic Eating (eating is based on inner cues).
2. Extrinsic Eating (eating is based on external influence such as mood, social, and food availability).
3. Anti-Dieting (eating is not based on diets, counting calories, or desire for weight loss).
4. Self-Care (body acceptance, taking care of body regardless of size).

Today, Tylka's IE scales are the most widely used in Intuitive Eating research. Of great significance, both of Tylka's IE assessment scales found that Intuitive Eaters have higher interoceptive awareness. This is really an important concept, because it's part of the scientific underpinning for the process of Intuitive Eating, so let's unpack it.

Interoceptive Awareness Is Your Superpower: *The Foundation for Intuitive Eating*

Interoceptive Awareness. Interoceptive awareness is the ability to perceive physical sensations that arise from within your body. It's a direct experience, a felt sense that happens in the present moment—it's not the past or future, it happens right now. It includes basic states like feeling a distended bladder, hunger and satiety cues, and the felt sense of every emotional feeling. Every emotion has a unique physical sensation in the body. When you perceive bodily sensations, it gives rise to powerful information to help get your psychological and biological needs met. In fact, there is a growing body of research that shows interoceptive awareness is profoundly implicated in your physical and mental well-being (Quadt et al. 2018).

In his seminal book, *How Do You Feel: An Interoceptive Moment with Your Neurobiological Self*, scientist A.D. (Bud) Craig describes the very moment of the felt sense as our *"global emotional moment,"* which is the current state of all our feelings that represent the *sentient self*. We think that's part of the reason people describe Intuitive Eating as life-changing—they get reconnected to their sentient self on a very deep level.

Ultimately, IE is a personal process of honoring health by listening and responding to the direct messages of the body in order to get your needs met. The principles of Intuitive Eating work either by enhancing interoceptive awareness, or by removing the obstacles to perceiving and responding to the felt sensations in the body. The obstacles are usually from the mind in the form of rules, beliefs, and thoughts. (See Table 1.)

The challenge in today's diet culture is that many people do not value, let alone trust, their body sensations. Instead, they eat based on externality—that is, eating according to rules and diet plans, which ultimately create confusion between mind and body. Interoceptive awareness is based on inner sensation, which is an inside job. That's why using external methods to eat—such as counting macros, calories, or points—does not help you connect to your body.

Interoceptive Sensitivity. An excellent study out of Germany asked an important question: How do we know if someone is capable of Intuitive Eating (Herbert et al. 2013)? Since interoceptive awareness is the key mechanism of Intuitive Eating, the researchers decided to use the gold standard objective measure of interoceptive sensitivity, which is the perception of heart rate test. The operative word here is "perception." The researchers hooked people up to electrodes, which independently monitored their heart rate. Meanwhile, they instructed the subjects to count their heart rate, by merely perceiving (no putting their fingers on their pulse). Indeed, those scoring higher on Intuitive Eating had higher accuracy at perceiving their heart rate. For those of you who want to read more about how to do this, we included a perceived heart rate activity in our *Intuitive Eating Workbook*. (An important caveat here: if you have experienced trauma and/or have been dissociated from your body, this will take more unpacking. It may be important to work with a specialist in trauma and Intuitive Eating, depending on your situation.)

Interoceptive Responsiveness. Body awareness itself is only one part of the process of becoming an Intuitive Eater. The way an individual values and responds to these body sensations is known as *interoceptive responsiveness*. Imagine your best friend pounding at your door to deliver helpful news. Although you hear the knocking, you don't bother to let them in. The issue at hand is responsiveness. A 2017 study found that Intuitive Eaters had more body appreciation and interoceptive responsiveness. It's all connected. Notably, body appreciation was the mitigating factor for people to respond to the messages of their body. The cultural challenge, however, is that weight stigma, combined with the influences of patriarchy and healthcare policy, has conditioned us to distrust our bodies and their cues.

When healthcare professionals or scientists are not familiar with our work (or the research), we find it helpful to first explain interoceptive awareness. It seems to get their attention and they see the connection to and validity of Intuitive Eating.

TABLE 1. INTUITIVE EATING PRINCIPLES AND INTEROCEPTIVE AWARENESS	
Improves Interoceptive Awareness	*Removes Obstacles to Interoceptive Awareness*
Honor your hunger. Respect your fullness. Discover the satisfaction factor. Movement—feel the difference.	Reject the diet mentality. Make peace with food. Challenge the Food Police. Cope with your emotions with kindness. Respect your body. Honor your health with gentle nutrition.

STUDIES INDICATE BENEFITS AND CHARACTERISTICS OF INTUITIVE EATING

General Benefits of Intuitive Eating

A recent meta-analysis review of twenty-four studies published between 2006 and 2015 found that Intuitive Eating was associated with the following benefits (Ricciardelli 2016):

- Greater body appreciation and satisfaction
- Positive emotional functioning
- Greater life satisfaction
- Unconditional self-regard and optimism
- Psychological hardiness
- Greater motivation to exercise, when focus is on enjoyment rather than guilt or appearance

Furthermore, IE was inversely related to: disordered eating, dieting, poor interoceptive awareness, and internalization of the thin ideal.

Adolescents

Sally Dockendorff and colleagues (2011) adapted Tylka's Intuitive Eating Scale for over five hundred middle school adolescents. Dockendorff's team identified another key component of Intuitive Eating—trust. As in trusting the body's innate hunger and satiety cues. In other words, it wasn't enough to be aware of hunger and satiety cues; Intuitive Eaters in this age group also trusted their bodies to tell them when and how much to eat. Given the growing demonization of food and weight stigma, cultivating trust may be a significant feature for Intuitive Eaters, regardless of age. Notably, Dockendorff reported findings similar to Tylka's results on college women (2006). Adolescents who scored high on Dockendorff's Intuitive Eating Scale had: (a) lower internalization of culturally thin ideals, (b) lower body dissatisfaction, and (c) fewer mood problems. Intuitive Eaters had better life satisfaction scores and experienced a greater positive mood. This is a noteworthy finding, as adolescents are particularly vulnerable to hormone fluctuations and peer pressure to fit in, which can influence mood and life satisfaction.

Health Properties of Intuitive Eaters' Food Choices

Some critics express concern about one of the key components of Intuitive Eating—unconditional permission to eat when hungry and to eat whatever food is desired. They assert that if people were "allowed" to eat whatever they wanted, it would result in unhealthy diets and weight gain. To address this contention, Smith and Hawks (2006) designed a study involving nearly 350 male and female college students and evaluated the health-related properties of the food choices made by Intuitive Eaters. Contrary to the expectation of critics, students scoring high on the Hawks Intuitive Eating Scale (2004a) ate a more diverse diet and had a lower body mass index. Furthermore, there was no association between Intuitive Eating and the amount of "junk food" eaten in the diet. In other words, Intuitive Eaters were not eating an unbalanced diet. Intuitive Eaters also reported taking more pleasure in their eating. Interestingly, more men than women were rated as Intuitive Eaters (173 and 124 students, respectively). A scholarly review evaluated the relationship between IE and health indicators and found that IE was associated with improved blood pressure, blood lipids, and dietary intake (Van Dyke & Drinkwater 2014).

A Note About the Body Mass Index (BMI): The BMI is fraught with problems because it does not accurately reflect health status—in fact, it is a poor determinant of health (which we describe in more depth on page 209).

Preliminary research indicates that Intuitive Eating is associated with weight stability (Tylka et al. 2019), which may be an important determinant of health. Conversely, weight cycling (the repeated gaining and losing weight) may increase the risk of developing heart disease or type 2 diabetes (Bacon and Aphramor 2011).

For some people, there may be a side effect of weight loss as a consequence of implementing the IE principles, especially if Intuitive Eating has helped them get their self-care needs met. Yet it would be a mistake to promote IE for weight loss, as it would undermine and interfere with the process, because IE is an internally based process, whereas a focus on body weight is externally based. It would also philosophically counter HAES, Health at Every Size, which we discuss in more detail on p. 214 and reinforce weight stigma. A recent three-year prospective study illustrates this problem. Women who were trying to lose weight had a *reduction* in their IES at year three, compared to their baseline scores (Leong and Gray 2016). Furthermore, these women had an increase in binge eating, which is consistent with the body of research linking dieting to binge-eating behaviors.

The main purpose of Intuitive Eating is to cultivate a healthy relationship with food, mind, and body. It is a weight-neutral model, meaning that the focus is not on body size, but rather on healing your relationship with food.

Health and Well-Being

Positive health psychology represents the more positive aspects of one's character, such as feeling upbeat, happy, and appreciative, and has been shown by several studies to predict future levels of health and well-being. Moreover, these effects accumulate and compound over time, making people healthier, more socially integrated, effective, and resilient. Also, there are documented physical health benefits of such states, which include lower levels of the stress chemical cortisol and less inflammation. A study by Tylka and Wilcox (2006) of 340 college women showed that two core constructs of Intuitive Eating, (1) eating for physical rather than emotional reasons and (2) reliance on internal hunger and satiety cues to determine when and how much to eat, uniquely contribute to psychological well-being, including: optimism, psychological hardiness (an indicator of resilience, or the ability to recover from adversity), unconditional self-regard, positive affect, proactive coping, and social problem-solving.

The study's findings highlight the importance of a person's ability to detect and attend to their emotions and their biological cues of hunger and satiety, as detection and awareness of these states are uniquely connected to well-being. These findings validate many of the Intuitive Eating principles (*honor your hunger, respect your fullness, cope with feelings with kindness, reject the diet mentality*).

Eating Disorders. A study from Germany looked specifically at the relationship between IE and individuals who had a range of eating disorders (Van Dyck et al. 2016). It provided the first evidence for reduced IE scores in individuals with eating disorders and suggested the IES could be a useful tool in monitoring recovery progress. This is consistent with other research, which indicates promise for using IE in the prevention and treatment of eating disorders. Similarly, a study on retired athletes indicates that IE may help reduce disordered eating and help athletes to relearn how to trust their bodies' signals about hunger and satiety once they leave their sport (Plateau et al. 2016).

The most promising study to date asked the question: Can patients with eating disorders learn to eat intuitively? (Richards et al. 2017). The study's finding was a resounding yes. This two-year pilot study found that the Intuitive Eating principles could be effectively taught in a residential treatment setting. There was improvement across the board in patients with anorexia nervosa, bulimia, and eating disorders not otherwise specified (EDNOS). It should be noted, however, that undernourished brains may have difficulty in sensing hunger signals, and slowed stomach emptying, which can lead to continual fullness, will not give an accurate end point to eating. With re-nourishment, these signals become more reliable and noticeable.

A 2019 study by a team of European researchers looked at eighty-six people—forty-four with anorexia nervosa and forty-two healthy controls to evaluate the relationships between Intuitive Eating, eating disorder recovery, and interoceptive sensitivity (which was measured by having both groups perceive their heart rate (a process described earlier in this chapter). There were a number of key findings from this study:

- The healthy controls who scored higher on Intuitive Eating had higher interoceptive sensitivity (not surprising, but good validation).
- As the patients with anorexia improved in their recovery, evidenced by better weight restoration with a longer stay in the hospital, they improved in both interoceptive sensitivity and Intuitive Eating assessment scores.
- In both groups, stronger interoceptive sensitivity meant stronger Intuitive Eating.

This is a very promising study for eating disorder recovery!

Diabetes. Emerging research suggests IE programs could be a valuable tool to improve blood sugar control (Wheeler et al. 2016; Willig et al. 2014). In children and adolescents with type 1 diabetes mellitus, there was an inverse relationship between hemoglobin A1c and IE scores. IE may have even more saliency with managing diabetes, because people with diabetes are at higher risk of developing eating disorders, and IE is associated with decreased risk of problematic eating.

Intervention Studies

In 2017, I (ET) was a guest on Christy Harrison's *Food Psych* podcast and shared that one of my personal motivations for writing the *Intuitive Eating Workbook* was to have a standardized method for researchers to use in intervention studies. Blair Burnette, from Virginia Commonwealth University, heard that interview and contacted me with a research idea using the IE workbook. Two years later, she finished the study, using the *Intuitive Eating Workbook* in college-aged women in both individual and group settings and got some exciting results:

- Decreases in body dissatisfaction, dietary restraint, frequency of binge eating and loss-of-control eating, and weight bias internalization.
- Increases in body appreciation, body functionality appreciation,

overall Intuitive Eating (and all subscales of the IES-2), intuitive exercise, and satisfaction with life!

A recent short-term study used a combination of IE with acceptance commitment therapy (ACT) (Boucher et al. 2016). ACT is a validated counseling process that cultivates psychological flexibility via mindfulness, based on a person's value system. Women who completed the three-month intervention improved in these areas: binge eating, general mental health, psychological flexibility, and IE.

A ten-week worksite wellness intervention program combined IE and mindfulness to address problematic eating behaviors, which is an unintended consequence of many traditional worksite wellness programs, because they focus on weight loss (Bush et al. 2014). The intervention group had improvements in body appreciation, IE, and problematic eating behaviors compared to the waitlisted control group. Notably, weight and BMI were not used as indicators of success, because focus on weight alone may trigger problematic eating.

FACTORS THAT PROMOTE OR INTERFERE WITH INTUITIVE EATING

Studies show that there are many factors that influence Intuitive Eating, such as comments and feeding practices by parents and other caregivers, self-silencing of thoughts and feelings, body acceptance and appreciation, and cultural westernization, including exposure to weight stigma and diet culture. These studies are described in the following section.

Parent/Caregiver Feeding Practices and Eating Messages

Parental Feeding Practices. Galloway and colleagues (2010) evaluated the impact of parental feeding practices on Intuitive Eating and body mass index with a novel study design. Nearly one hundred college-aged students and their parents completed retrospective questionnaires of parental feeding practices regarding the college students' childhood. Examples of the questions included: Did your parent keep track of _____:

- The sweets (candy, ice cream, cake, pies, and pastries) that you ate?

- The snack foods (such as potato chips) that you ate?
- The high-fat foods that you ate?

Next, the researchers measured the students' Intuitive Eating levels using Tylka's Intuitive Eating Scale. The results showed that parental monitoring and restriction of food intake had a significant impact on their college student's emotional eating and Intuitive Eating Scale scores.

Parents who monitored and restricted their daughters' eating had daughters who: (a) reported significantly more emotional eating and (b) were less inclined to eat for physical reasons of hunger and satiety. The association was different for the male college students. Parents who recollected restriction of their son's food intake did not report higher emotional eating. This might be due to the difference of social pressure for women to conform to the thin ideal. The researchers concluded that controlling feeding practices by parents has potentially long-term consequences and may contribute to the development of emotional eating.

Impact of Parent and Caregiver Eating Messages. Kroon Van Diest and Tylka (2010) report similar findings from a study on college-aged men and women. They created and validated a questionnaire that asked students to rate the degree to which their parents/caregivers emphasized the following types of behaviors while growing up:

- Told you that you shouldn't eat certain foods because they will "make you fat."
- Talked about dieting or restricting certain high-calorie foods.
- Commented that you are eating too much.

They found that high levels of critical and restrictive eating messages from caregivers were associated with low Intuitive Eating scores and higher body mass index scores.

These Intuitive Eating studies on parental feeding practices add to the body of research by L.L. Birch, which shows that when parents attempt to restrict children's eating, it backfires by disconnecting them from their natural hunger and satiety cues, ultimately creating the very problem they were trying to circumvent. These studies also support many principles of Intuitive Eating, including: *challenge the Food Police, honor your hunger, feel your fullness, and make peace with food.*

Self-Silencing. Self-silencing is the suppression of one's thoughts, feelings, or needs, and it is a gender phenomenon influencing women's mental health. Although it hasn't been documented in studies of gay men and people on the gender spectrum, we think that this is a strong possibility, and our understanding of the issue would benefit from further research. The process of self-silencing is thought to begin in adolescence, a vulnerable time when body dissatisfaction and social pressures emerge. When silencing their voices, young women may begin to ignore or suppress physiological or hunger cues that are inconsistent with societal ideas of thinness. Expression of thoughts, feelings, or needs appears to be a critical aspect of healthy eating behaviors. In a study that involved only women and not others on the gender spectrum, Shouse and Nilsson (2011) evaluated the relationship between disordered eating, Intuitive Eating, and self-silencing and found that Intuitive Eating is maximized when a woman has high levels of emotional awareness, combined with low levels of self-silencing.

However, when high emotional awareness was coupled with more self-silencing, participants had more disordered eating and less Intuitive Eating. The researchers believe that when women have clarity about their thoughts and feelings, but silence their voices, hunger signals may become confused, which may decrease trust of internal signals of hunger and satiation. The most intuitive and least disordered eaters in the study displayed high emotional awareness and low self-silencing. The results of this study validate the principles *challenge the Food Police* and *cope with your emotions with kindness*. (Note: More research needs to be done for folks on the entire gender spectrum.)

ACCEPTANCE AND BODY APPRECIATION

While the ability to eat intuitively is inborn, the likelihood of remaining an Intuitive Eater is influenced by the environment, which includes family, friends, and exposure to weight stigma and diet culture, as mentioned above. Intuitive Eating can be thwarted by an environment that lacks acceptance and/or imposes rigid rules for eating that ignore a person's inner experience (such as hunger or satisfaction). When people encourage others to be critical of their bodies, they learn to eat in a disconnected manner in an attempt to regulate their appearance instead of listening to their bodies. Additionally, pressure to lose weight from family members, friends, healthcare providers, and culture (in lieu of body acceptance) contributes to focusing on appearance-related eating. Many people are surprised to learn that body compliments can be a form of judging a person by their appearance, such as "You look great—how much weight did you lose?" or "I wish I had a body like yours."

Acceptance Model of Intuitive Eating

A series of studies by Tracy Tylka and colleagues (Avalos and Tylka 2006; Augustus-Horvath and Tylka 2011) of nearly six hundred college women and eight hundred women ages eighteen to sixty-five years old, respectively, found that placing emphasis on body function and body appreciation are key ways to translate body acceptance into Intuitive Eating behaviors. When women emphasize the functionality of their bodies over appearance, they are more inclined to eat according to their body's biological cues. Furthermore, they found that adopting an attitude of body appreciation predicted Intuitive Eating, because favorable body attitudes are associated with greater awareness of body signals, combined with a greater tendency to honor these signals. Their research indicates that it is important to promote a positive body orientation, which focuses on body appreciation and body functionality, rather than appearance, which in turn facilitates Intuitive Eating.

Tylka and colleagues found that body appreciation was uniquely and positively related to Intuitive Eating in a wide variety of age groups for women. They identified four hallmarks of body appreciation:

1. Possessing a favorable opinion of the body despite size and perceived imperfections.
2. Being aware of and attentive to the body's needs.
3. Engaging in healthy behaviors to take care of the body.
4. Protecting the body by rejecting unrealistic media body ideals.

Tylka and colleagues believe that it is important to challenge Western promulgation of the thin ideal stereotype and promote acceptance of a diversity of body sizes.

Objectification

Living in a culture where social media reigns supreme means that it's easier than ever for people to compare and critique the bodies of others.

This is a form of objectification, in which a person's self-worth is tied up in their appearance. This is a problem because it is linked to disordered eating, eating disorders, body image disturbance, and lower Intuitive Eating. A fascinating study of more than eleven hundred adolescent girls by a team of Chinese researchers found that higher exposure to these types of social media messages is linked with lower Intuitive Eating (Luo et al. 2019).

This study found that the more the teens experienced online objectification, the less they engaged in Intuitive Eating behaviors. Fortunately, the researchers found two key protective factors: (1) body appreciation and (2) broader conceptualization of beauty, which includes inner characteristics and a wider range of diverse sizes and appearances. Those who had more expansive definitions of beauty were associated with higher Intuitive Eating—even when online objectification was present.

Cultural Acceptance

A fascinating series of multicultural studies by Hawks and colleagues indicate that prior to and during the early stages of westernization, individuals from their native countries are natural Intuitive Eaters, but this process of eating is sacrificed at the expense of the westernized thin ideal (Hawks et al. 2004b, Madanat and Hawks 2004). During acculturation, the westernized standard of beauty becomes internalized, via the bombardment of unrealistic media images of thinness, and indigenous Intuitive Eating styles erode, while the focus shifts toward external cues of eating, both of which can lead to eating disorders. These acceptance studies support and validate principle 8, *respect your body*.

We would be mistaken, however, to blame Western acculturation on the media alone. A profound book by scholar Sabina Strings, *Fearing the Black Body: The Racial Origins of Fat Phobia,* describes how a combination of white supremacy and patriarchy are at the roots of fat phobia and weight stigma, originating in Europe, starting in the early 1500s.

Intuitive Eating Characteristics

Together the results from these studies show that Intuitive Eaters have many attributes associated with both physical and mental health, as summarized in table 2 on pages 16 and 17.

STUDIES ON BINGE-EATING TREATMENT AND EATING DISORDER PREVENTION

Up until recently, research on eating disorders has been pathology- and symptom-based, without considering positive eating behaviors. But in 2006, Tylka and Wilcox evaluated the constructs of Intuitive Eating and concluded that they were distinct and contributed uniquely to psychological well-being—and that Intuitive Eating is more than the absence of eating disorder symptoms. Furthermore, they recommended that Intuitive Eating be part of the educational process for treating eating disorders, as it could contribute to the patient's ability to flourish and thrive in recovery.

A recent study (Young 2011) found that the Intuitive Eating model is a promising approach for eating disorder prevention on college campuses. Intuitive Eating was found to have more appeal because it did not have the perceived stigma of "eating disorders," which is less threatening for voluntary student participation.

Binge-Eating Treatment

A promising study by Laura Smitham, from the University of Notre Dame, used an eight-week Intuitive Eating program (based on our book) for treating thirty-one women diagnosed with binge-eating disorder (Smitham 2008). The results of this study showed a significant reduction in binge eating; so much so that the women no longer met the diagnostic criteria for binge-eating disorder. A caveat of this study was that there was no control comparison group.

An eight-year longitudinal study followed nearly 1,500 subjects from adolescence to young adulthood, and measured Intuitive Eating, disordered eating, and psychological health (Hazzard et al 2020). They found higher Intuitive Eating scores at baseline in 2010, as well as a follow-up in 2018, were associated with *lower* odds of the following:

- Depressive symptoms
- Low self-esteem
- Body dissatisfaction
- Unhealthy weight control behaviors
- Extreme weight control behaviors
- Binge eating

These results indicate that IE longitudinally predicts better psychological and behavioral health across a range of outcomes. Notably, the strongest protective association was observed for binge eating. This study adds to a body of work that Intuitive Eating contributes uniquely to psychological well-being above and beyond the absence of dieting and disordered eating.

However, there were control comparison groups for two larger studies on binge eaters, using an approach similar to an Intuitive Eating process, which also resulted in a significant reduction in binge eating (Kristeller and Wolever 2011). The treatment process used was Mindfulness-Based Eating Awareness Training (MB-EAT), which was developed by Jean Kristeller, PhD, and it shares a significant number of features with Intuitive Eating, as shown in the chart below. Although the MB-EAT program does not have a specific *reject the diet* component, Kristeller agrees that dieting interferes with mind-body attunement.

Intuitive Eating: The Solution for Overall Health and Prevention of Eating Disorders

A body of research indicates that IE is a promising and comprehensive approach to healthy eating with physical and psychological health benefits. Because of the growing body of research indicating that Intuitive Eaters eat diverse foods, have better self-esteem, better psychological hardiness, and reduced eating disorder symptomatology, we believe that Intuitive Eating can be the solution for preventing the emergence of an eating disorder. It's time to empower our autonomy and bring the joy back into eating, while overcoming fear-mongering and worry.

In the next chapter, we'll explain why it's time to let go of the public health policies "fighting the war on obesity." It is a failed paradigm that causes harm, including weight stigma, and increases the risk of eating disorders, the hazards of which are documented in a position statement by the Academy for Eating Disorders.

Intuitive Eating Characteristics

The chart below summarizes the research findings of characteristics of Intuitive Eating.

Note: Keep in mind that the correlations of IE with fewer problems with eating, well-being, life satisfaction, and body appreciation are likely a reflection of the degree of exposure to weight stigma and diet culture itself.

Intuitive Eaters Have Lower	Intuitive Eaters Have Higher
Disordered eating	Self-esteem
Triglycerides	Well-being and optimism
Emotional eating	Variety of foods eaten
Self-silencing (suppressing one's thoughts, feelings, and needs)	Body appreciation and acceptance
	HDL (good cholesterol)
Loss-of-control eating	Interoceptive awareness
Binge eating	Pleasure from eating
Weight bias internalization	Proactive coping
Blood pressure	Psychological hardiness
Body dissatisfaction	Unconditional self-regard
	Life satisfaction

TABLE 2: SIMILARITIES BETWEEN MB-EAT AND INTUITIVE EATING PRINCIPLES	
Mindfulness-Based Eating Awareness Training Components	*Intuitive Eating Principles*
Hunger awareness training	Honor your hunger
Taste and enjoyment of eating	Discover the satisfaction factor
Awareness of fullness	Respect your fullness
Food choices based on liking and health	Satisfaction; make peace with food; honor health with gentle nutrition
Nonjudgmental awareness of eating	Challenge the Food Police
Meet emotional needs in a healthy way	Cope with your feelings with kindness
Acceptance and nonjudgment of body	Respect your body
Gentle exercise	Movement—feel the difference

Chapter 2

Hitting Diet Bottom

I just can't go on another diet, you're my last resort." Sandra had been dieting all her life and knew she could no longer endure a single diet. She'd been on them all: paleo, Whole 30, keto, gluten-free, dairy-free, sugar-free, Weight Watchers . . . diets too numerous to itemize. Sandra was a dieting pro. At first dieting was fun, even exhilarating. "I always thought, this diet would be different, *this time*." And so the cycle would recharge with each new diet or food plan, and every summer. But inevitably, the weight loss would eventually rebound.

Sandra had hit diet bottom. By now, however, she was more obsessed with food and her body than ever. She felt silly. "I should have had this dealt with and controlled long ago." What she didn't realize was that it was the exposure to weight stigma, the idea that her body was not okay, and the *process* of dieting to "fix" it, that had done this to her. *Dieting* had made her more preoccupied with food. *Dieting* had made food the enemy. *Dieting* had made her feel guilty when she wasn't eating diet types of foods (even when she wasn't officially dieting). *Dieting* had turned on her body's defense mechanism to thwart the self-induced famine by slowing her metabolism.

It took years for Sandra to truly know dieting doesn't work (yes, she was familiar with the concept that dieting doesn't work, but she always thought she would be different). While most experts and consumers accept the premise that fad diets don't work, it's tough for a nation of people who are influenced by weight stigma and, thus, obsessed with their bodies to believe that even "sensible dieting" is futile. Sandra had been hooked into modern-age social mythology—our cultural assignment to be "thin and healthy," the "big diet hope"—for most of her life, since her first diet at the age of fourteen.

By the age of thirty, Sandra felt stuck. While she couldn't bear the thought of another diet, she didn't realize that most of her food issues were actually *caused* by her dieting and various food plans. Sandra was also frustrated and angry: "I know everything about diets." Indeed, she could recite calories and macros like a walking nutritional database. That's the big caveat—diet failure is not usually a knowledge issue. If we didn't have the motivation to escape weight stigma, and all we needed to be comfortable in our bodies was knowledge about food and nutrition, most folks wouldn't turn to diets. The information is readily available. (Pick up any style or health magazine, or simply check out the internet to find diets and food comparisons galore.)

Also, the harder you try to diet, the harder you fall—it really hurts not to succeed if you did everything "right." The harder you try restricting the foods you eat, the more your body and mind adapt to surviving the self-imposed famine. As far as your cells are concerned, you are trying to kill them. Your brain finally sends out chemicals that send you to seek large amounts of food for survival. Cravings escalate, until you can't resist them, and for many people, the pressure to eat escalates to the point of loss-of-control eating. It's like holding your breath. You have the illusion of willpower to limit your breathing. But at some point, your body can't take it, because it needs air to survive. When you finally breathe, it's a profound gasp for dear life, rather than a polite inhalation.

SYMPTOMS OF DIET BACKLASH

Diet backlash is the cumulative side effect of dieting (or some type of food restriction for the purpose of shrinking your body)—it can be short term or chronic, depending on how long a person has been dieting. It may be just one side effect or several.

By the time Sandra came to the office, she had the classic symptoms of diet backlash. Not only diet weary, she was eating less food and hungry all the time—her body was starving, and her metabolism was crashing. Other symptoms included:

• *The mere contemplation of going on a diet brings on urges and cravings* for "sinful" foods, such as ice cream, chocolate, and cookies.
• *Upon ending a diet, going on a food binge and feeling guilty.* One study indicated that post-dieting binges occur in 49 percent of all people who end a diet.

• *Having little trust in yourself with food.* Understandably, every diet has taught you *not* to trust your body or the food you put in it. Even though it is the process of dieting that fails you, the failure continues to undermine your relationship with food.

• *Feeling that you don't deserve to eat,* because you believe that your body doesn't fit into diet culture's body hierarchy.

• *Shortened dieting duration.* The lifespan of a diet gets shorter and shorter. This inability to diet for prolonged periods of time may cause you to believe that you are bad at dieting. But diets create a setup that fails you, as mentioned above. Your body is very smart and wired to survive. It gets smarter and smarter with each self-imposed food restriction.

• *The Last Supper.* Most diets are preceded by consuming foods you presume you won't eat again. Food consumption often goes up during this time. It may occur over one meal or over a couple of days. The Last Supper seems to be the final step before "dietary cleansing"—almost a farewell-to-food party. For one client, Marilyn, *every* meal felt as if it were her last. She would eat each meal until she was uncomfortably stuffed, as she was terrified that she would never eat again. For good reason! She had been dieting since the sixth grade—over two-thirds of her life! She had attempted periods of fasting and a series of semi-starvation diets. As far as her body was concerned, a diet was always around the corner—so better eat while you can. Each meal for Marilyn was famine relief.

• *Social withdrawal.* Since it's hard to stay on a diet and go to a party or out to dinner, it just becomes easier to turn down social invitations. At first, social food avoidance may seem like the wise thing to do for the good of the diet, but it escalates into a bigger problem when people decide to return to the social scene. There's often a fear of not being able to stay in control. It's not uncommon for this experience to be reinforced by "saving up the calories or fat grams for the party," which usually means eating very little. But by the time the dieter arrives at the party, ravenous hunger dominates and eating feels very out of control.

• *Sluggish metabolism.* Each diet teaches the body to adapt better for the next self-imposed famine (another diet). Metabolism slows as the body efficiently utilizes each calorie as if it's the last. The more drastic the diet, the more it pushes the body into the calorie-pinching survival mode. This effect made headline news when a study on *Biggest Loser* contestants found that six years later, their metabolism was still blunted by an average of 700 calories per day. Worse yet, their muscle mass was lower than their baseline by over ten pounds (Fothergill et al. 2016). Fueling metabolism is like stoking a fire. Remove the wood, and the fire diminishes. Similarly, to fuel metabolism, we must eat a sufficient amount of calories, or our bodies will compensate and slow down. Part of that compensation is that the body will cannibalize its own muscle tissue to use as an energy source (as it has the ability to convert amino acids from the muscle protein into glucose through a process called gluconeogenesis).

• *Using caffeine to survive the day.* Coffee and diet drinks are often abused as management tools to feel energetic, while being underfed.

• *Eating disorders.* Finally, for some, repeated dieting is often the stepping-stone to an eating disorder with features of restricting, purging, and/or binge eating. Research shows that 35 percent of dieters will progress into disordered eating, and 30 to 45 percent of those dieters will progress into a full eating disorder (Shisslak and Crago 1995). Sadly, this study, published so long ago, has not been followed up on, because there is little to no interest from traditional weight researchers about the harms of dieting and its connection to disordered eating and eating disorders. Furthermore, very few weight loss studies evaluate the harmful consequences of food restriction.

Although Sandra felt she could never diet again, she still engaged in the Last Supper phenomenon. (We regularly encounter this when we see someone for the first time.) She literally ate higher quantities of food than usual and ate plenty of her favorite foods (she thought she would never see these foods again). It was as if she were getting ready for a long trip and was packing extra clothes. Just the thought of working on her food issues put her into the pre-diet mentality, a common occurrence.

While Sandra was just beginning to understand the futility of dieting, her desire to be thin had not changed—clearly a dilemma. She held on to the allure of diet culture's thin ideal, as a way to escape the problem of weight stigma.

THE DIETING PARADOX

In our society, the pursuit of thinness has become the battle cry of diet culture, under the sneaky guise of health and wellness. Eating a single morsel of any high-carbohydrate or so-called unhealthy food is punishable by a life sentence of "guilt" by association. You may be paroled, however, for "good behavior." Good behavior, in our society, means starting a new diet, or having good intentions to diet. And so begins the deprivation cycle of dieting—the battle of deprive and indulge. Rice cakes one week, Häagen-Dazs the next.

"I feel guilty just letting the grocery clerk see what I buy," lamented another client, who happened to have her cart stocked with fruits, vegetables, whole grains, pasta, and a small pint of *real* ice cream. It's as if we live in a Food Police state run by the food mafia. And there always seems to be a dieting offer you can't refuse. Exaggeration? No. There's a good reason for this perception—it's a confluence of factors.

Medicalization and the Politics of Body Weight

Up until the early 2000s the pursuit of shrinking your body was primarily in the purview of the beauty and fitness industries. But that changed with these key political events:

- In 2002 President Bush proclaimed the war on fat, resulting in what Sonya Renee Taylor calls "body terrorism" in her excellent book *The Body Is Not an Apology*.
- In 2010 Michelle Obama launched a campaign to solve the "epidemic" of childhood "obesity," which ushered in a new form of parental guilt.
- In 2013 the American Medical Association voted *against* its own scientific committee to declare that "obesity" is a disease—in spite of the fact that there was not enough evidence to support this assertion. Suddenly, body size alone became a disease, based on a popular vote and the financial incentives to be reimbursed for weight loss prescriptions, not science.

One of the strongest predictors of weight gain is dieting, regardless of the actual body weight of the dieter (O'Hara and Taylor 2018). This is a profound irony, given the medicalization of the pursuit of weight loss. Yet, if dieting were held to the same standards as prescription drugs, it would fail miserably, and wouldn't even be approved for use in the first place! There is a body of research that shows that food restriction for the purpose of weight loss is not effective in the long run, not sustainable, and moreover causes harm—*even if it's prescribed by a physician or dietitian!* In spite of this research, weight loss continues to be prescribed. This is a modern-day Semmelweis reflex, which is the rejection of new evidence because it contradicts established norms, beliefs, or paradigms. This cultural reflex is named after the physician who discovered that patients' lives could be saved if doctors washed their hands. But Dr. Semmelweis was summarily dismissed and scoffed at by his medical colleagues for his preposterous idea! He was later proven right, after his death. (See sidebar, "Dieting Increases Your Risk for Weight Cycling, p. 28.)

Consequently, by framing "obesity" as a disease and an epidemic, it legitimized the pursuit of thinness in the beauty, dieting, and fitness industries. Suddenly losing weight was a health and moral imperative. But the pursuit of weight loss in the name of health perpetuates weight stigma and weight cycling, increases the risk of eating disorders, and harms a person's relationship with food, mind, and body. Now, add in the popular media, which amplifies these messages with their uncritical reporting of flawed studies. Factor in social media, with its influencers and advertising—it's a giant mess. Here's a quick look:

Advertisements

A study published in *Eating Disorders: The Journal of Treatment and Prevention* in 1993 found that between 1973 and 1991 commercials for dieting aids (diet food, reducing aids, and diet program foods) increased nearly linearly. Given the growth of the dieting industry, this number has surely increased several-fold. In the United States alone, nearly half of Americans are dieting (Mundell 2018).

The researchers also noted a parallel trend in the occurrence of eating disorders. They speculated that the media pressure to diet (via commercials) is a major influence in the eating disorder trend.

Before cigarette ads were banned in the United States, subtle billboards aimed at women had slenderizing names, such as Ultraslim 100 and Virginia Slims. An ad for Kent "Slim Lights" cigarettes reads more like a commercial for a weight loss center than for a cigarette, by highlighting slender descriptions—"long," "lean," "light." It is no surprise that the Center for Disease Control (CDC) attributed an increase in smoking by women to their desire to be thinner. Sadly, we have heard women contemplate in our offices that they too have considered taking up smoking or vaping on e-cigarettes as a weight loss aid.

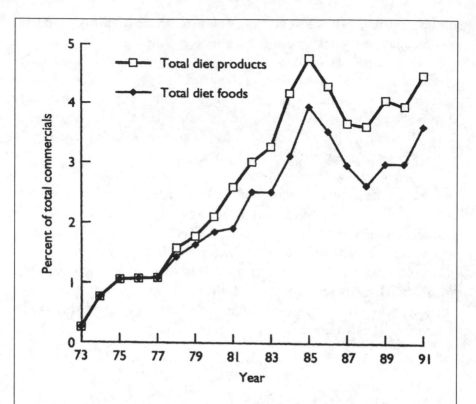

Total number of diet product commercials and total number of diet food commercials as a percent of total commercials, 1973–1991.

Reprinted with permission from: Wiseman, Claire et al. Increasing pressure to be thin: 19 years of diet products in television commercials. *Eating Disorders: The Journal of Treatment & Prevention.* 1(1):55, 1993.

Media

Magazine articles, social media, and movies also drive body dissatisfaction and the pressure to be slim. According to Beauty Redefined, a nonprofit devoted to promoting positive body image, the representations of women's bodies across all media have shrunk dramatically in the last thirty years.

But weight loss and body shape is not just a women's issue (although there's clearly added pressure on women). The proliferation of light beer commercials has planted the seed of body consciousness in men's minds as well—a lean belly is better than a beer belly. It's no coincidence that in the late '80s we saw the launch of magazines aimed at men, such as *Men's Fitness* and *Men's Health*.

While the pursuit of leanness has crossed over the gender barrier, sadly, we have given birth to the first generation of weight watchers. A disturbing dieting trend is affecting the health of U.S. children. Shocking studies have demonstrated that school-age children are obsessing about their weight—a reflection of a nation obsessed with diet and weight. Around the country, children as young as six years old are shedding pounds, afraid of being fat, and increasingly being treated for eating disorders that threaten their health and growth. Societal pressure to be thin has backfired on children.

In fact, in 2019, Weight Watchers introduced an app for children as young as age seven, with before and after pictures, called Kurbo, which was decried by health professionals and eating disorder organizations.

Dieting not only does not work, it, along with weight stigma, is at the root of many problems. While many may diet as an attempt to lose weight or for "health reasons," the paradox is that it may cause more harm. Here's what our nation has to show for dieting and weight stigma:

- Body weights are higher than ever in adults and children.
- The weight rebounds from weight cycling expose more people than ever to weight stigma.
- Eating disorders are on the rise. The prevalence of eating disorders has more than doubled from the 2000–2006 period to the 2013–2018 period, from 3.5 percent to nearly 8 percent (Galmiche et al. 2019).
- More than twelve hundred tons of fat were liposuctioned from 1982 to 1992. A recent study showed that only one year after having a liposuction procedure the fat returns, but to a different part of the body. Liposuction is the most frequently performed cosmetic surgery procedure in Western countries (Bellini et al. 2017).

DIETING CAN'T TRANSCEND BIOLOGY

Dieting is a form of short-term starvation. Consequently, when you are given the first opportunity to *really* eat, eating is often experienced at such intensity that it feels uncontrollable, a desperate act. In the moment of biological hunger, all intentions to stick with a food plan are fleeting and paradoxically irrelevant.

While intense eating may feel out of control, and unnatural, it is a normal response to starving and *dieting*. Yet so often, post-diet eating is viewed as having "no willpower," or a character defect. But when you interpret post-diet eating as such, it slowly erodes trust in yourself with food, diet after diet. Every diet violation, every eating situation that feels out of control lays the foundation for the "diet mentality," brick by brick, and diet by diet. You can't fight biology. When the body is starving, it needs to be nourished and allowed to heal.

So often a dieter laments, "If only I had the willpower." Clearly, this is not an issue of willpower. (Although glowing testimonials from weight loss clinics foster this misplaced blame on lack of willpower.) When underfed, you will obsess about food—whether from a self-imposed diet or from starvation.

Maybe you don't diet but eat vigilantly or eat "clean" in the name of health and fitness. This seems to be the socially accepted term for "dieting" in recent years. But for many, it's the same food issue—with the same symptoms. Avoiding carbohydrates, a trend that has circled back into fashion like a revolving door, at all costs, and subsisting on almost exclusively low-carbohydrate foods is essentially dieting, and often results in being underfed.

DIET CULTURE

We don't fault you for wanting to lose weight—there is no shame in having this desire. It's completely understandable, because it's a byproduct of our diet culture and a strategy to survive weight stigma. It's important to understand the influence of diet culture, because it is everywhere, embedded in our lives, and it can impact you in ways that are not obvious. The best definition of diet culture comes from Christy Harrison, a Certified Intuitive Eating Counselor* and host of the popular podcast *Food Psych*: *"Diet culture is a system of beliefs that:*

- Worships thinness and equates it to health and moral virtue, which means you can spend your whole life thinking you're irreparably broken just because you don't look like the impossibly thin "ideal."

---

* For information on becoming a Certified Intuitive Eating Counselor, see page 360.

• Promotes weight loss as a means of attaining higher status, which means you feel compelled to spend a massive amount of time, energy, and money trying to shrink your body, even though the research is very clear that almost *no one* can sustain intentional weight loss for more than a few years.

• Demonizes certain ways of eating while elevating others, which means you're forced to be hyper-vigilant about your eating, ashamed of making certain food choices, and distracted from your pleasure, your purpose, and your power.

• Oppresses people who don't match up with its supposed picture of "health," which disproportionately harms women, femmes, trans folks, people in larger bodies, people of color, and people with disabilities, damaging both their mental and physical health.

The impact of diet culture and weight stigma shows up in life like this:

• The five-year-old son who didn't eat his mother's homemade cookie packed in his lunch out of fear of what his kindergarten teacher would think.

• Weigh-ins in public schools, which trigger shame in kids.

• Strangers commenting on your food choices.

• Strangers heckling a marathon runner because she is in a higher-weight body.

• Exercise is framed as penance for what you eat or are about to eat.

• Pressure on new brides to lose weight for the wedding dress.

• Pressure on new mamas to "get their bodies back."

• Incessant talk of food plans and diet in nearly every social realm, from office cubicles to the church pulpit, from the schoolyard to weddings, as if it's normal.

• Nonstop dialogue and apologizing for your body and what you are about to eat.

• People in larger bodies are more dramatically affected by:
  • Inaccessible seating in public spaces and transit
  • Seatbelts on airplanes that don't fit
  • Lack of movement opportunities
  • Medical care withheld (infertility treatments, organ transplants, hip and knee replacement surgeries)

This incessant talk about food, nutrition, and body is reminiscent of the famous Minnesota Starvation Experiment, where college-age men who were Conscientious Objectors to the second world war and who had no previous eating or body image issues were put on a semi-starvation diet. Consequently, they talked obsessively about food (that's actually a symptom of undereating). In their writeup of the study, the scientists reported that one man could not stand this self-absorbed engrossment and called it "nutritional masturbation" (Keys et al. 1950). In our present diet culture, this type of talk has become normalized.

There's nothing wrong with wanting to be healthy and feel good. The problem is that sneaky diet culture has hijacked the word "health." Health has become synonymous with weight—losing weight or being lean, which ultimately restricts what you eat. The key will be shifting the focus to the practices that support health that are possible in a given person's life. Weight is not a practice or a behavior. Health is not a moral imperative or a requirement for being treated with dignity and respect.

There are many forms of dieting and many types of dieters. We will explore your dieting personality and meet the Intuitive Eater in the next chapter.

DIETING INCREASES YOUR RISK FOR WEIGHT CYCLING

If dieting programs had to stand up to the same scrutiny as medications, they would never be allowed for public consumption. Imagine, for example, taking an asthma medication that improves your breathing for a few weeks, but in the long run causes rebound asthma attacks and ultimately damages your lungs. Would you blame yourself for the medication not working, yet still continue to take it? Of course not! That's what the process of dieting is like, even if your healthcare professional prescribes it. Would you really embark on a diet (even a so-called sensible diet) if you knew that it would ultimately fail? The pursuit of weight is so problematic. It perpetuates weight cycling and harms your relationship with food, mind, and body. The relationship between dieting and gaining back more weight is so strong that an Australian National Health and Medical Research Council rated it level "A" evidence, which according to academic Fiona Willer is the scientific equivalent of smoking causing lung cancer!

Here are some sobering studies indicating that dieting promotes weight gain. (As a caveat: these facts about subsequent weight gain are not to imply, in any way, that we collude with weight stigma—they're simply scientific data, which confirm the absurdity of dieting.)

- A team of UCLA researchers reviewed thirty-one long-term studies on dieting and concluded that dieting is a consistent predictor of weight gain—up to two-thirds of the people regained *more* weight than they lost (Mann et al. 2007).
- Research on nearly seventeen thousand kids ages nine to fourteen concluded that "in the long term, dieting to control weight is not only ineffective, it may actually promote weight gain" (Field et al. 2003).
- Teenage dieters had twice the risk of gaining more weight, compared to nondieting teens, according to a five-year study (Neumark-Sztainer et al. 2006). Notably, at baseline, the dieters did not weigh more than their nondieting peers. This is an important detail, because if the dieters weighed more, it would be a confounding factor (which would implicate other factors, rather than dieting, such as genetics).
- A novel study on more than two thousand sets of twins from Finland, ages sixteen to twenty-five, showed that dieting itself, independent of genetics, is significantly associated with accelerated weight gain (Pieti-laineet et al. 2011). A dieting twin who embarked on just one intentional weight loss episode was nearly two to three times more likely to gain more weight, compared to their nondieting twin counterpart. Further-more, with each dieting episode, the risk of gaining weight increased in a dose-dependent manner.

The constant yo-yo dieting, or gaining and losing weight from dieting, is known as weight cycling. Weight cycling itself is an independent risk factor for cardiovascular disease, inflammation, high blood pressure, and insulin resistance, yet it is seldom controlled for in many large studies that associate weight with health issues (Bacon and Amphamor 2011). Two large studies showed that weight cycling accounts for all the excess mortality that had been linked to body size.

Studies aside—what has your own dieting experiences shown you? Many of our patients and workshop participants say their first diet was easy—the pounds just melted off. But that first dieting experience is the seduction trap

cont.

Cont.

that launches the futile pursuit of weight loss via dieting. We say futile because our bodies are very smart and wired for survival.

Biologically, your body experiences the dieting process as a form of starvation. Your cells don't know you are voluntarily restricting your food intake. Your body shifts into primal survival mode—metabolism slows down and food cravings escalate. And with each diet, the body learns and adapts, resulting in rebound weight gain. Consequently, many of our patients feel like they are a failure—but it is dieting that has failed them.

Chapter 3

What Kind of Eater Are You?

Perhaps you are still dieting and don't know it! There are many types of eating styles that are actually unconscious forms of dieting. Many of our patients have said they were *not* on a diet—but upon closer inspection of what and how they ate—they were still dieting! Diet culture and its sneaky ways have co-opted the language of health, lifestyle, wellness, and even mindfulness. It may be possible to be following some food plan in the name of health, but it's actually some form of food restriction with the goal of shrinking the body.

Here's a good example. Ted said that in his fifty years of living, he had only been on four serious diets. When perusing the book titles in the office (compulsive overeating texts, eating disorder books, and so forth), he stated: "You work with a lot of serious dieting problems . . . Well, I'm not one of those." Ted clearly did not see himself as a dieter, merely a careful eater. Yet it turned out that he was an unconscious dieter. Although Ted was not actively dieting, he was *undereating* to a level where he was nearly passing out in the afternoon. The reason—he had always been unhappy with his weight! In the mornings he would go for an intense hilly bike ride for one hour, come home, and eat a small breakfast. Lunch was usually a chicken salad with iced tea (while this may sound healthy, it's too low in carbohydrates). By suppertime, his body would be screaming for food. Ted was not only in a severe calorie deficit, but also carbohydrate-deprived. Evenings turned into a food fest! Ted had thought he had a "food volume" problem with a strong sweet tooth. In reality, he had an unconscious diet mentality that biologically triggered his night eating and sweet tooth.

Alicia also was not a conscious dieter. She came in because she wanted to increase her energy level. During the initial session, it became clear that she had complicated issues with food. She was asked if she had been dieting a lot. She looked astonished. "How did you know that I've been on zillions of diets?" While Alicia claimed to be okay with her body, she was still at war with food; she didn't trust herself with food. As it turns out, Alicia had been dieting since she was a child. Although she was not officially dieting, she retained (and expanded) a set of food rules with each diet that nearly paralyzed her ability to eat normally. We see this all the time, the hangover from dieting: avoiding certain foods at all costs, feeling out of control the moment a "sinful" food is eaten, feeling guilty when self-imposed food rules are broken (such as "Thou shall not eat past 6 p.m."), and so on.

Unconscious dieting usually occurs in the form of meticulous eating habits, which for some people evolves into disordered eating and ultimately an eating disorder. Notice how even the frozen diet foods such as Lean Cuisine and Weight Watchers are putting their emphasis on health rather than diet. Weight Watchers recently changed their name to WW and changed their meeting names to Wellness Workshops. Nice try, WW, we are on to you.

As long as you are engaged in some form of dieting or food restriction to shrink your body, you won't be free from food and body worries. Whether you are a conscious or an unconscious dieter, the side effects are similar—the diet backlash effect. This is characterized by periods of careful eating, "blowing it," and paying penance with more dieting or extra-careful eating.

In this chapter, we will explore the various dieting and eating styles to help see where you are now. Later, you will meet the Intuitive Eater and the Intuitive Eating style, the solution to living without diets.

THE EATING PERSONALITIES

To help you clarify your eating (or dieting) style, we have identified the following key categories of eaters that exhibit characteristic eating patterns: the Careful Clean Eater, the Professional Dieter, and the Unconscious Eater. These eating personalities are exhibited even when not officially dieting. It's possible to have more than one eating personality, although we find that there tends to be a dominant trait. Events in your life can also influence or shift your eating personality. For example, one client, a tax attorney, was normally a Careful Clean Eater, but during tax season he became the Chaotic Unconscious Eater.

You may find yourself occasionally possessing the eating characteristics described under the three core eating personalities. Take note of this, and if your eating exists in one of these domains most of the time, it can be a problem.

Read through each eating personality and see which one best reflects your eating style. By understanding where you are now, it will become easier to learn how to become an Intuitive Eater. For example, you may find you have been engaged in a form of dieting and not even have been aware of it. Or you may discover traits that work against you without you knowing it.

The Careful Clean Eater

Careful eaters are those who tend to be vigilant about what foods they put into their bodies. Ted was an example of a Careful Clean Eater (by day). On the surface, Careful Clean Eaters appear to be "perfect" eaters. They are highly nutrition conscious. Outwardly, they seem health- and fitness-oriented (noble traits admired and reinforced in our society). Today, we know that they may actually have a condition called orthorexia.

Eating Style. There is a range of food behaviors that the Careful Clean Eater exhibits. At one extreme, the Careful Clean Eater may anguish over each morsel of food allowed into the body. Grocery shopping trips are spent scrutinizing food labels. Eating out often means interrogating the server—what's in the food, how is the food prepared—and getting assurances that the food is prepared specifically to the Careful Clean Eater's liking. What's wrong with this? Aren't label reading and assertive restaurant ordering in the health interest of some people? Possibly, but the difference is the intensity of the vigilance and the ability to let go of an any guilt in regard to your eating choice. Careful Clean Eaters tend to be very rigid and monitor the quantity and quality of food eaten.

The Careful Clean Eater can spend most of their waking hours planning out the next meal or snack, often worrying about what to eat. While the Careful Clean Eater is not officially on a diet, their mind is—chastising themselves for every "unhealthy" fatty or sugary food eaten. The Careful

Clean Eater can run the fine line between being genuinely interested in health and eating carefully for the sake of body image.

Sometimes the Careful Clean Eater is guided by time or events. For example, some Careful Clean Eaters are meticulous during the weekdays, so that they earn their "eating right" to "splurge" on the weekends or for an upcoming party. But weekends account for 104 days of the year—the splurges can backfire with disconnected eating. Consequently, it's not unusual for a Careful Clean Eater to contemplate going on a diet or the latest food plan.

The Problem. There's nothing wrong with being interested in the well-being of your body. The problem occurs when diligent (bordering on militant) eating affects a healthy relationship with food—and negatively impacts your body. The problem is rigidity. A Careful Clean Eater, upon closer inspection, resembles an evangelist, wanting to convert anyone who will listen to their way of eating. It's their identity and source of pride. They may not diet, but they scrutinize every food situation, including the food choices of the people around them.

The Professional Dieter

Professional dieters are easier to identify; they are perpetually on some food plan. They have usually tried the latest commercial diet, diet book, or new weight loss gimmick. Sometimes dieting takes the form of fasting, or "cutting back." Professional Dieters know a lot about portions of foods, calories, and "dieting tricks," yet the reason they are always on another diet is that the original one never worked. Today, the Professional Dieter is also well versed in counting macros.

Eating Style. Professional Dieters also have careful eating traits. The difference is that chronic dieters guide every eating choice for the sake of losing weight, often in the guise of health. (Although with the ever-pervasive diet culture, this line is getting very blurry, because for many people, thin is equated to health.) When the dieter is not officially on a diet, they are usually thinking about the next diet that can be started. They often wake up hoping this will be a good day—the new beginning (again).

While Professional Dieters have a lot of dieting knowledge, it doesn't serve them well. It's not unusual for them to binge or engage in Last Supper eating the moment a forbidden food is eaten. That's because chronic dieters truly believe they will not eat this food ever again, for tomorrow they start a new food plan, tomorrow they start over with a clean slate. Better eat now; it's the last chance. Not surprisingly, the Professional Dieter gets frustrated by the futility of the vicious cycle. Diet, lose weight, gain weight, intermittent binges, and back to dieting.

The Problem. It's hard to live this way. Chronic undereating usually results in overeating or periodic binges.

For some Professional Dieters, the frustration of losing weight becomes so intensified that they may try laxatives, diuretics, and diet pills, which can become very dangerous. And because these "diet aids" do not work, they may try other extreme methods, such as chronic restricting, in the form of anorexia nervosa, or purging (such as throwing up after a binge), in the form of bulimia. While anorexia and bulimia are multifactorial and rooted in psychological issues (and many other issues—genetic, societal, familial, and so on), a growing body of research has demonstrated that chronic dieting is a common stepping-stone to an eating disorder. One study in particular found that by the time dieters reach the age of fifteen, they are eight times as likely to suffer from an eating disorder as nondieters.

The Unconscious Eater

The Unconscious Eater is often engaged in paired eating—which is eating and doing another activity at the same time, such as watching television and eating, or reading and eating, or the growing favorite, using the cell phone and eating—be it playing games, checking social media, or surfing the internet. Because of the subtleties, and lack of awareness, it can be difficult for a person to identify this eating personality. There are many subtypes of unconscious eaters.

The Chaotic Unconscious Eater. The Chaotic Unconscious Eater often lives an overscheduled life, too busy, too many things to do. The chaotic eating style is haphazard; whatever's available will be grabbed—vending machine fare, fast food, it'll all do. Nutrition is often important to this person—just not in the *critical moment* of the chaos. Chaotic Unconscious Eaters are often so busy putting out fires that they have difficulty identifying biological hunger until it's fiercely ravenous. Not surprisingly, the Chaotic Unconscious Eater goes long periods of time without eating.

The Refuse-Not Unconscious Eater. This eater is vulnerable to the mere presence of food, regardless if hungry or full. Candy jars, food lying around at meetings, food sitting on a kitchen counter will not usually be passed up by the Refuse-Not Unconscious Eater. Most of the time, however, Refuse-Not Unconscious Eaters are not aware that they *are* eating, or how much they are eating. For example, the Refuse-Not Unconscious Eater may pluck up a couple of candies on the way to the restroom without being aware of it. Social outings that revolve around food, such as cocktail parties and holiday buffets, are especially challenging for the Refuse-Not Unconscious Eater.

The Waste-Not Unconscious Eater. This eater values the food dollar. Their eating drive is often influenced by getting as much food as you can for the money. The Waste-Not Unconscious Eater is especially inclined to clean the plate (and others' plates as well). It's not unusual for a Waste-Not Unconscious Eater to eat the leftovers from their children or partner.

The Emotional Unconscious Eater. The Emotional Unconscious Eater uses food as the predominant way to cope with emotions, especially uncomfortable emotions such as stress, anger, and loneliness. While Emotional Unconscious Eaters view their eating as the problem, it's often a symptom of a deeper issue. Eating behaviors of the Emotional Unconscious Eater can range from grabbing a candy bar in stressful times to chronic compulsive binges of vast quantities of food.

The Problem. Unconscious Eating in its various forms is a problem if it results in chronic overeating (which can easily occur when you are eating and not quite aware of it).

Keep in mind that somewhere *between* the first and last bite of food is where the lapse of consciousness takes place. As in, "Oh, it's all gone!" For example, have you ever bought a large box of candy or popcorn at the movies and begun to eat it only to discover your fingers *suddenly* scraping the bottom of the empty box? That's a simple form of Unconscious Eating. But Unconscious Eating can also exist at an intense level, in a somewhat altered state of eating. In this case, the person is not aware of what is being eaten, why they started eating, or even how the food tastes. It's zoning out with food.

WHEN YOUR EATING PERSONALITY WORKS AGAINST YOU

Eventually, the eating styles of the Careful Clean Eater, the Professional Dieter, and the Unconscious Eater become an ineffective way of eating. The solution for the frustrated eater: try harder with a new food plan or diet! At first, the new diet seems exhilarating and hopeful, but eventually it doesn't work, once again. Dieting gets more difficult, and even when you resume your baseline eating personality, it may feel more uncomfortable than before. This is because with each diet the inner food rules get stronger. These food rules often perpetuate feelings of guilt about eating even when you are not officially dieting. Also, the biological effects of dieting (as detailed in chapter 6) make it increasingly difficult to have a normal relationship with food.

The Intuitive Eater personality, however, is the exception. It is the one eating style that doesn't work against you and can help you end the war with your body, food, and mind.

INTRODUCING THE INTUITIVE EATER

Intuitive Eaters march to their inner hunger signals and eat whatever they choose in a satisfying way, without experiencing guilt or an ethical dilemma. The Intuitive Eater is an unaffected eater. Yet it is increasingly difficult to be an unaffected eater in today's diet culture, when you consider the bombardment of nutrition, food, and weight messages from commercials, social media, and health professionals.

When we've described the basic eating traits of the Intuitive Eater to our clients, it's amazing how often we'll hear the response, "That's how my wife eats" or "That's how my boyfriend eats." When we ask how that person's relationship to food and body are, the response is, "No problem!"

Consider toddlers. They are the natural Intuitive Eaters—virtually free from societal messages about food and body image. Toddlers have an innate wisdom about food, if you don't interfere with it. They don't eat based on dieting rules or health, yet study after study shows that if you let a toddler eat spontaneously, they will eat what they need when given free access to food. (This is probably the toughest thing for a concerned parent to do—to let go and trust that kids have an innate ability to eat! (See chapter 16 for more information on raising Intuitive Eaters.)

A landmark study, led by Leann Birch, PhD, and published in the *New England Journal of Medicine*, confirmed that preschool-age children have an innate ability to regulate their eating according to what their bodies need for growth. This holds true even when, meal by meal, the little tykes' eating appears to be a parent's nightmare. Researchers found that at a given meal, calorie intake was highly variable, but it balanced out over time. Yet many parents assume that their young children cannot adequately regulate their food intake. Consequently, parents often adopt coercive strategies in an attempt to ensure that the child consumes a nutritionally adequate diet. But previous research by Birch and her colleagues indicates that such *control* strategies are counterproductive.

Similarly, Duke University psychologist Philip Costanzo, PhD, found that higher weights in school-age children were highly associated with the degree to which parents tried to restrain their children's eating. Even well-meaning parents interfere with Intuitive Eating. When a parent tries to overrule a child's natural eating cues, the problem gets worse, not better.

A parent who feeds a baby whenever a hunger signal is heard and who stops feeding when the baby shows that they've had enough can play a powerful role in the initial development of Intuitive Eating. It's one of the reasons we are so excited about baby-led weaning (see chapter 16).

Unfortunately, parents have been affected by diet culture too. Due to weight stigma, parents worry that if they have a larger-bodied child, it will reflect badly on them. Consequently, well-meaning parents pressure their kids about the types and amounts of food they eat. But groundbreaking work by therapist and dietitian Ellyn Satter has shown that if you get the parents of these kids to back off, and let them eat without parental pressure, the kids will eventually eat *less*. Why? The child begins to hear and understand their own inner signals of hunger and satiety. The child also knows that they will have access to food. According to Satter, "Children deprived of food in an attempt to be thin become preoccupied with food, afraid they won't get enough to eat, and are prone to overeat when they get the chance." We have found this to be true for adult dieters as well. Only for adults, the Intuitive Eating process has been buried for a long time, often years and years. Instead of having a parent loosen up the pressure, this loosening of pressure needs to come from within—against diet culture's distorted body worship.

Fortunately, *we all, for the most part, possess the natural Intuitive Eating ability*; it's just been suppressed, especially by dieting. This book is devoted to showing you how to awaken the Intuitive Eater within.

HOW YOUR INTUITIVE EATER GETS BURIED

As toddlers get a little older, the mixed messages begin to creep in—from the early influences of the Saturday-morning food commercial, to the well-meaning parent who coaxes their child to "Clean your plate." The assault does not stop after childhood. There are several external forces that influence our eating, which can further bury Intuitive Eating.

Dieting. You have already seen the damage that chronic dieting plays, including but not limited to:

- Increased binge eating
- Decreased metabolic rate
- Increased preoccupation with food
- Increased feelings of deprivation
- Increased sense of failure
- Decreased sense of willpower

This only serves to erode your trust with food and urges you to rely on *external* sources to guide your eating (a food plan, a diet, the time of day, food rules, and so forth). The more you go to external sources to "judge" if your eating is in check, the *further* removed you become. Intuitive Eating relies on *your* internal cues and signals.

Eat-Healthy-or-Die Messages. Messages about eating healthfully are everywhere, from nonprofit health organizations to food companies touting the health benefits of their particular product. The inherent message? What you eat can improve your health. Conversely, take one wrong move (bite) and you're one step closer to the grave. Is this an exaggeration? No! Here are some recent headlines found in a Google search:

- "12 Foods That Can Kill You," in *Men's Journal* magazine
- "16 Foods You Didn't Know Could Kill You," in *Cosmopolitan* magazine

- "Bad Diets Kill More People Around the World than Smoking, Study Says," in the *Washington Post*

That kind of message can easily leave you feeling guilty for eating the "wrong" kind of food and feeling confused about what you should eat.

Are we saying that you should ignore the value of healthful eating? Of course not. However, when you have a dieting mindset, the barrage of "healthy eating" messages can make you feel guiltier about the food you choose to eat. Consider these statistics:

- A 2015 Harris Poll of more than two thousand Americans found that nearly eight out of ten women and seven out of ten men in the United States suffer from food guilt.
- In 2013, the *Guardian* reported that three-quarters of women in the U.K.—24 million—say they often feel guilty about how much they eat.

Women may be especially guilt-ridden. An American Dietetic Association Gallup poll showed that women feel guiltier than men about the food they eat (44 percent versus 28 percent). Could this be because women diet more frequently than men? Or because women are usually the target of health messages and food ads (consider the number of women's magazines)? Women are the key decision makers for the healthcare for the family and are usually the gatekeepers of food and nutrition issues as well; they serve as a prime target.

Honestly, unless you killed the chef or the farmer, there should be no guilt about your eating choices. Guilt certainly robs the joy of eating. This guilt factor is one of the reasons that establishing nutrition or healthy eating as an *initial* priority in the Intuitive Eating process is counterproductive. In the beginning we *ignore* nutrition, because it interferes with the process of relearning how to become an Intuitive Eater. Nutrition heresy? No. It's possible to respect and honor nutrition. It just can't be the first priority when you've been dieting all your life. Look at it this way: If you have focused all your attention on nutrition, has it helped? The most nutritious eating plan (including counting macros) can become embraced as another form of diet. In fact, we have witnessed folks unwittingly try to turn Intuitive Eating into a diet!

To get an idea of whether you are already an Intuitive Eater, or where you might need some further work, see the "Intuitive Eating Assessment Scale" on page 42. It is adapted from research that defines Intuitive Eating characteristics.

You can recapture Intuitive Eating, but first you have to get rid of the diet mentality rules that keep the Intuitive Eater buried. In the next chapter, we will briefly introduce you to the core principles of Intuitive Eating. The remainder of the book will show you, step by step, how to become an Intuitive Eater.

SUMMARY OF EATER STYLES		
Eater Style	Trigger	Characteristic
Careful Clean Eater	Fitness and health	This person appears to be the perfect eater, yet anguishes over each food morsel and its effect on the body. On the surface this person seems health- and fitness-oriented.
Professional Dieter	Shrinking the body	This person is perpetually dieting, often trying the latest commercial diet or diet book.
Unconscious Eater	Eating while doing something else at the same time	This person is often unaware that they are eating or how much is being eaten. To sit down and simply eat is often viewed as a waste of time. Eating is usually paired with another activity to be productive. There are many sub-types.
Chaotic Unconscious Eater	Overscheduled life	This person's eating style is haphazard—gulp'n'go when the food is available. Seems to thrive on tension.

(Cont.)

SUMMARY OF EATER STYLES

Eater Style	Trigger	Characteristic
Refuse-Not Unconscious Eater	Presence of food	This person is especially vulnerable to snacks or food present in meetings or sitting openly on the kitchen counter.
Waste-Not Unconscious Eater	Free food	This person's eating drive is often influenced by the value of the food dollar and is susceptible to all-you-can-eat buffets and free food.
Emotional Unconscious Eater	Uncomfortable emotions	Stress or uncomfortable feelings trigger eating—especially when alone.
Intuitive Eater	Biological hunger	This person makes food choices without experiencing guilt or an ethical dilemma. Honors hunger, respects fullness, enjoys the pleasure of eating.

INTUITIVE EATING ASSESSMENT SCALE—2

This quiz will assess whether you are an Intuitive Eater, or perhaps where you might need some work. It is adapted from Tracy Tylka's research on our model of Intuitive Eating [1,2]. This updated assessment was validated for use with both men and women, and includes a new category, Body—Food Choice Congruence, which reflects Principle 10 of Intuitive Eating—Honor Your Health with Gentle Nutrition.

Directions: *The following statements are grouped into the three core characteristics of Intuitive Eaters. Answer "yes" or "no" for each statement. If you are unsure of how to respond, consider if the description usually applies to you—is it mostly "yes" or "no"?*

SECTION 1. UNCONDITIONAL PERMISSION TO EAT

Yes No

☐ ☐ 1. I try to avoid certain foods high in fat, carbs, or calories.

☐ ☐ 2. If I am craving a certain food, I don't allow myself to have it.

☐ ☐ 3. I get mad at myself for eating something unhealthy.

☐ ☐ 4. I have forbidden foods that I don't allow myself to eat.

☐ ☐ 5. I don't allow myself to eat what food I desire at the moment.

☐ ☐ 6. I follow eating rules or diet plans that dictate what, when, and/or how to eat.

SECTION 2. EATING FOR PHYSICAL RATHER THAN EMOTIONAL REASONS

Yes No

☐ ☐ 1. I find myself eating when I'm feeling emotional (anxious, sad, depressed), even when I'm not physically hungry.

☐ ☐ 2. I find myself eating when I am lonely, even when I'm not physically hungry.

☐ ☐ 3. I use food to help me soothe my negative emotions.

☐ ☐ 4. I find myself eating when I am stressed out, even when I'm not physically hungry.

☐ ☐ 5. I am not able to cope with my negative emotions (i.e., anxiety and sadness) without turning to food for comfort.

☐ ☐ 6. When I am bored, I eat just for something to do.

☐ ☐ 7. When I am lonely, I turn to food for comfort.

☐ ☐ 8. I have difficulty finding ways to cope with stress and anxiety, other than by eating.

SECTION 3. RELIANCE ON INTERNAL HUNGER/SATIETY CUES (TRUST)

Yes No

☐ ☐ 1. I trust my body to tell me *when* to eat.

☐ ☐ 2. I trust my body to tell me *what* to eat.

☐ ☐ 3. I trust my body to tell me *how much* to eat.

☐ ☐ 4. I rely on my hunger signals to tell me when to eat.

☐ ☐ 5. I rely on my fullness (satiety) signals to tell me when to stop eating.

☐ ☐ 6. I trust my body to tell me when to stop eating.

cont.

Cont.

SECTION 4. BODY—FOOD CHOICE CONGRUENCE

Yes No

☐   ☐   1. Most of the time, I desire to eat nutritious foods.

☐   ☐   2. I mostly eat foods that make my body perform efficiently (well).

☐   ☐   3. I mostly eat foods that give my body energy and stamina.

Scoring:

- Sections 1—2: Each "yes" statement indicates an area that likely needs some work.
- Section 3—4: Each "no" statement indicates an area that likely needs some work.

Source:

1. Tylka, Tracy L. (2006). Development and psychometric evaluation of a measure of intuitive eating. *Journal of Counseling Psychology* 53(2), Apr:226—240.
2. Tylka, T.L. (2013). A psychometric evaluation of the Intuitive Eating Scale with college men. *Journal of Counseling Psychology*, Jan;60(1):137—53.

Chapter 4

Principles of Intuitive Eating: Overview

Only when you vow to discard dieting and replace it with a commitment to Intuitive Eating will you be released from the prison of yo-yo dieting and food obsessions. In this chapter, you will be introduced to the core principles of Intuitive Eating—a snapshot of each concept, with a case study or two. The most significant achievement of each client mentioned was gaining a healthy relationship with food and their body. By following the ten principles of Intuitive Eating, you will normalize and heal your relationship with food. And, please keep in mind that these ten principles are simply guidelines and not new rules that can be turned into a new diet. Any desire for weight loss must be put on the back burner, or it will sabotage your process of healing your relationship with food, your mind, and your body. Intuitive Eating is an inside job—it's about listening to the messages of the body through interoceptive awareness. When you focus on weight, it interferes with the process of becoming an Intuitive Eater. Focusing on the scale or your weight immediately introduces an external factor, creating a wedge between your inner wisdom and eating choices. We are not against people losing weight as a byproduct or side effect of Intuitive Eating—we have seen many folks get this important perspective wrong, including the media and health professionals!

Later in the book, each principle will be discussed step by step in great detail. You may find it useful to return to this chapter for a quick reference.

PRINCIPLE 1:

REJECT THE DIET MENTALITY

Throw out the diet books and magazine articles that offer you the false hope of losing weight quickly, easily, and permanently. Get angry at diet culture that promotes weight loss and the lies that have led you to feel as if you were a failure every time a new diet stopped working and you gained back all of the weight. If you allow even one small hope to linger that a new and better diet or food plan might be lurking around the corner, it will prevent you from being free to rediscover Intuitive Eating.

James dieted most of his life, starting with the little diets his mother put him on and ending with a liquid protein fast, which gave him his most recent short-lived "success." By the time he came to the office, James complained that he weighed more than he ever had in his life. He knew he was incapable of ever going on another diet but felt guilty because he thought he "should." *Rejecting the diet mentality* was a key milestone for James. He discovered that he was not a failure, but that the system of dieting itself created the setup for failure.

Today, James is a committed ex-dieter who found his way back through Intuitive Eating. He no longer feels that he "should" be on a diet. He has made peace with his body and is pleased and amazed that he has satisfaction in his eating without guilt, while eating everything he likes. Ironically, James sadly watches his boss go from diet to diet, while truly knowing that dieting is the quickest way to short-circuit a healthy relationship with food.

PRINCIPLE 2:

HONOR YOUR HUNGER

Keep your body biologically fed with adequate energy and carbohydrates. Otherwise you can trigger a primal drive to overeat. Once you reach the moment of excessive hunger, all intentions of moderate, conscious eating are fleeting and irrelevant. Learning to honor this first biological signal sets the stage for rebuilding trust in yourself and in food.

A critical step to becoming an Intuitive Eater for Tim, a busy physician, was learning to honor his hunger. Tim dieted all through medical school, while trying to keep up with a frenetic schedule, working over eighty hours a week. He felt hungry most of the time but ignored these signals, because he didn't think he deserved to eat because of his body size. By mid-afternoon, his eating was out of control, with snack attacks at the vending machine. Not surprisingly, he felt low in energy most of the time from his chaotic eating.

Today, Tim has learned to pay attention to his biological signals of hunger and to honor them by taking the time to feed himself. He knows, now, that if he doesn't listen to his growling stomach and eat breakfast before he leaves for work, he can't concentrate on what his patients are saying during their morning appointments. Tim has learned to *honor his hunger*.

As a result of becoming an Intuitive Eater, Tim feels full of energy throughout the day. He has ended the cycles of restriction and overeating that plagued him for twenty years and feels confident that this futile cycle is gone forever.

PRINCIPLE 3:

MAKE PEACE WITH FOOD

Call a truce; stop the food fight! Give yourself unconditional permission to eat. If you tell yourself that you can't or shouldn't have a particular food, it can lead to intense feelings of deprivation that build into uncontrollable cravings and, often, bingeing. When you finally "give in" to your forbidden foods, eating will be experienced with such intensity it usually results in Last Supper overeating and overwhelming guilt.

Nancy is a server whose battleground was the gourmet restaurant where she worked. This restaurant offered an array of delicious, rich foods. Before becoming an Intuitive Eater, Nancy would valiantly refrain from all of the tempting foods available at the restaurant. She would leave each night, physically tired and with haunting visions of the foods she thought she shouldn't have. Her restraint was consistent, until making her first appointment. Suddenly in the week prior to coming in, all she wanted to do was eat. And eat, she did!

Nancy experienced the Last Supper effect that accompanies intense food deprivation. She had an eating backlash from not allowing herself to touch her favorite foods. Nancy believed any nutritionist would confirm that she had to give up these foods for good *and* follow a rigid meal plan. She acknowledged feeling scared and angry about her future food choice loss and automatically went into a phase of overeating, especially of foods that she perceived would be forever forbidden.

Now that Nancy is an Intuitive Eater, she eats whatever appeals to her at the restaurant (and elsewhere). She no longer restricts the foods she likes, nor does she feel guilty when she occasionally overeats. She discovered that some of the foods that looked wonderful didn't even taste good! Nancy has *made peace with food* and loves the freedom that comes with it.

PRINCIPLE 4:

CHALLENGE THE FOOD POLICE

Scream a loud no to thoughts in your head that declare you're "good" for eating minimal calories or "bad" because you ate a piece of chocolate cake. The food police monitor the unreasonable rules that diet culture has created. The police station is housed deep in your psyche, and its loudspeaker shouts negative barbs, hopeless phrases, and guilt-provoking indictments. Chasing the food police away is a critical step in returning to Intuitive Eating.

As an adolescent, Linda had been a competitive track sprinter and went on to qualify for the Olympic trials. Linda's coach had been a strong influence in her life, and to this day, her coach's voice reverberates, "To be competitive, you must diet to get rid of body fat." She can also hear her mother's voice chiming in about which foods are "good" and "bad."

Years of yo-yo dieting and weight cycling resulted from obeying the monotonous diet tapes droning in her head. These inner tapes originated from her well-meaning coach and numerous diets, only to be reinforced with negative messages that her mother doled out. Linda's food police strengthened with each diet, each coachly admonishment, and each motherly chastisement.

Linda's breakthrough came when she discovered how to *Challenge the Food Police*. Linda learned to talk back to the inner critical voices that tried to restrict her food choices. She learned to give herself nurturing messages and make nonjudgmental decisions about her eating. The voice of the Intuitive Eater was allowed to reemerge once the food police were silenced. Linda is guilt-free about her eating, her weight is no longer cycling up and down, and her "good" and "bad" thoughts about food have vanished.

PRINCIPLE 5:

DISCOVER THE SATISFACTION FACTOR

Japanese have the wisdom to keep pleasure as one of their goals of healthy living. In our compulsion to comply with diet culture, we often overlook one of the most basic gifts of existence—the pleasure and satisfaction that can be found in the eating experience. When you eat what you really want, in an environment that is inviting, the pleasure you derive will be a powerful force in helping you feel satisfied and content.

Denise is a production assistant who was surrounded by a variety of "forbidden" foods each day when she went to the set. Instead of giving herself permission to eat what she really wanted, she would ignore her preference signals. If she wanted French fries, she would "nobly" substitute an austere baked potato, unadorned. If cookies beckoned, she'd settle for fruit. Rather than stopping at her substitute food choice, however, she'd continue to seek out food after food, trying to find satisfaction in unsatisfying foods.

Once Denise realized that all of these alternate food choices were only fillers, that none of them led her to feel satisfied, she decided to experiment and eat what she was craving. She was delighted to find that not only did she get true pleasure from the food, but she stopped eating when she was comfortably full, sometimes even leaving some behind! She was satisfied, content—not needing to seek out yet another replacement for her "phantom food." Denise *discovered the satisfaction factor* in eating. She rarely continues eating after she's full and has experienced the benefits of our motto, "If you don't love it, don't eat it, and if you love it, savor it."

PRINCIPLE 6:

FEEL YOUR FULLNESS

In order to honor your fullness, you need to trust that you will give yourself the foods that you desire. Listen for the body signals that tell you that you are no longer hungry and observe the signs that show that you're comfortably full. Pause in the middle of eating and ask yourself how the food tastes, and what your current hunger level is.

Jackie was a party girl. She loved to go out to eat with her friends every night after work and felt that weekends were not complete without a party. Jackie loved life and loved to eat. But she also didn't know how to stop eating when she began to feel full. (Rather, she often did not recognize feeling full until she was uncomfortably satiated, stuffed.) The morning after each social event she made the same vow: "I never want to eat again. I feel sick and stuffed and bloated, and I hate how my body feels."

Learning to *feel fullness* was a key element in Jackie's journey to Intuitive Eating. She began to pay attention to the transition from an empty stomach to a slightly full stomach. She soon learned to sense the signals of fullness that were starting to emerge in the midst of her meals.

It was easier for Jackie to honor her body's satiety signals when she truly knew she could eat again if hungry (even within the hour) and eat her favorite foods. (What starving person would stop at comfortable fullness if they thought they were never going to eat again, or have access to a particular food?) Jackie made an interesting observation while feeding alley cats during one of her out-of-town parties: the starving alley cat will eat until the bowl is licked clean, but house cats know they will be fed again, so they can easily turn up their tails and leave food in their dish. House cats can honor fullness because they know they will eat again.

Jackie also discovered that by honoring satiety signals and pushing her plate away (when *she* was ready), she felt that she was showing more respect for herself. After becoming an Intuitive Eater, Jackie felt that she had it all. She could still go out with her friends whenever she liked, and she could wake up the next morning feeling great!

PRINCIPLE 7:

COPE WITH YOUR EMOTIONS WITH KINDNESS

First, recognize that food restriction, both physically and mentally, can, in and of itself, trigger loss of control, which can feel like emotional eating. Find kind ways to comfort, nurture, distract, and resolve your issues. Anxiety, loneliness, boredom, and anger are emotions we all experience throughout life. Each has its own trigger, and each has its own appeasement. Food won't fix any of these feelings. It may comfort for the short term, distract from the pain, or even numb you. But food won't solve the problem. You'll ultimately have to deal with the source of the emotion.

Marsha was a writer who did most of her work at home. She loved her work, but sometimes found that she would have mini periods of writer's block. To relieve her tension about finding the right word to put on the computer, she would visit the kitchen many times during the day to get a snack. Marsha was *using* food to help her get her work done.

Lisa was a fourteen-year-old who would come home after school and plop herself down in front of the TV with a bag of potato chips. Lisa was *using* food to procrastinate about doing her homework.

Cynthia's children were grown; she had an illness that depleted her energy, not allowing her to go to work, and her husband didn't pay much attention to her. Cynthia found food to keep her occupied when she was bored and to soothe her lonely soul.

Using food to cope with emotions comes in degrees of intensity. For some, food is simply a means of distraction from boring activities or a filler for empty times. For others, it can be the *only* comfort they have to get through a painful life.

Before becoming Intuitive Eaters, Marsha, Lisa, and Cynthia were coping with the problems of their lives by using food as a distracter, comforter, and calmer. But they soon learned to savor the foods they had chosen, eat in an inviting environment, and honor their biological hungers. Increased gratifying eating experiences allowed each to let go of using food as a coping mechanism. These experiences also offered clarity—it was easier to distinguish an eating urge from an emotional urge.

These women discovered that food never tasted as good or was as satisfying when they weren't really hungry or hadn't figured out what they
really wanted to eat or when they bolted the food down without respecting
fullness. Marsha, Lisa, and Cynthia found coping mechanisms and appropriate outlets for their emotions. Now they save their eating for the times
it gives them true satisfaction and are in tune with the quantities of food
their bodies need.

PRINCIPLE 8:

RESPECT YOUR BODY

Accept your genetic blueprint. Just as a person with a shoe size of eight
would not expect to realistically squeeze into a size six, it is equally futile (and
uncomfortable) to have a similar expectation about body size. But mostly, respect your body so you can feel better about who you are. It's hard to reject
the diet mentality if you are unrealistic and critical of your body size or shape.
All bodies deserve dignity.

One of the most important goals that Andrea made while working
toward becoming an Intuitive Eater was to *respect her body*. She was
fifty years old, had given birth to four children, and was a valuable
member of the community. Her body had gotten her through childbirth,
traveling, working, and exercise. It was a body to respect, rather than
belittle. Yet Andrea spent many of her waking hours criticizing her
body and pining for the days when she was younger and thinner. The
more she made negative comments to herself, the more despair she felt.
She would go to food when she wasn't hungry to console herself for her
misery. She also found herself overeating as a way to punish herself for
looking so "bad."

Once Andrea stopped comparing herself to every other woman she
knew and started to respect and honor her body, she began to eat less, and
to take better care of herself. Andrea became an Intuitive Eater, took pride
in her achievements, and stopped trying to have the "perfect" body!

Janie, a twenty-five-year-old publicist, also played the "body-check"
game. Every time she was at a party, she silently compared herself to other
women, only to feel that she didn't match up. Janie felt mortified every

time and would vow that night to begin a diet the next day. Only when Janie began to focus on respecting her body and its inner cues, rather than external forces (what other people look like, what other people are doing), did she make a significant breakthrough.

PRINCIPLE 9:

MOVEMENT—FEEL THE DIFFERENCE

Forget militant exercise. Just get active and feel the difference. Shift your focus to how it feels to move your body, rather than the calorie-burning effect of exercise. If you focus on how you feel from working out, such as energized, it can make the difference between rolling out of bed for a brisk morning walk or hitting the snooze alarm.

Miranda had all the accoutrements of a regular exerciser—a membership in a gym, a stationary bike at home, athletic clothes and shoes. There was just one problem—she was *not* exercising. Miranda was burned out. She had tried almost as many new exercise programs as she had diets. It was a vicious cycle—begin a diet and simultaneously begin working out, and then quit both the diet and the exercise. That was precisely the problem. Miranda never really felt the pleasure of moving her body. Part of the problem was that when she was underfeeding her body (dieting), she had little energy, if any, to exercise—and that *does not feel good*. Consequently, exercising was always a struggle. It was only the initial enthusiasm and momentum of the diet that would carry her through a monotonous workout. But because dieting was short-lived, so too was exercise.

When Miranda began feeding her body (by *honoring her hunger*), she felt better and entertained the idea of beginning a walking program. She discovered that by reframing the purpose of exercise from a weight loss tool to *feeling* good and beginning to think of it as movement instead of exercise, she began to actually enjoy walking.

For the first time in her life Miranda has consistently included movement in her life and *enjoys* it. She also knows that she will continue to be consistent, because she enjoys the payoff—which includes knowing that she's taking such great care of herself.

PRINCIPLE 10:

HONOR YOUR HEALTH—GENTLE NUTRITION

Make food choices that honor your health and taste buds while making you feel good. Remember that you don't have to eat perfectly to be healthy. You will not suddenly get a nutrient deficiency or become unhealthy from one snack, one meal, or one day of eating. It's what you eat consistently over time that matters. Progress, not perfection, is what counts.

Louise, like so many of our clients, had dieted all her life. She had been enlightened by the anti-dieting movement and was ahead of the game with a reject-dieting mentality. But Louise had been meticulously counting macros like a dieter counting calories—in essence, she was still dieting. She was using nutrition information militantly to keep herself in check. Her food choices were primarily low-carb foods; they were safe and healthy, she reasoned. Yet Louise couldn't understand why she was still bingeing. When Louise realized that she was using nutrition as a dieting weapon, rather than as an ally for health, she began to change the way she chose her foods. Louise began to honor her taste buds and listen to her body with respect to how food made her feel. When Louise was finally able to relax and eat with less rigidity, she discovered that it was possible to honor both the pleasure of taste and her health. And by doing this, not only was she more satisfied with eating, but her binges ceased completely.

A PROCESS WITH GREAT REWARDS

All of the clients mentioned in the previous examples had been dissatisfied with their relationship with food and their bodies. Each had tried either formal or informal dieting and had felt failure and despair. By learning the principles of Intuitive Eating and putting them to work, each found a deepening of the quality of life and eating satisfaction. You can too!

Chapter 5

Awakening the
Intuitive Eater: Stages

The journey to Intuitive Eating is like taking a cross-county hiking trip. Before you even strap on your hiking boots, you'd want to know what to expect during your journey. While a map is helpful, it doesn't describe what you'll need to be adequately prepared, such as trail conditions, climate, special sightseeing spots, what kind of clothes to wear, and so forth. The purpose of this chapter is to help you understand what to expect during your journey to Intuitive Eating.

Whether it's hiking or relearning a more satisfying eating style, you will go through many stages along the way. The amount of time that you need to stay in any particular stage is variable and highly individualized. For example, traversing new hiking trails depends on how physically fit you are, how you deal with fear of new trails, how much time you have to hike, and the availability of hiking trails. Similarly, your journey back to Intuitive Eating depends on how long you've been dieting, how strongly entrenched your diet thinking is, how long you've been using food to cope with life, and how willing you are to trust yourself. It equally depends on how willing you are to make learning to become an Intuitive Eater the primary goal, while accepting that a focus on weight loss will sabotage your Intuitive Eating process. You will begin to hold self-compassion for your desire to lose weight, as you learn that it has been a result of being conditioned by diet culture to believe in its significance as a measure of your worth.

Sometimes you'll move back and forth among the stages. If you accept that this is a normal part of the process, it will help you to keep going without feeling that you are backsliding or not making progress.

Consider this scenario: You are on a hiking trail and encounter a fork in the road that is hard to decipher with your trail map. Do you go to the right or left? You ponder for a while and decide to go left. While walking, you spot something you've never seen before, a bright-green caterpillar shimmying up a purple flower. A few steps ahead, you discover an unusual bird. But a few steps beyond these glories of nature is a big boulder signaling that you chose the wrong path. You turn around, go back to the fork, and take the other path. Was this detour a waste of time? No! Similarly, on the path to Intuitive Eating, you will take many turns and experiment with new thoughts and behaviors. You may even find that after making noticeable progress, you go back to old ways that are uncomfortable and unfulfilling. But like taking the "wrong" path on the scenic hiking trail, you'll discover that excursions into old eating patterns can be used as learning experiences. (Most hikers would not chide themselves for being unsure of which path to take; instead, they'd be grateful for the discoveries of nature that a blocked path offered.) It's important to be kind to yourself and appreciate the learning that comes out of the experience. This process involves coming from a place of curiosity rather than a place of judgment, so whatever you do, don't beat yourself up mentally!

Intuitive Eating is very different from dieting. Dieters usually get frustrated when they don't follow the diet plan exactly as prescribed. We have seen many a chronic dieter merely take a perceived wrong turn at one meal, be critical for that mistake, and "blow" the diet for that day or weekend or even longer!

Keep in mind that the journey to Intuitive Eating is a *process* complete with ups and downs, unlike dieting, when the common expectation is linear progress.

The road to Intuitive Eating is like investing in a long-term mutual fund. Over time, there will be a return on the investment, in spite of the daily fluctuations of the stock market. It is normal and expected. How ironic that we have been taught that, in economics, the day-to-day changes in the stock market are normal, and seldom is there a get-rich-quick fix, yet, in the multibillion-dollar-a-year weight loss business, "get thin fast" is the only goal for success. We are invested, instead, in helping you bring peace to your relationship with food and body. You will receive more satisfaction from eating and feel more in tune with your body's signals. On the path to this goal, keep in mind Webster's definitions of "process": "a continuing development involving many changes" and "a particular method of doing something, generally involving a number of steps or operations."

As with any process, it's important to stay focused in the present and grow from the many experiences you will encounter. If you focus on the end result, it can make you feel overwhelmed and discouraged and end up sabotaging the process. Instead, if you acknowledge small changes along the way and value the learning experiences (which can sometimes be frustrating), it will help you stay on the Intuitive Eating path and move forward. Once you truly become an Intuitive Eater, you will consistently tune in to your inner wisdom, and you will feel better in mind, body, and spirit.

At this point, we feel it is important to clarify the pursuit of the weight loss issue. We understand that you may be feeling uncomfortable in your body and that you believe that weight loss will allow you to have all of the life experiences you may be avoiding. We have tremendous compassion for you as you experience the pressure that diet culture puts on you to meet unrealistic goals of achieving society's culturally thin ideal. Our goal is to help you find the richest life you can, regardless of your size or shape, and to help you focus on the behaviors that have kept you from feeling the best you can, both physically and emotionally. Remember, focusing on the goal of weight loss will interfere with your ability to make choices based on your body's signals.

Once you've given up on the futility of dieting forever, you'll find yourself eating the amount of food that your body actually needs, and a desire to experience regular movement in your life. You'll find that your body feels so much better when your stomach isn't under- or overfilled. You will also find that as your thoughts about your eating and body begin to change, you will experience a more peaceful feeling, rather than the chronic background anxiety that looms with every food choice. However, if you continue to focus on weight loss as the goal, you'll get tied up in the old diet mentality, which does not serve you.

Over the years, we have seen that our patients go through a five-stage progression in learning how to become an Intuitive Eater. The following section will help you get an idea of what to expect in your own personal journey.

STAGE ONE:
READINESS — HITTING DIET BOTTOM

This is where most people begin. You are painfully aware that every attempt to lose weight has ended in "failure." You are tired of valuing each day based on whether the scale is up or down a pound or two (or if you overate the day before). You think and worry about food all the time. You talk the restrictive food talk—"if only I didn't have to watch my weight, I could eat that," or "I had two cookies—I was really bad today."

At the present time, you're very focused on your weight, as you've likely been losing and gaining weight as frequently and rapidly as you wash your clothes and they get dirty once again!

You have lost touch with biological hunger and satiety signals. You have forgotten what you really like to eat and instead eat what you think you "should" eat. Your relationship with food has developed a negative tone, and you dread eating the foods you love, because you're afraid it will be hard to stop. When you give in to the "temptation" of forbidden foods, it's not unusual to overeat them, because you feel guilty. Yet you sincerely vow you will never eat them again.

It's not unusual to find that you eat to comfort, distract, or even numb yourself from your feelings, as your primary coping mechanism. If that's the case, you will sense that the quality of your life has been clouded by obsessional thinking about food and by disconnected eating.

Your body image is negative—you don't like the way you look and feel in your body, and self-respect is lessened. You have learned from your own experience that dieting does not work—you have hit diet bottom and feel stuck, frustrated, and discouraged.

This stage continues until you decide that you are unhappy eating and living this way—you are ready to do something about it. Your first thoughts may veer toward finding a new diet to solve your problems. But almost immediately, you realize that you just can't do that one ever again. If this is where you find yourself, then you are ready for the process that will bring you back to eating intuitively.

STAGE TWO:
EXPLORATION — CONSCIOUS LEARNING AND PURSUIT OF PLEASURE

This is a stage of exploration and discovery. You will go through a phase of *hyperconsciousness* to help reacquaint yourself with your intuitive signals: hunger, taste preferences, satisfaction, and satiety.

This stage is a lot like learning how to drive a car. For the novice driver, just getting the car out of the driveway requires a lot of conscious thinking, complete with a mental checklist: put the key in the ignition, make sure the gear is in park or neutral, turn on the engine, check the rearview mirror, remove the hand break, and so forth. This hyperconsciousness is necessary to lock in all of the steps needed just to get that car into drive! In the same sense, you will be zooming in on details of eating that have evolved without your conscious thought. (But this is necessary to reclaim the Intuitive Eater in you.)

It may seem awkward and uncomfortable, even obsessive. However, hyperconsciousness is different than obsessive thinking. Obsessive thinking is pervasive and is characterized by worry. It fills your mind during most of the day and keeps you from thinking of much else. Hyperconsciousness is more specific. It zooms in when you're ready to eat but goes away when the eating experience is over. And just like the steps required to drive a car become autopilot for the experienced driver, Intuitive Eating will eventually be experienced without this initial awkwardness.

You may feel that you are in a hyperconscious state much of the time during this stage. This may feel uncomfortable at first and perhaps even strange. Remember, much of your previous eating was either mostly disconnected or diet-directed.

In this stage, you'll begin to *make peace with food* by giving yourself unconditional permission to eat. This part may feel scary, and you may choose to move slowly (within your comfort level). You will learn to get rid of guilt-induced eating and begin to discover the importance of the satisfaction factor with food. The more satisfied you are when eating, the less you think about food when you are not hungry—you will no longer be on the prowl.

You will experiment with foods that you may not have eaten for a long time. This includes sorting out your *true* food likes and dislikes. You may even discover that you don't like the taste of some of the foods you've been dreaming of! (Keep in mind that years of dieting, or eating what you "should," only serve to disconnect you from your internal eating drive and true food preferences.)

You will learn to *honor your hunger* and recognize your body signals that indicate the many degrees of hunger. You will learn to separate these biological signals from the emotional signals that might also trigger eating.

In this stage, you may find that you are eating larger quantities of foods than your body needs. It will be difficult to *respect your fullness* at this stage, because you need time to experiment with the quantity it takes to satisfy a deprived palate. It also takes time for you to develop trust with food again and know that it's truly okay to eat. How can you honor fullness, if you are not completely sure it's okay to eat the particular food, or if you fear it won't be there tomorrow?

If you have been eating as your predominant way to comfort yourself, you may find that you will begin to *feel* your feelings and may experience discomfort, sadness, or even depression at times.

The bulk of your eating may be foods that have previously been forbidden, although you may have been eating large quantities of these foods secretly or with guilt. *It is unlikely that the way you eat during this stage will be the pattern that you will establish or want for a lifetime.* You will notice that your nutritional balance is off-kilter and you may not feel physically on top of things during this time. This is all normal and expected. You must let yourself go through this stage for as long as you need. Remember, you are making up for years of deprivation, negative self-talk, and guilt. You are rebuilding positive food experiences, like a strand of pearls. Each food experience, like each pearl, may seem insignificant, but collectively they make a difference.

STAGE THREE:
CRYSTALLIZATION

In this stage, you will experience the first awakenings of the Intuitive Eating style that has always been a part of you but was buried under the debris of dieting. When you enter this stage, much of the exploration work from the previous stage begins to crystallize and feels like solid behavior change. Your thoughts about food are no longer obsessive. You hardly need to maintain the hyperconsciousness about eating that was originally needed. Consequently, your eating decisions don't require quite as much directed thought. Instead, you find that your food choices and responses to biological signals are mainly intuitive.

You have a greater sense of trust—both in your right to choose what you really want to eat and in the discovery that your biological signals are dependable. You are more comfortable with your food choices and will start to notice increased satisfaction at your meals.

At this point, you *honor your hunger* most of the time, and it's easier to discern what you feel like eating when you are hungry. You continue to *make peace with food*.

What feels new in this stage is that it's easier to take a time-out in the midst of your meal to consciously gauge how much your stomach is filling up. You will be able to take note of your fullness and respect the presence of that signal, although you may find that you often eat beyond the fullness mark. Just like when an archer takes aim at a new target, it often requires shooting many arrows before learning how to reach the bull's-eye. You may still be choosing previously forbidden foods most of the time, but you will find that you don't need as much of them to satisfy you.

If you've been an emotionally cued eater, you'll become quite adept at separating biological hunger signals from emotional hunger. Because of this clarity, more often than not, you will be experiencing your feelings and finding ways to comfort and distract yourself without the predominant use of food.

Remember to put weight loss on the back burner (which in and of itself is a practice resulting from the insidiousness of diet culture). What is most important at this stage is the sense of well-being and empowerment that begins to take place. You won't feel helpless and hopeless anymore. You will begin to respect your body and understand that if you've been eating more than your body needs, it's as a result of the dieting mentality, rather than lack of willpower.

Stage Four:
The Intuitive Eater Awakens

By the time you reach this stage, all of the work you have been doing culminates in a comfortable, free-flowing eating style. You consistently choose what you really want to eat when you are hungry. Because you know that you can have more food of your choosing, whenever you are hungry, it's easier to stop eating when you feel comfortably full.

You may begin to find that you choose more nutrient-dense foods, not because you think you should, but because you *feel* better physically when you eat this way. The urgent need to prove to yourself that you can have previously forbidden foods will have diminished. You truly know and trust that these foods will always be there, and if you really want to eat them, you can—so they lose their alluring quality. Chocolate starts to take on the same emotional connotation as a peach. You won't need to test yourself anymore, and your deprivation backlash with food will be gone.

When you do choose the foods you used to restrict, you will get great pleasure and be more acutely in touch with satisfaction, without feeling guilt. (When you feel guilty eating a food, it takes away the pleasure from eating.)

If coping with your feelings had been difficult for you, you will be less afraid to experience them, and become more adept at sitting with them. Finding diverse alternatives to distract and comfort yourself when necessary will become natural for you.

Your food talk and self-talk will be positive and noncritical. Your peace pact with food is firmly established, and you will have released any conflict or leftover guilt about food choices that you have carried around.

You have stopped making disrespectful comments about your body. You respect it and accept that there are many different sizes and shapes in the world and begin to appreciate that your inner qualities hold much more value than a number on the scale.

STAGE FIVE:
THE FINAL STAGE — TREASURE THE PLEASURE

At this point your Intuitive Eater has been reclaimed. You will trust your body's intuitive abilities—it will be easy to *honor your hunger* and *respect fullness*. Finally, you will feel no guilt about your food choices or quantities. Because you feel good about your relationship to food and treasure the pleasure that eating now gives you, you will, for the most part, discard unsatisfying eating situations and unappealing foods. Bear in mind that being able to respect fullness and experience satisfaction with food can only come with knowing you have food security. Intuitive Eating is a privilege that is not felt for those who don't have food security.

You will want to experience eating in the most optimal of conditions and not taint it with emotional distress. You will feel an inner conviction to let go of using food to cope as your primary coping skill, if that has been your dominant habit. When emotions become too overwhelming, you will find that you would much rather deal with your feelings or distract yourself from them with something other than food.

Because your eating style has become a source of pleasure rather than an affliction, you will experience nutrition and movement in a different way. The *burden* of exercise will be removed, and moving your body will begin to feel enticing to you. Exercise will no longer be used as a driving force to burn more calories; rather, you become committed to movement as a way to *feel* better, physically and mentally. Likewise, nutrition will no longer be another mechanism to make you feel bad about the way you eat; instead, it becomes a path to feeling good physically and will be part of your journey toward self-care.

When you reach the final stage, your concerns about weight will diminish as you appreciate the other qualities that make you the unique person that you are. You will feel free from the call of diet culture and the burden of dieting. And you will be an Intuitive Eater once again. While many of you will feel empowered and protected from outside forces telling you what and how much to eat, and how your body should look—it is important to acknowledge that this personal Intuitive Eating work does nothing to get rid of the root of oppressive forces, which occur at the systemic level (such as racism, anti-semitism, transphobia, homophobia, ableism, poverty, classism, and weight stigma).

YOU CAN DO IT!

These stages and the changes that occur with your eating and thoughts may seem impossible. Or they might seem scary. For example, the thought of giving yourself unconditional permission to eat may seem terrifying—and you might fear that you will never stop eating. The remainder of the book explains in great detail how to implement each principle, why it is needed, and the rationale behind it. You will also find how other chronic dieters became Intuitive Eaters and how it changed their lives. By the time you finish reading this book, you will know that you too can become an Intuitive Eater and stop the futility of dieting.

Chapter 6

PRINCIPLE 1:

Reject the Diet Mentality

Throw out the diet books and magazine articles that offer you false hope of losing weight quickly, easily, and permanently. Get angry at diet culture that promotes weight loss and the lies that have led you to feel as if you were a failure every time a new diet stopped working and you gained back all of the weight. If you allow even one small hope to linger that a new and better diet or food plan might be lurking around the corner, it will prevent you from being free to rediscover Intuitive Eating.

If you're like most clients we see, the idea of *not* dieting or following some food rules can be scary (even when you know that you can't choke down one more food plan or drink). It's normal to feel panicky about letting go of dieting, especially when it seems everyone around you is on some diet or some "lifestyle" plan to shrink the body. It has been the only tool you have known to (attempt to) lose weight (albeit temporarily).

Hitting diet bottom is a paralyzing feeling—damned if you diet and damned if you don't. Many of our clients feel stuck between two conflicting fears: "if I continue dieting, I'll continue to feel like a failure" and "if I stop dieting, I'll feel lost." Other common fears that we hear are:

FEAR: If I stop dieting, I won't stop eating.

REALITY: Dieting is often the *trigger* for overeating. Of course, it's hard to stop eating when you've been undereating and restricting food. It's a normal response to starvation (you'll learn more about that in the next chapter)! But once your body learns (and trusts) that you will not be starving it anymore (through dieting or some restricted food plan), the intense drive for overeating will decrease.

FEAR: I don't know how to eat when I'm not dieting or following an eating plan.

REALITY: When you banish food plans and become an Intuitive Eater, you will be eating in response to inner signals, which will guide your eating. This is like learning how to swim for the first time. The feeling of being surrounded by water can be terrifying to the novice swimmer, especially when totally submerged. Similarly, being surrounded by food can be terrifying to the chronic dieter, who is learning how to eat again. But you will not learn how to swim by merely standing at the edge of the pool (even while believing that learning how to swim is a good thing). You begin by getting your feet wet and learning how to breathe when you're in the water. Eventually you will put your head in the water when you are ready—and you get more comfortable.

FEAR: I will be out of control.

REALITY: Control is not an issue in Intuitive Eating. Instead, you will be relying on your internal signals, rather than on external factors, social media influencers, and authority figures (whom you're bound to defy). Nobody can be the expert of "you." Only *you* know your thoughts, feelings, and experiences. And you also won't be reacting to the deprivation that goes hand in hand with dieting. You will learn to trust your internal wisdom and will learn to listen to and honor your inner cues (both physical and emotional), all of which feels empowering.

THE DIET VOID

For many people dieting has been a way to cope with life, from filling up time, to serving as a symbol of control over your life. Think of the times in your life in which you started a diet or a food plan. How often did your diets coincide with difficult times or transitions in your life? It's not unusual to begin a diet during the following life transitions: passing from childhood to adolescence, leaving home, marrying, starting a new job, or when experiencing marital difficulties. While dieting may have been futile, it offered excitement and hope—the exhilaration of quick weight loss and the excitement of watching the scale inch downward. The hope—that this diet will be it. It's similar to going to a hairstylist for a new cut, with the expectation that it will revolutionize the way you look and feel about yourself and maybe change your life. But when you say goodbye to the thrill and excitement of dieting, you'll also be letting go of the false hope and disappointments from dieting.

There's a social element to dieting that you may miss, *diet bonding.*

When you decide to give up dieting, you might be surprised how often new diets and dieting are the topic of conversation at parties, with
friends, at work—and now you won't be playing *that* game. It might feel
like a must-see movie everyone is talking about, only you haven't seen
it and have no plans to view it either. You might feel a little left out,
detached.

Remember, as long as there is money to be made, there will always be
a new gimmick or diet for a quick weight loss fix. At one point, the manu-
facturer of a product called "Sleepers Dieter" claimed to help people attain
greater weight loss while sleeping. Talk about dreaming! The manufac-
turer was fined by the FTC for making unsubstantiated claims. But people
still shelled out money for this gimmick.

THE ONE-LAST-DIET TRAP

The initial step to becoming an Intuitive Eater is to reject the diet mentality. Yet even when you come to terms with the futility and harm that
dieting unleashes on the body (and mind), it can be a difficult first step, as
described in a letter below from a client, Lisa:

> *I have been in the dieting dilemma all my life. Every diet I've ever
> been on has worked for me, at least what I thought of as worked.
> Worked in the past was losing a certain number of pounds, never
> considering the reality of regaining the weight, plus more, with each
> and every diet I went on. At age thirty-six, I came to a point in my
> life where I was dieted-out. I knew there had to be another way. Yet
> my first thought was to let myself find one more diet for the last time,
> and I would make a promise to myself to never gain the weight back
> through a change in lifestyle.*

Lisa's letter represents a common conflict. You've hit diet bottom, you
know dieting doesn't work, but you're desperate—just one more diet, just
this time, "I'll be good." And so begins the familiar chronic dieter's plea:
just let me lose the weight now, and *after* I lose the weight, I'll figure it out.
But as long as you cling to a small hope that a quick little diet will turn
your weight around, or jump-start you into a new person, you won't be free
from the tyranny of diet culture. Giving in to just-one-more-diet is one of

the biggest traps, because it doesn't face the reality—diets do not work. So how could another diet truly be part of the solution?

Jack, another client, had been consistently dieting since the age of twelve. By the time he came in, Jack thought he was ready to give up dieting. Jack made a lot of progress in three months. For the first time, he began to have a normal relationship with food rather than constant food worry and obsession. But he wanted to take a break from our work together. Five months later, Jack called—he desperately needed to come back. Jack said that he "finally got it." He knew once and for all that dieting creates *more* problems. Jack revealed that during his initial work with Intuitive Eating, he had secretly hoped that a little diet was all he needed. He thought losing some quick pounds would allow him to work on his "real food issues," without worrying about his body, and then he would have more patience. It was part of his reason for leaving.

When Jack left, he dabbled with two serious quickie diets, which resulted in disaster. The first included juice fasting and intense exercise. The second was a detox cleanse. He was so "motivated" that he thought his problems would be over. Jack couldn't have been further from the truth. He became more obsessed with food and began bingeing. He ended up being more frustrated and had less trust in himself with food.

Every diet is like a Hula-Hoop flung onto your body. At first, it's effortless to keep the hoop in motion. But multiple Hula-Hoops disrupt normal rhythm and become binding. You cannot rotate the Hula-Hoops—you can't even move. To get yourself out of the last-chance-diet trap, you need to come to terms with the fact that dieting doesn't work and can, in fact, be harmful. We believe that if people (including healthcare professionals) really accepted that they are actually promoting weight stigma, they would not go down the futile dieting path.

Perhaps you're inclined to argue, however, that you'll *feel* better about yourself *when* you lose the weight. But studies have shown that improvements in psychological well-being associated with weight loss are just as temporary as the pounds lost and regained. The "good feelings" diminish with regained weight, and existing issues of self-worth and general psychological function return to initial levels when the weight is regained. And of equal importance, a focus on weight loss and dieting only keep you stuck in the belief that your weight is a measure of "who you are." Remember, you are much more than your weight!

PSEUDO-DIETING

Many of our clients state, "I've given up dieting," but they still have trouble shaking the diet mentality. They may be physically off of a diet, but the food-restrictive thoughts remain. The problem is that dieting thoughts usually translate into diet-like behaviors, which becomes *pseudo-dieting* or unconscious dieting. Consequently, these clients will still suffer the side effects of dieting, but it's much harder to spot (and then they really feel out of control with their eating). *Pseudo-dieting* behaviors are not usually apparent to the person engaged in them. Keep in mind that eating is so universal that it's hard to be objective. It can be difficult to find the loopholes in your own eating mentality and behavior if you don't know what you are looking for. To the surprise of our clients, they often don't discover that they have been pseudo-dieting until *together* we review their Intuitive Eating journal. Here are some examples of pseudo-dieting:

• *Meticulously counting carbohydrate grams or macros* is the modern version of counting calories. While being conscious of what you eat has its merits, the act of counting carbohydrate grams to control weight is really no different than counting calories. Many of our chronic dieters are pros at rationing their carbohydrate grams for the day—and they are stuck.

• *Eating only "safe" foods.* This usually means sticking with fat-free, carb-free, and/or low-calorie foods, beyond counting fat or carbohydrate grams. For example, thinking it was unhealthy, one client would not eat any food that listed more than one gram of fat on the food label, regardless of what her total fat and energy intake for the day was. Remember, however, that one food, one meal, or one day will not make or break your health.

• *Eating only at certain times of the day*, whether or not you are hungry, is a common leftover habit from dieting, especially *not* eating after a certain time of night, such as after 6 p.m. Reality check: our bodies do not punch time clocks; we do not suddenly turn off our need for energy at a certain time. This can especially be a problem for a dieter who exercises after work, comes home, and decides it's too late to eat. While it is reasonable to not want to go to bed on a full stomach, because it would be uncomfortable, to deny a hungry body *any* food or energy is unreasonable.

• *Paying penance for eating perceived "bad" foods* such as cookies, cheesecake, or ice cream. The penalty can include skipping the next meal, eating less, vowing to be "good" tomorrow, or doing *extra* exercise.

• *Cutting back on food,* especially when clothes feel tight or when a special event such as a wedding or class reunion comes up. It's amazing how often this gets acted out in the form of unconscious *undereating.* Remember, undereating usually triggers overeating.

• *Pacifying hunger by drinking coffee or diet soda.* This is a common dieting trick to assuage hunger pangs without eating or calories.

• *Limiting carbohydrates.* We are struck by the number of clients who profess they know of the importance of consuming this form of fuel, yet eat an *inadequate* amount of carbohydrates, such as bread, pasta, and rice, because they are afraid they will gain weight.

• *Putting on a "false food face" in public.* You only eat what is "proper" in front of other people—this is also known as performative eating, eating to please the expectations of other. One client, Alice, ate an enjoyable meal with friends. When the dessert tray came around, she really wanted a piece of pie, but fought the urge, because she wanted to appear to be the "health-conscious" eater. However, on her way home, the urge for the pie swelled into an uncontrollable craving. Alice stopped at the store, bought a whole pie, and ate one-fourth of it—*more* than she would have eaten had she honored her true food preference! This social dieting behavior of putting on a false food face backfired (and it often does).

• *Competing with someone else who is dieting,* feeling obligated to be equally "virtuous" (if not more so). Because dieting is viewed as virtuous in our society, it is not unusual that you would get sucked in. This can easily occur when friends, family, or a significant other is dieting.

• *Second-guessing or judging what you deserve to eat* based on what you've eaten earlier in the day, rather than on hunger cues. One client, Sally, ate two large bowls of puffed rice cereal for breakfast after running for one hour. She thought that was too much food, and later in the midmorning did not allow herself to eat, although she was ravenous. Sally thought, "How could I be hungry only two hours after I ate a big breakfast?" The reality for Sally was that while her volume of food in the morning was larger than her norm, it was still *inadequate* for the amount of exercise she did. Her body was trying to tell her, "I need more fuel." Yet Sally felt guilty for being hungry. She also felt guilty for eating a "big" breakfast, until she realized that in actuality, she had *undereaten.* Just because a meal or snack does not fit the "standard" portion size from your dieting days, it does not mean you are overeating!

• *Becoming a vegetarian/vegan or eating a gluten-free diet only for the purpose of losing weight.* A vegetarian lifestyle can be a healthy way of eating and living, but if it is embraced with a diet mentality, it becomes merely another diet. For example, Karen began eating meatless to lose weight. But a month into her vegetarian eating, she began craving meat. Never before had she experienced meat cravings! Karen realized she never really intended to become a vegetarian. She wasn't interested in vegetarian eating for health or ethical reasons, only as a vehicle to lose weight, and so her diet backfired. And there are others, who do not have Celiac disease or an extreme gluten sensitivity, who also go down this path, attempting to disguise their desire for weight loss.

• *It's a lifestyle.* Thanks to diet culture influence we have worked with folks who are counting or eliminating foods for the purpose and expectation of weight loss. But because they believe the rhetoric of "it's a lifestyle," they don't view it as a diet. Counting macros is not a lifestyle. Counting points is not a lifestyle. Nice try, diet culture, we're on to you!

• *Rigidly healthy.* Inflexible eating in the name of health.

THE DIETER'S DILEMMA

Whether you are engaged in bona fide dieting or pseudo-dieting, any form of dieting is bound to lead to problems. The inherent futility of dieting is explained in the Dieter's Dilemma model created by psychologists John P. Foreyt and G. Ken Goodrick, shown below. The Dieter's Dilemma is triggered by the desire to be *smaller*, which is programmed by diet culture and leads to dieting. That's when the dilemma unfolds. Dieting increases cravings and urges for food. The dieter gives in to the craving, overeats, and eventually regains any lost weight. They are back to where they started, with the original weight—or higher. And once again the dieter has the desire to shrink their body . . . and so another diet begins. The Dieter's Dilemma is perpetuated and gets worse with each turn of the cycle, making the dieter feel more out of control with eating.

How do you break the futile Dieter's Dilemma? You must simply make the decision to let go of dieting. Although the anti-dieting movement is growing in popularity, there is always a new diet or program around the corner. Diet culture is sneaky!

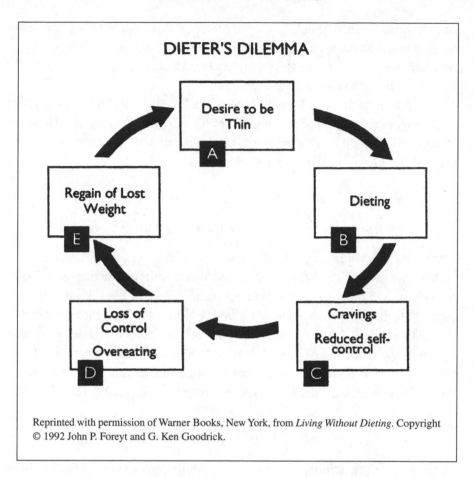

DIETER'S DILEMMA

Reprinted with permission of Warner Books, New York, from *Living Without Dieting*. Copyright © 1992 John P. Foreyt and G. Ken Goodrick.

HOW TO REJECT THE DIET MENTALITY

To let go of the dieting myth and the dieting mentality, our minds require a new frame of reference. In his bestselling book *The 7 Habits of Highly Effective People,* Stephen Covey popularized the concept of paradigm shifts. A paradigm is a model or frame of reference by which we perceive and understand the world. In the world of "weight management," dieting is the cultural paradigm by which we attempt to control our weight. A paradigm shift is a break with tradition, with old ways of thinking, with old paradigms. We must change our paradigm to reject dieting; only then can we build a healthy relationship with food and our bodies.

While Covey's work is aimed at the business community, he hits upon an issue that rings true for chronic dieters. He believes that people are often drawn to remedy the problem without regard to the long-term implications of this "quick fix." He feels that this approach actually exacerbates the problem rather than permanently solving it. He points to the physical body as a prized asset that often is ruined, while one is in the race for rapid results and short-term benefits.

Several researchers and health professionals are calling for a paradigm shift away from weight-focused healthcare (O'Hara and Taylor 2019; Hunger et al. 2020). Weight is not a behavior! Here are the steps to begin your paradigm shift of rejecting the diet mentality.

STEP 1:
RECOGNIZE AND ACKNOWLEDGE THE DAMAGE THAT DIETING CAUSES

There is a substantial amount of research on the harm that dieting causes. Acknowledge that the harm is real, and that continued dieting and food restriction will only perpetuate your problems. Some of the key side effects gleaned from major studies are described below, in two categories, biological and emotional. As you read, take a personal inventory, and ask yourself which of the problems you are already experiencing. Recognizing that dieting is *the* problem will help you break through the cultural myth that diets work. Remember, *if dieting is the problem, how can it be part of the solution?*

Damage from Dieting: Biological and Health-Related

In every century, famine and human starvation have existed. Sadly, this is still true today. Survival of the fittest in the past meant survival of the fattest—only those with adequate energy stores (fat) could survive a famine. Consequently, our bodies are still equipped in this modern age to combat starvation at the cellular level. As far as the body is concerned, dieting is a form of starvation (even though it's voluntary).

- *Chronic dieting teaches the body to retain more fat when you start eating again.* Low-calorie diets double the enzymes that make and store fat in the body. This is a form of biological compensation to help the body store more energy, or fat, after dieting.
- *Dieting decreases metabolism.* Dieting triggers the body to become more efficient at utilizing calories by lowering the body's need for energy. (Recall the *Biggest Loser* study, which showed that this effect persisted for six years!)

- *Dieting increases binges and cravings.* Both humans and rats have been shown to overeat after chronic food restriction. Food restriction stimulates the brain to launch a cascade of cravings to eat *more,* because the body on a cellular level is trying to survive the self-imposed famine.
- *Dieting increases the risk of premature death and heart disease.* A thirty-two-year study of more than three thousand men and women, the Framingham Heart Study, has shown that *regardless of initial weight,* people whose weight repeatedly goes up and down—known as weight cycling or yo-yo dieting—have a higher overall death rate and twice the normal risk of dying of heart disease. These results were independent of cardiovascular risk factors and held true regardless of a person's weight. (Lissner et al. 1991)

Similarly, results of the Harvard Alumni Health Study show that people who lose and gain at least eleven pounds within a decade or so don't live as long as those who maintain a stable weight. (Lee et al. 1992)

- *Dieting causes satiety cues to atrophy.* Dieters usually stop eating due to a self-imposed limit rather than inner cues of fullness. This, combined with skipping meals, can condition you to eat meals of increasingly larger size.
- *Dieting causes body shape to change.* Yo-yo dieters who continually regain the lost weight tend to regain weight in the abdominal area. This type of fat storage increases the risk of heart disease.

Other documented side effects include headaches, menstrual irregularities, fatigue, dry skin, and hair loss.

Damage from Dieting: Psychological and Emotional

Decades ago, psychological experts reported the following adverse effects at the landmark 1992 National Institutes of Health Weight Loss and Control Conference:

- *Dieting is linked to eating disorders.* In an unrelated study, dieters were eight times as likely to suffer from an eating disorder by the age of fifteen than non-dieters.

- *Dieting may cause stress or make the dieter more vulnerable to its effects.*
- *Dieting is correlated with feelings of failure, lowered self-esteem, and social anxiety,* independent of body weight itself.
- *The dieter is often vulnerable to loss of control, overeating* when violating "the rules" of the diet, whether there was an actual or *perceived* transgression of the diet! The mere perception of eating a forbidden food (regardless of actual calorie content) is enough to trigger overeating.

In a separate report, psychologists David Garner and Susan Wooley make a compelling case against the high cost of false hope from dieting. They conclude that:

- *Dieting gradually erodes confidence and self-trust.*
- Many folks in larger bodies assume they could not have become large unless they possessed some *fundamental character deficit.* Garner and Wooley argue that while many larger individuals may experience binge eating and depression, these psychological and behavioral symptoms are often the *result of dieting.* But these folks easily interpret these symptoms as further evidence of an underlying problem. Yet people in larger bodies do not have inordinate psychological disturbances compared to people in smaller-size bodies.

STEP 2:
BE AWARE OF DIET-MENTALITY TRAITS AND THINKING

The diet mentality surfaces in subtle forms, even when you decide to reject dieting. It's important to recognize common characteristics of the diet mentality; it will let you know if you are still playing the dieting game. Forget about willpower, being obedient, and failing. The general traits of how the dieter versus the non-dieter view eating, exercise, and progress are summarized in a chart at the end of this section.

Forget willpower. While no doctor would expect a patient to "will" blood pressure to normal levels, physicians frequently expect their larger patients to "will" their weight loss by restricting their food, according to Susan Z. Yanovski, MD. This is also a prevailing attitude among our clients and many Americans—all you need is willpower and a little self-control. In a 1993 Gallup poll, the most common obstacle cited to losing weight by women was willpower. It's still a common belief!

For example, Marilyn is a highly successful lawyer who climbed to the top of the corporate ladder. She credits her success to her determination, willpower, and self-discipline. Yet when she tried to use these exemplary principles in her dieting attempts, she always failed. Whatever success she had achieved in her professional life was dulled by her sense of failure with her eating.

Why was Marilyn able to be so disciplined in one area of her life but not in the other? The word "discipline" is derived from the word "disciple." According to Stephen Covey's work, if you are a disciple to your own deep values that have an overriding purpose, it's likely that you'll have the *will* to carry them out. Marilyn believed deeply that writing exacting contracts and keeping immaculate records were requisites to building confidence with her clients and her law firm. But, somehow, hearing that bread was wrong on one diet and anything with sugar was wrong on another did not engender the same kind of deep beliefs. Try as she might, she couldn't really believe that chocolate chip cookies were that evil!

"Willpower" can be defined as an attempt to counter natural desires and replace them with proscriptive rules. It also implies the ability to do unpleasant tasks that are not essential. The desire for sweets is natural, normal, and quite pleasant! Any diet that tells you that you can't have sweets is going against your natural desire. The diet becomes a set of rigid rules, and these kinds of rules can only trigger rebellion.

Willpower does not belong in Intuitive Eating. As Marilyn became an Intuitive Eater, she found that listening to her personal signals reinforced her natural instincts, rather than countering them. She had no one else's proscriptive rules to follow or to rebel against. Marilyn has stopped fighting the phantom willpower battle and has made peace with food and her body.

Forget being obedient. A well-meaning suggestion, by a spouse or significant other, such as "Honey, you *should* have the broiled chicken" or "You *shouldn't* eat those fries," can set off an inner food rebellion. In this type of food combat, your only arsenal to fight back becomes a double order of fries. Our clients call this "*forget-you* eating."

In physics, resistance always occurs as a reaction to force. We see this principle in action in society—riots often erupt when the force of authority becomes too great. Similarly, the *simple act of being told* what to do (even if it's something you want to do), can trigger a rebellious chain reaction. Just like "terrible two-year-olds" or teenagers who revolt to prove they are independent, dieters can initiate rebellious eating in response to the act of dieting, with its set of rigid rules. And so, it's not surprising to hear from our clients that breaking the rules of a diet makes them feel just like they did when they were defiant teens.

But take heart: rebellion is a normal act of self-preservation—protecting your space, or personal boundaries.

Think of a personal boundary as a tall brick wall surrounding you, with only one gate. Only you can open that gate, if you choose. Therefore, no one is allowed inside, unless you invite the person in. Within your fence reside private feelings, thoughts, and biological signals. People who *assume* they know what you need and tell you what to do are picking the lock to your gate or invading your boundaries. Remember, nobody can be the expert of "you." Only *you* know your thoughts, feelings, and experiences. No one could possibly know what's inside, unless you tell them by inviting them in.

What diet or social media influencer can possibly know when you are hungry or how much food it will take to satisfy you? How can anyone but you know what texture and taste sensations will be pleasing to your palate? In the world of dieting, personal boundaries are crossed at many levels. For example, you are told what to eat, how much of it to eat, and when to eat it. These decisions should all be personal choices, with respect for individual autonomy and body signals. While food guidance may come from elsewhere, *you* should ultimately be responsible for the *when, what,* and *how much* of eating.

When a diet doctor or a diet plan invades your boundaries, it's normal to feel powerless. The longer you follow the food restrictions, the greater the assault to your autonomy. Here is where the paradox lies. When dieting, you will likely rebel by eating more—to restore your autonomy and protect your boundaries. But the act of rebelling can make you feel as out of control as a city riot. Instead, you have an inner food fight on your hands. But once the food rebellion is unleashed, its intensity reinforces feelings of lack of control and the belief that you don't possess willpower. Ultimately you begin to drown in a sea of self-doubt and shame. *What begins as a psychologically healthy behavior ends in disaster.* Ultimately, a healthy relationship with food and your body is sabotaged, as a result of this natural rebellion. With Intuitive Eating there will be no need to rebel, because you become the one who is finally in charge!

Boundaries are also invaded when someone makes comments about your weight or how you should look. Again, you are bound to rebel by reactive eating. It's a way of saying, once again, "Forget you. You have no right to tell me what to weigh."

Rachel is an artist who had dieted all her life. She was married to a successful lawyer who wanted to show off his wife to all of his colleagues. He'd continually make subtle remarks that she wasn't as thin as she could be. He would even go so far as to give her dirty looks when she would reach for a rich dessert at a party. Rachel rebelled against her husband by sneaking foods behind his back (free from his evil eye). While going through the Intuitive Eating process, Rachel discovered that she was actually sneakeating and eating more than she wanted as the ultimate form of rebellion against her husband.

But instead of feeling strong and powerful from her rebellion, she found that she actually felt weak, out of control, and miserable. She knew that she would feel better if she ate according to her body's hunger and fullness signals, but "something" kept making her turn to the hidden extra foods. Rachel had been trapped in a game of control, boundary invasion, and rebellion all her life. Her husband and diet culture had been trying to control this free-spirited woman. To protect her boundaries, she would fight the diets by overeating and fight her husband's inappropriate demands to be in a smaller body.

Eventually Rachel stood up to her husband and told him that he had no right to make comments about her food or her weight. Although initially resistant, he began to respect her boundaries. She also made a firm commitment to give up dieting. As a result, Rachel was shocked to find that her secret eating disappeared, as did her self-doubt, and she began to eat what her body needed, by listening to her intuitive signals.

Forget about failure. All of our chronic dieters walk into our offices feeling as if they are failures. Whether they are highly placed executives, prominent celebrities, or straight-A students, they all talk about their food experiences shamefully, and they doubt whether they'll ever be able to feel successful in the area of eating. The diet mentality reinforces feelings of success or failure. You can't fail at Intuitive Eating—it's a learning process at every point along the way. What used to be thought of as a setback will instead be seen as a learning experience. When you are able to learn from a perceived setback, it will help you let go—and you'll see this as progress, not perfection.

Dieters rely on external forces to regulate their eating, sticking to a regimented food plan, eating because it's time, or eating only a specified (and measured) amount, whether hungry or not. This is not body autonomy! Dieters also validate progress by external forces—primarily the scale, asking, "How many pounds have I lost? Is my weight up or down?" It's time to throw out your dieting tools. Get rid of the meal plans, tracking apps on your phone, and the food and bathroom scales.

The scale as false idol. "Please, please, let the number be . . ." This wishful number prayer is not occurring in the casinos of Las Vegas, but in private homes throughout the country. But just like a desperate gambler waiting for his lucky number to come in, so is it futile for the dieter to pay homage to the "scale god." In one sweep of the scale roulette, hopes and desperation combine to form a daily drama that will ultimately shape what mood you'll be in for the day. Ironically a "good" or "bad" scale number can *both* trigger overeating—whether it's a congratulatory eating party or a consolation party.

The scale ritual sabotages body and mind efforts; it can in one moment devalue days, weeks, and even months of progress, as illustrated with Connie.

Connie had been working very hard at Intuitive Eating and refrained from weighing herself, which in itself had been a feat since she originally weighed in daily, and sometimes even twice a day at home. But Connie felt she had made so much progress in three months that she stepped on the scale. The momentary brush with the scale, with its focus on weight loss, boomeranged Connie right back to the diet mentality. That week, Connie cut back her food intake, which resulted in a large binge. Stepping on the scale was a step back into the diet mentality. It was no surprise that Connie countered her scale experience with a dieting approach. She also thought, "I must be doing something wrong." Her newfound trust began to erode—all with a single trip to the scale.

So much power is given to the almighty scale that it ultimately sabotages our efforts. But in the case of Sherry, she found the weighing process to be so humiliating that she had postponed going to the doctors for fifteen years! At the age of fifty-five, Sherry had not had a mammogram or other essential physical exams because she did not want to be weighed at the doctor's office. In this case the scale was getting in the way of Sherry's health; she was at risk for breast cancer, because it ran in her family. Getting the mammogram was more important than any number on the scale, but Sherry couldn't face the routine admonishments from the nursing staff. It was standard procedure—weigh the patient regardless of the reason for the appointment. Sherry did not realize that she had the right to refuse to be weighed. She finally got the courage after our work together. She made a doctor's appointment and refused to be weighed, since it was not an essential component of her medical care at the moment. Fortunately, her physical exam results were healthy.

We have found that the "weigh-in" factor usually detracts from a person's progress. In the "old days" when we used to weigh all patients, we found that sessions were often spent on why the weight went up or did not move at all, and they became scale-counseling sessions. Our patients also dreaded the weighing-in part as much as we did. We certainly regret those days!

When a pound is not a pound. Many factors can influence the number on the scale, so deifying the scale to give you the power to feel good or bad about yourself is falling prey to the influence of false facts. The number on the scale is affected by water retention or release of water. Anytime the scale suddenly rises or falls, it is usually because of a fluid shift in the body. Many factors can influence fluid retention—hormones, excessive sodium intake, and even the weather! Yet how easily chronic dieters believe they did something wrong. Conversely, a rapid drop on the scale immediately after an hour of aerobics is mostly water loss from sweat.

Also, muscle is made up of mainly water (70 percent). When a hungry body is not given enough calories, the body cannibalizes itself for an energy source. The prime directive of the body is that it must have energy, at any cost—it's part of the survival mechanism. The protein in muscles is converted to valuable energy for the body. When a muscle cell is destroyed, water is released and eventually excreted. The whittled-away muscle contributes to lowering your metabolism. Muscles are metabolically active tissue—generally the more muscle we have, the higher our metabolic rate.

That's one of the reasons men burn more calories than women—they have more muscle mass.

Increased muscle mass, while metabolically more active, weighs more than fat. A chronic dieter often gets frustrated by the rising, or unchanging, number on the scale. *The scale does not reflect body composition—* just like weighing a piece of steak at the butcher's does not tell you how lean the meat is.

Weighing in on the scale only serves to keep you focused on your weight; it doesn't help with the *process* of getting back in touch with Intuitive Eating. Constant weigh-ins can leave you frustrated and impede your progress. Best bet: let go of weighing yourself.

STEP 4:
BE COMPASSIONATE TOWARD YOURSELF

When everyone around you is dieting and euphoric about how weight is melting away as a result of the latest diet craze, it's understandable that you can get pulled in. But this pull is more than just aesthetics.

In her book *The Religion of Thinness*, Harvard-trained theologian and scholar Michelle M. Lelwica makes a compelling argument about how the endless pursuit of thinness, through dieting, fulfills a spiritual hunger. The pursuit of dieting serves as an "ultimate purpose" by:

- Providing a set of myths to believe regarding the "rewards" of thinness
- Offering rituals to organize the daily lives of women
- Creating a moral code of which to live and eat by
- Creating a common bond and a community for women

Although Lelwica refers specifically to women, these outcomes can apply to anyone on the gender spectrum.

When you consider these covert "benefits" of dieting, it's no wonder you can get seduced by the "rewards" of dieting. Don't beat yourself up for entertaining fantasies of trying one more diet or just wanting to diet. It takes a while to let go of this desire, even when you intellectually understand that the pursuit of dieting is truly futile. Self-compassion and kindness are so important on the path to becoming an Intuitive Eater. Remember, unlike dieting, this process is not pass or fail. It's a journey of self-discovery.

Intuitive Eating Tools

The tools of the Intuitive Eater are internal cues—not outside forces telling you what, when, and how much to eat. But to acquire and understand these internal cues, you need a new set of power tools—or rather, *empowerment* tools—which will be discussed in the following chapters.

SUMMARY: THE DIET MENTALITY VS. THE NONDIET MENTALITY		
Issue	Dieting Mentality	Nondiet Mentality
Eating/food choices	• Do I deserve it? • If I eat a high-calorie food, I try to find a way to make up for it. • I feel guilty when I eat high-calorie foods or foods high in carbs. • I usually describe a day of eating as either good or bad. • I view food as the enemy.	• Am I hungry? • Do I want it? • Will I feel deprived if I don't eat it? • Will it be satisfying? • Does it taste good? • I deserve to enjoy eating without guilt.
Movement benefits	• I focus primarily on the calories burned. • I feel guilty if I miss a designated exercise day.	• I focus primarily on how movement makes me feel, especially the energizing and stress-relieving factors.
Progress is viewed as	• How many pounds did I lose? • How do I look? • What do other people think of my weight? • I have good willpower.	• My weight is not my primary goal or an indicator of my progress. • I have increased trust with myself and food. • I am able to let go of "eating indiscretions." • I recognize inner body cues.

REJECT THE DIET MENTALITY: A DIET IS A DIET IS A DIET

Diet culture is so sneaky that the weight loss industry is moving away from overt dieting terms to healthy-sounding descriptions such as "lifestyle," "healthy," and "wellness." But whatever name they call it—if it's about shrinking your body and following food rules, it's still a diet. If you are counting calories, macros, or points, it's a diet. Unbelievably, the weight-stigmatizing television show *The Biggest Loser* announced in 2019 that it's rebooting with a wellness angle, which followed on the heels of Weight Watchers' rebranding.

Weight Watchers changed its name to WW in 2018, but it's still a dieting program. People often express surprise when they hear that counting points is a dieting behavior. That's when we will gently ask, "What do you do if you are hungry, and your points are used up?" The reply to this question is usually "Ohhh. How did you know?"—which is followed by a deep sigh.

Deconstructing Weight Watchers. Any way you look at it, WW is a diet in every aspect. Here are seven examples:

1. The focus on points pulls one away from internal signals of hunger and fullness.
2. The points become obsessional. For years after someone gets off of Weight Watchers, the points stay embedded in the brain to haunt them.
3. It encourages overeating. If you can eat as much as you want of vegetables (in the old days) and fruits (now), it promotes eating to push away feelings, eating of foods that give false fullness signals, and substituting these foods for foods that might be more satisfying.
4. It promotes the concept of "good" and "bad" foods. Foods that have a low number of points become the good foods, and foods with a high number become the bad.
5. If there are points left over at the end of the day, the person will be apt to eat beyond need, because they don't want to waste the points.
6. If a person is hungrier one day than the allowed points, they either have to "starve" or eat beyond their points. This promotes feeling guilty for going beyond, and/or the intention to make up the points the next day. If able to do this, it leads, once again, to semi-starvation, restricting, or not being able to restrict, which leads to more guilt.

7. Before and after pictures are shown in their social media and/or ads. Bodies come in diverse sizes. These type of pictures that focus on "after" smaller bodies are a form of diet culture. (Recall that these types of pictures are used in the Kurbo app for kids as young as seven.)

Here are some other dieting examples that might not be so obvious:

- Drinking a weight loss beverage for breakfast and lunch, followed by a "sensible" dinner.
- Detox fast, which usually consists of some type of liquid fast, in order to "remove toxins" from your body. Our bodies are built with an amazing inner cleansing system—the liver, kidneys, and digestive system.
- Colon cleanse, which involves a process of forcing the colon to empty its contents (ultimately resulting in diarrhea). The process may be via laxatives, enemas, or colon irrigation, known as a high colonic.
- Sipping diet or detox teas. These teas are usually laced with laxatives, so you may be spending a lot of time on the toilet.

Diet culture is even starting to co-opt Intuitive Eating to sell its weight loss products. If there are any food rules, counting of macros, or cheat days— that is most certainly not Intuitive Eating. It's marketing hype.

Chapter 7

PRINCIPLE 2:
Honor Your Hunger

Keep your body biologically fed with adequate energy and carbohydrates. Otherwise you can trigger a primal drive to overeat.
Once you reach the moment of excessive hunger, all intentions of
moderate, conscious eating are fleeting and irrelevant. Learning
to honor this first biological signal sets the stage for rebuilding
trust with yourself and food.

A dieting body is a starving body. Drastic comparison? No. While a
dieting body may not *look* like a starving person, the "symptoms" from
dieting exhibit a striking resemblance to the starvation state. The body
does not know that there is a McDonald's on every corner as you embark
on a diet. As far as the body is concerned it is living in a famine state and
adapts. Our need for food (energy) is so essential and primal that if we are
not getting enough energy, our bodies naturally compensate with powerful
biological and psychological mechanisms.

The power of food deprivation was keenly demonstrated in the landmark starvation study conducted by Dr. Ancel Keys during World War II,
mentioned earlier in the book, designed to help famine sufferers. The subjects of the study were thirty-two healthy men who were selected because
they had superior "psychobiological stamina"—superior mental and physical health.

During the first three months of the study the men ate as they pleased,
eating their typical quantity of food. The next six months was the semi-
starvation period, at which time calories were cut nearly in half. The
effects of the semi-starvation were startling, and strikingly mirror the
symptoms of chronic dieting:

- Metabolic rate decreased 40 percent.
- The men were obsessed with food. They had heightened food cravings and talked of food and collecting recipes.
- Eating style changed—vacillating from ravenously gulping to stalling out the eating experience. Some men played with their food and dawdled over a meal for two hours.
- The researchers noted, "Several men failed to adhere to their diets and reported episodes of bulimia." One man was reported to have suffered a complete loss of "willpower." Another subject "flagrantly broke the dietary rules" and ate several sundaes and malted milks and even stole penny candy.
- Some men exercised deliberately to obtain increased food rations.
- Personalities changed, and in many cases there was the onset of apathy, irritability, moodiness, and depression.

During the refeeding period, when the men were once again allowed to eat at will, hunger pangs became more intense, and hunger was insatiable. In spite of being able to eat abundantly, some of the men developed an irrational fear that food would not be available.

The men found it difficult to stop eating. Weekend binges added up to 8,000 to 10,000 calories. It took the majority of men an average of five months to normalize their eating, and some never fully recovered.

It's important to remember that during the era of this classic study, there were no celebrity trainers, no Food Network on TV, no national fitness and food divas. Nutrition research was just in its infancy. Yet these men experienced a primal obsession with food that was not media driven or society driven; rather it was triggered by a biological survival mechanism. Such behavior was never observed in these men prior to their food deprivation encounter! Although this is a classic starvation study, the caloric level is representative of a modern weight loss diet for men. It's notable that these men still experienced marked physical and psychological symptoms. Imagine if the same study were conducted under today's pressures to be thin.

We have had several clients read highlights of the classic Minnesota starvation study, and they are struck by how similar their own experiences were to those of the semi-starved men. Mary, for example, noted that after completing her second liquid fast program, she was more obsessed with food than ever before. She bought several cookbooks and major cooking appliances—a waffle maker, a bread maker, and a food processor. The biggest paradox Mary noted was that she doesn't like to cook and did not use her new appliances or cookbooks!

Dan was put on a diet at age four and has been on some type of food plan ever since. He described his "irrational fear" that each time he sat down for a meal, he truly felt that it would be his last opportunity to eat. (This is actually a form of food insecurity, which has been linked to binge eating disorders).

Jan had dieted most of her life. But the more she dieted, the more she got interested in food. She collected magazine and newspaper recipes of all kinds, from rich gourmet to spartan spa cuisine, and read them as if they were engaging novels. Yet she would never dare prepare the scrumptious recipes; instead they were her food fantasy and food escapism.

Of mice and men. Rats are certainly not exposed to the social pressures and nuances of eating that humans are, yet when deprived of food, rats will also overeat. In one study, rats were divided into two groups, one food-deprived and one control group. The food-deprived rats went without food for up to four days, and then were allowed to eat again until they gained their weight back. Both groups of rats were then given free access to a "palatable diet"—beyond the ordinary rat chow staples, like five-star dining in the rodent world. While both groups gained weight, those in the food-deprived group gained more weight, *in direct proportion to the length of their prior deprivation.*

PRIMAL HUNGER

The psychological terror of hunger is profound, notes Naomi Wolf in her book *The Beauty Myth.* Even after hunger has ended, the nagging terror of it remains. She cites how hungry orphans adopted from poor countries often cannot control their compulsion to smuggle and hide food, even after living for years in a secure environment. A 2000 study showed that a disproportionate number of concentration camp survivors suffer from binge eating disorder.*

Food insecurity or food scarcity is a form of trauma, the effects of

* Favaro, A., Rodella, F. C., & Santonastaso, P. (2000). *Binge eating and eating attitudes among Nazi concentration camp survivors. Psychological Medicine, 30(2), 463–466.*

which are emerging in the research on eating disorders. Bulimia nervosa and binge eating are increased in people with food insecurity history.

Research historians have documented that during times of famine or food shortages, food becomes an overriding preoccupation, resulting in societal problems: breakdown of social behavior, abandonment of cooperative effort, and loss of personal pride and a sense of family ties. While this preoccupation with food has been observed during times of food deprivation, these actions also mirror dieting behavior at the individual level. How often have you become more socially isolated while on a diet, turning down a party invitation, for instance, because you didn't want to deal with the food, or not going out altogether until you are through with your diet?

While the hunger and food obsession from dieting may not be experienced as a terrifying event, it does leave a lasting mark, especially if it began in childhood.

Peter had been on several medically supervised fasts over his lifetime and became frightened of experiencing hunger. To him, hunger *was* terrifying and often resulted in out-of-control eating, which reinforced his fear of hunger. Therefore, Peter always kept himself in a "fed" state between diets, never able to really experience gentle biological hunger. He only knew what *extreme* hunger felt like with all of its voracious intensity. To avoid hunger, he was constantly eating, but the persistent eating caused Peter to feel uncomfortable in his body, so he would start a new diet or fasting program and the vicious cycle would continue—hunger from dieting, followed by overeating.

MECHANISMS THAT TRIGGER EATING

Whether or not you are a chronic dieter, powerful biological mechanisms are triggered when your body does not get the energy from food that it needs. It's no accident that food is included as one of the fundamental needs in Maslow's hierarchy of needs—a model that ranks human needs, suggesting that certain basic needs must be met before you can go on to fulfill more complex ones. Food and energy are so essential to the survival of the human species that if we don't eat enough we set off a biological fuse that turns on our eating drive, both physically *and* psychologically. The hunger drive is truly a mind-body connection. Eating is so important that the nerve cells of appetite are located in the hypothalamus region of the brain. A variety of biological signals triggers eating. What many people believe to be an issue of willpower is instead a *biological drive*. The power and intensity of the biological eating drive should not be underestimated. The neurochemicals from the brain coordinate our eating behavior with our body's biological need. Through a complex system of chemical and neural feedback, the brain monitors the energy needs of all our body systems, moment to moment. And it makes very emphatic chemical directives as to what we should eat. Fasting or restricting is particularly counterproductive to appetite. It simply turns on the neurochemical switches that induce us to eat.

Many studies have shown that dieting makes no sense metabolically or to our brain chemistry. In fact, it's counterproductive. The biological chemicals that regulate appetite also directly affect moods and state of mind, our physical energy, and our sex lives.

Most researchers agree that there are both complex biological *and* psychological mechanisms that influence our eating. In this chapter, we will focus on the profound biological mechanisms that turn on our desire to eat, especially if we have been food-deprived or dieting:

Heightened Digestion

In food-deprived individuals, research has shown, the body gets biologically primed for the moment of eating, like a sprinter crouched in a ready position for an explosive start, the moment the starting pistol is triggered.

- Salivation increases with increases of food deprivation, even when there is no food present or suggestion of eating! This has been demonstrated in studies both on dieters and normal (nondieting) individuals.
- Increased digestive hormones have been found in dieters both before and after eating.

The Carbohydrate Craver: Neuropeptide Y

Neuropeptide Y (NPY) is a chemical produced by the brain that triggers our drive to eat carbohydrates, the body's primary and preferred source of energy. While most of what we know about NPY comes from research on rats, there is a lot of evidence that shows that this brain chemical can have a profound impact on human eating behavior as well, by increasing both the size and duration of carbohydrate-rich meals.

Food deprivation or undereating intake drives NPY into action, causing the body to seek more carbohydrates. When the next meal or eating opportunity rolls around, it can easily turn into a high-carbohydrate binge—not because you lack willpower or are out of control; it's your biology (rather NPY) screaming, "Feed me."

NPY is revved up after any imposed period of food deprivation, including an overnight fast from dinner to breakfast. NPY's levels are naturally the highest in the morning because of the short-term food deprivation from an overnight fast. The elevated NPY levels are part of the biological basis for eating in the morning! During an overnight fast, your body's stores of carbohydrates (in the liver) are drained and need refilling. You literally wake up on empty in the morning. But if you skip breakfast, you are likely to pay for it with increases in NPY level, which can lead to midafternoon gorging.

The brain also makes more NPY when carbohydrates are being burned as fuel and under times of stress. Eating carbohydrates turns off NPY through its effect on serotonin, another brain chemical. As we eat more carbohydrates, it helps to increase the production of serotonin, which in turn shuts off the production of NPY and puts a halt to the desire for carbohydrates.

The more you deny your true hunger and fight your natural biology, the stronger and more intense food cravings and obsessions become. Fasting or restricting especially revs up the NPY and drives the body to seek more carbohydrates. So, by the time the next eating opportunity occurs, it can *easily* become a high-carbohydrate binge.

Why is there such a chemical drive for carbohydrates? Let's look briefly at the critical role carbohydrates play in the body—it will help you understand the primal hunger drive.

The importance of carbohydrates. Carbohydrates are the preferred source of food energy to the body. Cells function best when they receive a certain level of carbohydrates, in the form of glucose, and even small decreases can cause problems. The brain, nervous system, and red blood cells rely *exclusively* on glucose for fuel. Because of the importance of glucose, the levels of it in the blood are closely regulated by two hormones, insulin and glucagon.

There is a very limited amount of carbohydrates stored in the liver, in the form of glycogen, that help supply more glucose to the blood when levels get too low. Yet this precious fuel reserve ordinarily lasts only three to six hours. (Except at night, when liver glycogen lasts longer because the need for energy is lower.) How does it get replaced? Eating. Eating carbohydrate-rich foods, that is.

If carbohydrates are inadequate in the diet, the body has to turn to creative fueling mechanisms to supply vital energy to the body. Protein mainly from muscle will get taken apart and converted to energy, primarily in the form of glucose. It's like taking wood from the framework structure in your house to use as fuel in your fireplace. The wood will burn and provide necessary fuel, but it does so at a high price. You begin to lose the integrity of your structure! (The *Biggest Loser* study showed that the participants lost over twenty-four pounds of *lean mass* by the end of the show; and six years later, their lean body mass was still down by over ten pounds, compared to their baseline before they started the competition.)

If you think that eating a high-protein diet will prevent this dismantling from occurring, it's not so. When you eat an inadequate amount of energy or carbohydrates, the protein from the diet will *also* be diverted to be used as energy. Therefore this "high-protein diet" is no insurance. Instead, the protein is used as an expensive source of fuel, rather than for its intended use in the body. It's like having a building supplier provide lots of wood to rebuild your house. If you are constantly using that wood pile to make bonfires, instead of repairing your home, you are still left with a weak structure. Similarly, protein is needed to maintain and build muscles, hormones, enzymes, and cells in the body. When carbohydrates and energy are lacking, protein is shifted from its primary role to provide fuel.

Many of our clients believe that when we don't have enough energy, our bodies will finally start burning fat. It doesn't work that way. Remember, the brain and other parts of the body need carbohydrates exclusively for fuel. Only a very small component (5 percent) of the stored fat can be converted to a carbohydrate fuel. On the other hand, the body has plenty of enzymes to convert protein to glucose.

One reason people lose weight so quickly on low-carbohydrate or fasting diets is that they are devouring their own protein tissues as fuel. Also, with each pound of body protein, three or four pounds of associated water are lost. If your body were to continue to consume itself at this rate, death would occur within about ten days. Even the vital heart muscle is burned as fuel. Sadly, this is part of the reason that people on low calorie diets have died—because of cardiac wasting. Even when the heart muscle is deteriorating, it still has to keep up the same amount of work, with *less* power and at a slower heart rate. In essence the cannibalized heart muscle has to work harder with a smaller, faulty engine; pumping performance is not reduced in proportion to the amount of heart tissue lost.

Eventually, the body can convert stored fat to a usable energy form for the brain and nervous system, called ketones. This is known as ketosis. Ketosis is an adaptation to prolonged fasting or carbohydrate deprivation. The bottom line? Adequate carbohydrates and energy are important!

A note about the keto craze. There will always be some new diet boasting to be the latest and greatest. Yet never in our wildest imagination would we have predicted that the keto diet would become popular, let alone be called a "lifestyle." While this diet has utility for treating epilepsy in children, it has many side effects, including kidney stones, osteoporosis, hyperlipidemia, and impaired growth. New research on keto shows some disturbing trends that could negatively impact your health:

- In a twenty-year prospective study, a low-carbohydrate diet high in animal proteins and fats was associated with a twofold risk for type 2 diabetes in men (deKoning et al 2011).
- In animal studies, a keto diet increases fat accumulation in the liver and increases insulin resistance (Kosinski & Jornayvaz 2017).
- A keto diet decreases exercise performance in adult men and women (Wroble K et al. 2018).
- In a case report on a twenty-two-year-old woman who was sent to the hospital emergency department for vomiting, nausea, and abdominal cramping, the woman was diagnosed with lactation ketoacidosis from eating a low-calorie diet while breastfeeding her baby and toddler (Seaton et al. 2018). This has been documented in other cases when there is both insufficient carbohydrate stores (glycogen) combined with an inadequate intake of carbohydrates.

THE POWERHOUSE CELL THEORY

Hunger signals are not affected by low carbohydrates alone. According to the work of cellular researchers Nicolaidis and Even (1992), the hunger signal is generated by the overall energy need of the cell. When cellular power is low, it will produce a signal that induces hunger. While cells primarily get their energy from carbohydrates, protein and fat are factored into the cellular power equation, which could trigger hunger. For example, even if one of your household appliances runs on pure electricity, it could also get its energy from batteries, or a gasoline-powered generator. They all provide energy but have different costs and efficiencies. All nutrients that provide energy (carbohydrates, protein, and fat) eventually get converted to one universal energy denomination used by the cell-ATP. ATP is the chemical energy that powers the cells, and thus our bodies. Nicolaidis and Even propose that the hunger signal is triggered by the overall ATP need of the cell.

To sum up—we need energy. Energy comes from food.

Second-Guessing Your Biology

In spite of the complex and elegant biological systems that help ensure that our bodies get enough energy (food), all too often the chronic dieter tries to outthink biology. Rather than eating when hungry, eating is often tied in to a cognitive set point, based on the dieter's set of rules: Is it time? Do I deserve it? Is it carb-free? And so forth. For example, on the days Alice exercised early in the morning, she would get mad at herself for eating a larger (but appropriate) breakfast. She was worried that her body did not deserve the "extra" portion of food, so her solution was to skip lunch. Skipping lunch was easy, because Alice was a busy executive assistant, with never enough hours in the day to get her work done. Her busyness took precedence over any afternoon hunger that would surface. But by the time Alice arrived at home in the evening, she would be so hungry she would overeat at dinner and often late into the night. Or if she were eating out at a restaurant, she would devour the breadbasket and clean her plate, feeling stuffed and guilty by the end of her meal.

Even non-dieters who go too long without eating will often overeat. (Remember, even rats overeat when food-deprived.) You are also likely to buy more food impulsively when you are in a ravenous state, regardless of your health and dieting intentions.

The problem with consistently denying your hunger state is twofold. First, it usually crescendos into a period of overeating. Second, when the mind gets so used to ignoring hunger signals, they begin to fade and you don't hear them anymore. Or you can only "hear" hunger in extreme, ravenous states, which can be adverse. This further conditions you to believe that you can't be trusted with food, because ravenous hunger often triggers rebound eating. This is explained in part by the Boundary Model for the Regulation of Eating, developed by C. Peter Herman and Janet Polivy, psychological experts in chronic dieting. This model considers both the biology and psychology of eating.

The boundary model explains how dieters, through their cognitive set point, push their normal biological cues of hunger and satiety to the extremes. The gentle sensations of hunger are atrophied for a dieter who is constantly trying to suppress them. Instead, the dieter might only feel extreme, ravenous hunger—or be so disconnected that the feeling of hunger is difficult to identify. Similarly, for this individual, it can be increasingly difficult to know what comfortable satiety feels like. Instead the dieter hovers in a gray zone of what Herman and Polivy call "biological indifference." In the zone of biological indifference, there is no clear hunger or satiety cue. This zone is so wide for the chronic dieter that instead of eating based on internal eating cues, food thoughts and judgments prevail and tell the dieter what to do.

PRIMAL FOOD THERAPY: HONOR YOUR HUNGER

The first step to reclaiming the world of normal eating, free of dieting and food worry, is to *honor your biological hunger.* Your body needs to *know* consistently that it will have access to food—that dieting and deprivation have halted, once and for all. Otherwise, your biology will always be on call, ready to avert a self-imposed food deprivation.

Your body needs to be biologically reconditioned. Diet after diet has taught your body that personal famines are frequent, so it should stay on guard. Remember, famines and food shortages have always existed, even in our modern times. Our bodies are still biologically equipped to survive famines through lowering our energy requirements, increasing biological chemicals that trigger our eating drive, and so on.

It is much easier to stop eating when you truly know you will be able to eat again. For example, imagine you are in a room and offer a *starving* child a plate of cookies. You tell the child that they can have only one cookie. You exit the room and leave the child alone with the whole plate. What would the hungry child do? Eat *all* the cookies (and lick the crumbs), of course. The same is true for dieters.

For example, Barbara usually kept herself in a hungry state. She only allowed herself to eat when extremely ravenous. By her own definition, if she allowed herself to eat when simply hungry, *but not ravenous,* she thought she was overeating. Yet because her definition of "normal" hunger was being ravenous, her eating would vacillate from feast to famine cycles.

HUNGER SILENCE

What if you don't feel hunger anymore, or never really knew what the gentle sensation of hunger feels like? Can you get it back? Yes. But first let's look at a couple of reasons why hunger may be silenced.

• *Numbing.* Many people have learned over the years to quell or avert hunger pangs by turning to calorie-free beverages, such as diet sodas, coffee, and tea. The liquid in the stomach temporarily tricks the gastric mechanism into a sense of fullness.

• *Dieting.* Dieters get so used to denying their hunger that it becomes easy to tune it out. Eventually, when hunger comes knocking on their inner door and there is no response, the knocking, or rather the stomach rumbling, stops.

• *Chaos.* It's very easy to suppress hunger or ignore it when you are busy putting out the fires in your life or job. If this is a chronic pattern, hunger may slowly fade.

• *Trauma history.* You need to feel safe in order to feel hungry. If you have a history of trauma, you might need to engage in nourishment as self-care, while you are working with a trauma specialist.

• *Skipping breakfast.* Some of our clients skip eating in the morning, because they say it keeps them from feeling hungry the rest of the day. Yet hunger is a normal, welcomed body signal that should be embraced. It's a sign that you are getting back in touch with your body's needs. But because these clients are afraid of their hunger, especially when it becomes overwhelming in the evening, as a result of not eating early in the day, they respond by not eating breakfast the next morning—which repeats the vicious cycle of hunger silence.

• *Stress.* The biological cascade from the stress response can cause a temporary blunting in the felt sense of hunger.

• *Basic needs aren't being met.* This follows under the category of self-care. If you are not getting the basics, like enough sleep or enough down-time or breathing room (which may be beyond your control), it can disrupt your connection to your body.

HOW TO HONOR BIOLOGICAL HUNGER

It's too hard to hear hunger if you are never listening for it. The first step to honoring your biological hunger is to begin to listen for it. The hunger symphony has many sounds that are varied for different people. Just as an orchestra conductor can distinguish the sounds of each instrument in a symphony, you will eventually be able to key in to specific bodily sensations and what they mean. In the beginning, you may be able to recognize overt ravenous hunger, but have difficulty recognizing gentle hunger pangs. Similarly, to the untrained musical ear, loud cymbals might be easy to identify, but it will take time and listening to pick up on the subtler voices of the bassoon or oboe.

Each time you eat, ask yourself: Am I hungry? What's my hunger level? If the feeling of hunger is hard to identify, ask yourself: When was the last time I *ever* felt hungry? How did my stomach feel? How did my mouth feel? Any combination of the following can be experienced as hunger sensations or symptoms (ranging from gentle to ravenous):

- Mild gurgling or gnawing in the stomach
- Growling noises
- Lightheadedness
- Difficulty concentrating
- Uncomfortable stomach pain
- Irritability
- Feeling faint
- Headache

The ebb and flow of your hunger might not match other people's—that's okay; it's individual. Take care not to get overly hungry or ravenous. If this is difficult for you to gauge, a *general* guideline is to *go no longer than five waking hours without eating.* This is based on the biology of fueling up your carbohydrate tank in the liver, which runs out every three to six hours. We have observed that clients who go longer than five hours without eating tend to overeat at the next eating opportunity. (For some people, this can happen even after three or four hours without eating.)

To get in touch with the nuances of hunger, it helps to check the pulse of hunger at regular intervals. Check in with your body, and simply inquire, What's my hunger level? It's helpful to do this every time you eat, and between eating occurrences. Remember, although this may seem hyperconscious, it's a focused step of awareness to get you reacquainted with your body and its biology.

We have used a variety of tools to help our clients check in with their hunger, but we developed a new one, which is particularly helpful and is a little less exacting. Our brains naturally organize subjective feelings as pleasant, unpleasant, or neutral. So we decided to use those qualitative sensation ratings to help you connect with hunger and satiety cues. We find that if you start first, with those descriptions, you are less likely to get hung up on numbers.

The classic rating system of 0 to 10 is still very useful, where 0 = painful hunger and 10 = painful fullness. It's just that some folks tend to attach themselves to numbers as being right or wrong, when this is merely a system to help you connect. See table 3: "Qualitative Description of Hunger and Fullness Sensations."

Monitor your hunger levels each time you eat, before and after, using the Hunger Discovery Scale Journal (page 99). What pattern do you see emerging? Is there a certain time interval when you eat? Is there any relationship between how much you eat and the length of time between eating occurrences?

You may discover that your eating style leans toward nibbling or grazing. Don't be alarmed. If you eat small amounts of food such as a snack or mini-meal, you may find that you are hungry more often, such as every two, three, or four hours. Not only is this normal, it may have metabolic advantages. Nibbling studies (in which people are given multiple snacks or mini-meals) have shown that the release of insulin is lower in people fed nibbling diets compared to larger traditional meals of *identical* calories.

Sometimes our clients get worried when they suddenly feel more hungry than usual—as if something is wrong. However, on closer inspection, they usually find that a couple of days prior, they had an unusually light day of eating—not dieting, but just not a lot of food. The body plays catch-up on its own terms, not yours. Most of our clients have difficulty remembering what they ate one day ago, let alone two days ago. Research on children has shown that they make up for their needs in an average of time such as a week or couple of days. Why would adults be any different? In fact, new research is beginning to indicate that the same is true for adults. The body may do some of its energy fine-tuning over a period of days, rather than from hour to hour. We find this is especially true if you still have a tendency to eat diet types of food, such as low-calorie frozen dinners or salads without dressing. You may feel full, but the lack of energy catches up with you. The body wants to compensate.

Other Voices of "Hunger"

A common mistake with our newer clients is that they initially embrace the *honor your hunger* concept in the form of a diet mantra, "Thou shall eat only when hungry." The problem here is that this rigid interpretation can leave you feeling as if you have broken a "rule" or failed, if you eat for any other reason than hunger. When you feel like you have broken a rule, you get pulled right back into the diet mentality.

• *Taste hunger.* Sometimes people may eat simply because it sounds good or because the occasion calls for it. We call this *taste hunger.* The average eater can accept this—they don't view it as a big diet violation. In nearly every culture, food plays important roles in rites of passages and celebratory events. Would you chastise a bride or groom for eating a piece of wedding cake when they were not hungry? Yet it's not unusual for diet- ers to feel bad about *any* perceived food transgression, and then feel like they might as well throw in the towel. And that's when *overeating* often takes place.

• *Practical "hunger"—planning ahead.* While it's important to eat pri- marily based on your biological hunger, it's also important to be practical and not rigid. For instance, let's say you are attending a play with friends that lasts from 7 to 10 p.m. and your opportunity to eat dinner is at 6 p.m. You may not be hungry then, but you certainly will be later. Do you sit there at the restaurant and *not* eat, and let hunger roll in right in the middle of the play, only to culminate in ravenous hunger by the final act? No. Eat- ing a light meal or snack is a sensible solution.

• *Emotional hunger.* Once you are truly able to identify and distinguish biological hunger, it becomes easier to clarify *why* you want to eat. It is not unusual for a number of our clients to eat because of *emotional* hunger— to quench uncomfortable feelings (such as loneliness, boredom, or anger). Ironically, many of our patients are often amazed that what they assumed to be emotional eating was, in many instances, primal hunger eating. But the out-of-control feeling of eating is nearly identical, whether it was trig- gered emotionally, biologically, or as a result of cognitive distortion. A dis- cussion of how to distinguish the sources of hunger is found in chapter 12.

TABLE 3. DESCRIPTION OF HUNGER AND FULLNESS SENSATIONS

	Rating	Hunger and Fullness Sensations	Overall Quality of Sensation		
			Pleasant	Unpleasant	Neutral
Over-hungry	0	Painfully hungry. This is primal hunger, which is very intense and urgent.		X	
Over-hungry	1	Ravenous and irritable. Anxious to eat.		X	
Over-hungry	2	Very hungry. Looking forward to a hearty meal or snack.	X		
Normal Eating Range	3	Hungry and ready to eat, but there is no urgency. It's a polite hunger.	X		
Normal Eating Range	4	Subtly hungry, slightly empty.			X
Normal Eating Range	5	Neutral. Neither hungry nor full.			X
Normal Eating Range	6	Beginning to feel emerging fullness.			X
Normal Eating Range	7	Comfortable fullness, which feels satisfied and content.	X		
Over-full	8	You are beginning to feel a little too full. It's not pleasant, but it has not quite emerged into an unpleasant experience.		X	
Over-full	9	Very full, too full. You feel uncomfortable, as if you need to unbutton your pants or remove your belt.		X	
Over-full	10	Painfully full, stuffed. May feel nauseated.		X	

Adapted with permission from The Intuitive Eating Workbook *(New Harbinger, 2017).*

TABLE 4. HUNGER DISCOVERY SCALE JOURNAL

Before you eat your meal or snack: First, check the quality of your hunger as pleasant, unpleasant, or neutral. Place an X in the box that applies to you. Next, circle the number that best reflects your hunger level, where 0 = unpleasant/painful hunger and 10 = unpleasant/painful fullness.

Time	Quality of Hunger			Hunger Rating											Meal/Food Eaten
	Pleasant	Unpleasant	Neutral												
				0	1	2	3	4	5	6	7	8	9	10	
				0	1	2	3	4	5	6	7	8	9	10	
				0	1	2	3	4	5	6	7	8	9	10	
				0	1	2	3	4	5	6	7	8	9	10	
				0	1	2	3	4	5	6	7	8	9	10	

Adapted with permission from The Intuitive Eating Workbook *(New Harbinger, 2017).*

STUDIES SHOW: EATING IN RESPONSE TO INITIAL HUNGER IMPROVES HEALTH

A promising series of studies from an Italian research team in Florence shows that researchers were able to train people to predict when blood glucose is low by attending to their subjective experience of hunger (Ciampolini and Bianchi 2006).

There are two unique aspects to their approach. First, the focus of the training is distinguishing *initial hunger* from the uncomfortable signs that occur when hunger is prolonged. Second, a biofeedback technique, well known to diabetic educators, was utilized to train people how to make this distinction via blood glucose monitoring, using glucometers. (Note: These people did not have diabetes or impaired glucose tolerance.)

Initially, people were instructed to measure their blood sugar at the earliest feelings of hunger or discomfort. Next, if glucose was under 85 mg/dL, subjects were instructed to remember their physical feelings and to proceed to eat their meal. (The glucose level of 85 mg/dL was chosen based on previous studies, indicating that it represents the upper limit of homeostatic control of feeding.)

If blood sugar was higher than 85 mg/dL, subjects were instructed to delay the meal. They were then asked to wait for the spontaneous development of novel hunger feelings for at least one hour, before making further blood glucose measurements.

Two other studies using this initial hunger recognition technique demonstrated that people trained in this method had improved insulin sensitivity, compared to the nontrained controls (Ciampolini et al. 2010; Ciampolini, Lovell-Smith, and Sifone 2010). When insulin is less effective in your body, it is called "insulin resistance," which is related to chronic health problems.

The research team concluded that restoring and validating hunger and training people to recognize initial hunger could help in the prevention and treatment of diabetes and associated disorders.

Chapter 8

PRINCIPLE 3:

Make Peace with Food

Call a truce, stop the food fight! Give yourself unconditional permission to eat. If you tell yourself that you can't or shouldn't have a particular food, it can lead to intense feelings of deprivation that build into uncontrollable cravings and, often, bingeing. When you finally "give in" to your forbidden foods, eating will be experienced with such intensity, it will usually result in Last Supper overeating and overwhelming guilt.

When I was on the grapefruit diet, all I wanted was bananas, and when I was on a low-carbohydrate diet all I did was dream of eating bread and potatoes," said Laurie, an inveterate dieter. Does that sound ironic? Familiar? What may seem like irony is actually the natural reaction that is triggered by the limitation and deprivation that comes with most diets. Cravings run rampant as soon as we're restricted from any kind of substance—whether it is clothing, fresh air, scenery, or especially food. Scientists living in the Biosphere 2, an airtight glass-enclosed terrarium, coveted something as basic as fresh air, after being deprived of an open environment for two years. But fresh air was not the only fantasy of these researchers—so was the food they had sorely missed. After they emerged from this self-imposed captivity, the research team had more to say about food than science at their press conference. The scientists described cravings for food that began to occupy their thoughts—and led one of them to write a cookbook!

These scientists are not unlike the dieter who has been told certain foods are forbidden. Even though they were not on a diet, the scientists were still preoccupied with food cravings as a result of lack of availability. They dreamed about desserts that were nonexistent and obsessed about dinners, which were of limited variety. As cooking chores rotated, it became vitally important not to spoil the day's meal for the others. Common foods like salmon, berries, and coffee took on a heightened allure.

THE DEPRIVATION SETUP

Why would Biosphere scientists or the healthy men in the Minnesota Starvation study (described in the previous chapter) exhibit behaviors so unlike their normal eating patterns? Deprivation. These people had not been tainted by the dieting trap, yet their reactions to deprivation were virtually identical to those of dieters. While you have already seen the effects of *biological* deprivation in the last chapter, you should not underestimate the effect of deprivation *psychologically*. This effect is the focus of this chapter.

When you rigidly limit the amount of food you are allowed to eat, it usually sets you up to crave *larger* quantities of that very food. In fact, being restricted from anything in life sets it up to be extra special, regardless of age. (Oh, maybe not in the beginning, when you are in the initial stages of diet euphoria, but the craving builds with each "dieting day.") For example, if you put a two-year-old on the floor with several brand-new toys and tell them that they can play with any one of them except for the simple oatmeal carton, which do you think they'll choose? You guessed it—the plain oatmeal carton.

One client revealed that when they were young, they had little money and the thought of buying a new car gave them a deep thrill. Yet now that they're successful, they can buy *any* car they want at any time. Cars are no longer a big deal, no thrill. Food has replaced the thrill that buying a new car used to provide. Paradoxically, food is the one thing out of their reach, forbidden, when dieting. The forbidden object is elevated to an overvalued level of specialness.

Psychologist Fritz Heider states that depriving yourself of something you want can actually heighten your desire for that very item. *The moment you banish a food, it paradoxically builds up a "craving life" of its own that gets stronger with each diet and builds more momentum as the deprivation deepens.* Deprivation is a powerful experience both biologically and psychologically. You already saw in the last chapter how food deprivation sets off a biological drive. Psychological forces wreak havoc with your peace of mind, triggering cravings, obsessive thoughts, and even compulsive behaviors.

When a diet dictates that a particular food is forbidden or should be avoided it makes you crave that food even more! If you are someone who has experienced deprivation in areas outside of food, such as love, attention, material wants, and so on, the deprivation connected to dieting may be felt even more intensely for you. Bonnie is a client who grew up in a home where her father was never home, and her mother was emotionally distant. As a young child, she learned to use food as a way to substitute for the love and attention she wasn't getting. As an adult on a diet, she found that food deprivation evoked these deep feelings of deprivation from childhood. For Bonnie, this became a double whammy, which was hard to overcome. For the chronic dieter, the combination of biological changes (from undereating), psychological reactions, and cognitive distortions create just the right mix to set off the dynamite of rebound eating.

DEPRIVATION BACKLASH–REBOUND EATING

Meet Heidi. Her experience with chocolate typifies what can happen when you deprive yourself of a particular food. Heidi had been on every known diet, each forbidding one type of food or another, and chocolate was usually on the "do not eat" list. Heidi was a self-described chocoholic. She complained that the moment chocolate crossed her lips, she couldn't stop eating it. Her way of managing her chocolate problem was simply to not allow herself to eat it. But this was a vicious cycle. It was not uncommon for Heidi to consume large bags of chocolate in spite of her attempts to eliminate it from her life. The moment a box of chocolate was opened, she couldn't resist eating it to completion. Heidi's chocolate binges were triggered by the food rule she had created—"I am not allowed to eat chocolate." This meant that each time she "succumbed" and ate it, she truly believed that it was for the last time. Each chocolate episode would become a "farewell to chocolate," with all the sadness and mourning that goes along with saying goodbye to anything special in life. Since Heidi "knew" she was never, *ever* going to eat chocolate again (despite her experience demonstrating otherwise), she would consume large amounts of it as a last hurrah, or "get it while you can." When Heidi's chocolate binges occurred, she would feel guilty and as if she did not deserve to eat any food. She would compensate for her chocolate feasts by undereating or semi-fasting, which would set her up for ravenous hunger and more out-of-control eating.

Today Heidi eats chocolate but is often satisfied with a piece or two and can easily even pass it up! To Heidi, this is a miracle. How did she overcome her chocolate problem? Heidi's solution was to learn to make peace with food—especially with chocolate—an idea that she was terrified to try in the beginning. No wonder; her only experience with chocolate was eating it in massive quantities, then feeling out of control. For Heidi, making peace with chocolate was a brave and risky step.

Last Supper Eating

The mere *perception* that food might become banned can trigger overeating. Just thinking about going on a diet can create a sense of panic and send you on a trail of eating every food that you think won't be allowed. As we explained in chapter 2, this is Last Supper eating. It is triggered by the sincere belief that you will never get to eat a particular food (or foods) again. The threat of deprivation becomes so powerful that all reason is lost, and you find yourself eating whatever is to be forbidden, even if you are not hungry.

Clients will often overeat right before their first session. Although we make it clear that we use an anti-diet approach, they figure that we have something up our sleeves, a diet of sorts—after all, we are both registered dietitian nutritionists and nutrition therapists! For example, Paul ate in an out-of-control fashion the night before his first appointment. Why? Paul was sure that he would be advised to give up most of his favorite foods, and to start eating a diet of carrots and cottage cheese. His fear increased during the week leading up to his session, and so did his intake of French fries, hamburgers, and donuts. This experience was not new to Paul—in fact, he had engaged in Last Supper eating before *every* diet he started. Likewise, nearly all of our clients engage in this pre-dieting ritual of saying goodbye to favorite foods. In fact, some of our clients tell us that Last Supper eating is one of their favorite parts of dieting—it's almost an entitlement.

For some of our clients, however, there is such an intense sense of urgency with Last Supper eating that a period of frantic gorging ensues. One client described it as, "Hurry and get all the food while you can, and time is short, so get it all now!" The overeating that follows falsely gives "proof" that you need to diet, as you watch in horror your inability to "control" yourself.

Each impending diet brings with it more fear of deprivation—with the knowledge that you won't get "enough" or get what you want. Then comes more overeating, loss of self-control, and, finally, erosion of self-esteem. How could you possibly feel good about yourself if you truly believe that it's possible to eliminate certain foods, only to find yourself bingeing and failing on yet another diet?

Rebound Eating: Subtle Forms

Food competition. Have you ever shared a bowl of cherries or a piece of dessert with someone who eats faster than you? Watch how quickly you dig in because you're concerned that you won't get enough. Or see what happens when you hear that your favorite brand of cereal is to be discontinued; it's not unusual to buy every last box on the shelf because of fear of deprivation. Or some parents find themselves gobbling down the cookies before the kids can get their hands on them and eat them all.

Eating in a large group of people can instill a sense of future food-deprivation worry. To prevent this from occurring, there is a tendency to eat quickly, grab it while you can, or there won't be any food left. For example, Joshua was one of nine children in a family of moderate means. As a child he was worried that he wouldn't get enough food at mealtime, although in actuality there was an adequate amount of food to go around. This fear of food deprivation taught him to grab what he could. As an adult, he continued this behavior, regularly eating far more food than his body told him he needed to feel comfortable.

Returning home syndrome. When they return from having been away, people often overeat because they felt deprived of familiar foods while away. Kids returning home from summer camp or from their college dorms find themselves emptying the refrigerator, gorging on home cooking, or visiting their favorite local restaurants excessively. A number of years ago, I (ER) came home to find my stepson's friend, who had just returned from Thailand, methodically eating everything in the kitchen that he hadn't seen in three years. When he began to eat the cream cheese by the forkful (without a bagel), I knew how deprived he had been! Any food will take on a heightened allure when one is returning from a journey in which it wasn't available. For example, clients have described unusual cravings for salads after a two-week camping trip or trip abroad where it's been advised *not* to eat the fresh produce.

The empty cupboard. If there is consistently no food in the house because grocery shopping is chaotic, eating often vacillates between feast and famine, with emphasis on the former. Food in the pantry or refrigerator takes on extra specialness.

For example, Gayle is a teenager who exhibits a tendency to eat every bite of food in a meal regardless of how she feels. Gayle's parents work many hours, seldom shop for food, and eat most of their meals out. Gayle usually comes home from school to an empty house—no food or parents. With food haphazardly available, Gayle feels greatly deprived. She feels a compulsion to finish whatever food she gets, as she doesn't know where or when her next meal will appear.

Captivity behavior. Various accounts of released hostages have reported obsessive thinking about food and cravings while "in captivity." On a somewhat lighter level, my (ER) son described his "captivity" behavior during a survival training camp out in the wilderness in Montana. To occupy his lonely hours, he would write lists of all the foods he wasn't getting. Yet normally he is not preoccupied with food or cravings.

Depression-era eating. People who went through the Great Depression hold food in special regard; it's cherished. There is a pervasive sense that there won't be enough food, or certain foods may become unavailable. And like a precious metal, you dare not throw food away or otherwise waste it. "Clean your plate" takes on special meaning and is passed on with other family traditions and values.

Once in a lifetime. Eating a meal in a special restaurant while on vacation can stimulate a sense of future deprivation. For example, if you are in Paris eating a superb French meal, the thought of leaving even a forkful seems an impossible feat. After all, this is likely to be the one and only time you'll ever experience these particular tastes in this particular setting! You might eat until uncomfortably full, just because you're already feeling future deprivation.

One last shot. A similar experience can occur when eating a delicious meal at the home of a friend or tasting cookies that have been sent as a gift. The notion that this is your only shot at these foods drives you to eating every last bit of the meal or food.

Anticipation of food restriction. For many dieters, just the mere anticipation of starting yet another food plan with forbidden foods is enough to trigger overeating of the forbidden food, a farewell-to-food feast. A study on chocolate lovers illustrates this issue. When the chocolate aficionados were told that they would be restricted from eating their beloved chocolate for a period of three weeks, it triggered an increase in their chocolate intake before and after the restriction (Keeler et al. 2015). In a similar study on the allure of restricted food, a researcher told a group of children that they could eat as many of the yellow M&M chocolate candies as they wanted. But they were not supposed to eat the red ones. (Same candy, just a different color.) Guess which candies got eaten the most? The red ones! (Jansen et al. 2007).

HOW IS DIETING POSSIBLE?

If deprivation backlash is so powerful, how do dieters actually diet at all? Aren't the biological and psychological forces too compelling? Chronic dieters adapt by changing both their mindset and their responsiveness to inner body cues. This adaptation is known as *restrained eating*. Unfortunately, these changes work against them. In the long run, deprivation backlash still prevails.

Restrained eaters, in essence, are chronic dieters who are preoccupied with dieting and weight control. To stay in control with their food, restrained eaters set up rules that dictate how they should eat, rather than listening to their bodies. Forget *honor your hunger*; instead they calculate what to eat, choosing foods with their mental brakes on, and second-guessing the needs of their bodies. Their eating appears to be fine until one of their sacred rules is violated. When a rule is broken, so is their restraint—and, wham, overeating begins. This has been described as the *what-the-hell effect* by leading researchers in this field Janet Polivy, PhD, and C. Peter Herman, PhD, from the University of Toronto. And it is *that* phrase, rather than the term "restrained eating," that most of our clients relate to! Here's what it means in eating terms:

- The moment a forbidden food is eaten, overeating takes place.
- The moment a calorie level is exceeded, overeating takes place.
- The mere *perception* of breaking a food rule or eating a forbidden food triggers overeating.

Restrained Eating Studies

Studies on restrained eaters have shed a lot of psychological light in the world of dieting. They show how ineffective outlawing particular foods can be and how it sets you up for overeating. Most restraint studies follow this core procedure:

A short ten-question test, called the Restraint Scale, is given to identify who the restrained eaters are. (Questions include frequency of dieting, history of weight loss and gain, weekly weight fluctuations, emotional effect of weight fluctuations, effect of "others" on eating, obsessional thinking about food, and guilt feelings about eating.) Then a "preload" is given—that is, the subjects are "loaded up" with food *before* the real experiment begins. The preload is a calculated amount of food—and it's usually some sort of setup to see how the dieters versus non-dieters respond in various eating situations. Then the "real" experiment begins. Here are a couple of particularly significant studies on restrained eaters:

Mind games: The counterregulation effect. One of the classic studies involved fifty-seven female college students at Northwestern University. The students were led to believe that the goal of the study was to evaluate the *taste* of several ice cream samples. The actual purpose of the study was to determine how diet thinking might affect eating after drinking milkshakes. The women were arbitrarily divided into three groups, based on the number of eight-ounce milkshakes given (none, one, and two shakes). After drinking the shakes, the subjects were asked to taste and rate three flavors of ice cream. They were allowed to eat as much ice cream as they wanted, and "taste-tested" in privacy to guard against self-consciousness. The researchers saw to it that ample ice cream was provided so that substantial amounts could be eaten without making an appreciable dent in the supply!

Here's what happened. The non-dieters naturally regulated their eating; they ate less ice cream in proportion to the amount of milkshakes consumed. The dieters, however, had a dramatic, *opposite* behavior. Those who drank two milkshakes ate the *most* ice cream—a "counterregulation" effect. The researchers concluded that forcing the dieters to overeat or "blow their diet" caused them to release their food inhibitions. With inhibition banished, restraint was eliminated, and the dieters overate the ice cream.

Perception affects eating. Another similar study examined the notion of how dieters perceive calories. All subjects were given snacks of chocolate pudding with a substantial calorie difference. One group was given a high-calorie pudding, and another was given a lower-calorie version. But within each of these groups, half of the subjects were told that the pudding was high in calories, and half were told that it was low. Then the subjects were given a pseudo taste test. The dieters who *thought* the pudding was high in calories ate more than the dieters who *thought* the pudding was low in calories, by 61 percent! This study illustrates how much power thoughts and perception can have on eating behavior. And once again, when the dieter "blew the diet" (whether actual or perceived), overeating ensued.

The Seesaw Syndrome: Guilt Versus Deprivation

The longer foods are prohibited, the more seductive they become. Consequently, eating these "illegal" foods brings with it a compelling sense of guilt for most dieters. And as the guilt increases, so does the quantity of food intake. The more deprived you become from dieting and from specific foods, the greater the deprivation backlash. We see this all the time—we call it *the seesaw syndrome.*

When it comes to dieting, feelings of deprivation and guilt work in an opposing manner; like two kids on a seesaw—"what goes up must come down."

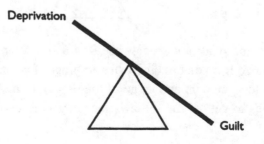

When dieting, as you restrict foods that you enjoy eating, deprivation becomes higher and higher. Meanwhile, in tandem, guilty feelings go down—because you haven't eaten any "bad" foods. But there's a limit to how high the seesaw can climb. The level of deprivation rises to its highest point, where you can't bear one more meal, let alone one more day of restrictive eating. Meanwhile, guilty feelings are at their lowest, because you have not eaten any forbidden foods; you've been "good." Since you have no buildup of guilt, you're wide open to allow some forbidden foods into your life and able to tolerate the beginning feelings of guilt that these foods engender. As you eat the first forbidden food, you begin to feel guilt. That guilt triggers feelings of being "bad," which lead you to more food (the what-the-hell effect), with its accompanying guilt. Now the seesaw looks like a tug-of-war:

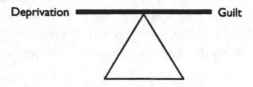

After a while, the guilt continues to build, and in tandem, deprivation begins to recede. As the days go by, you feel worse about breaking your diet rules, and guilt rises to its highest point. Deprivation feelings are virtually nonexistent, because you've been eating all the foods that weren't allowed on the diet. Now the seesaw looks like the following diagram:

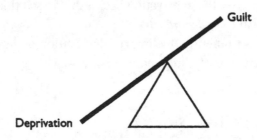

At this point the syndrome repeats itself—up and down, up and down—every time you go from diet to binge, diet to binge. The only way to get off this seesaw is to lighten up and let go of the deprivation. And just as when one kid decides to get off the seesaw, the other is forced to stop playing;

when you give yourself permission to not be deprived, you simultaneously let go of the guilt! By giving yourself permission to eat, you stop playing the futile seesaw game.

THE KEY: *UNCONDITIONAL* PERMISSION TO EAT

The key to abolishing the pattern of restraint and subsequent rebound overeating is to give yourself *unconditional* permission to eat. This means:

- Throwing out the preconceived notion that certain foods are "good" and others are "bad." No one food has the power to make you healthy or not.
- Eating what you *really* want. Yes, what you want.
- Eating without obligatory penance. ("Okay, I can have the cheesecake now, but tomorrow I diet.") These kinds of personal food deals are *not* unconditional.

When you truly free your food choices, without any hidden agenda of restricting them in the future, you eliminate the urgency to overeat. Yet it's an unsettling prospect to most of our clients, even more frightening than the initial idea of giving up diets.

The Peace Process

Making peace with food means allowing *all* foods into your eating world, so that a choice for chocolate becomes emotionally equal to a choice for a peach. It also means that your food choices do not reflect your character or morality. While for years many health professionals have agreed that there should be no forbidden foods, very few will go the distance and say you should eat *whatever* you want. Eventually there is a limit imposed. And knowing there is a limit can still impart a food lust of sorts—better eat it now!

Paradoxically, once you truly know you can eat whatever you want, the intensity to eat greatly diminishes. The most effective way to instill this belief is to experience eating the very foods you forbid! It becomes self-evident proof that you can "handle" these foods, or better yet that they have no magic hold on you or your "willpower." Ironically, once again, many of our clients discover that the very foods that they had prohibited and craved are no longer desirable once they can be eaten freely. Over and over, we hear stories of how when they were truly allowed to eat certain foods, they discovered, to their surprise, that they really didn't like them to begin with! For example, Molly had relished bakery birthday cakes, but tried not to eat them. She would, however, eventually relent, especially at a party, and power through two or more pieces. But when she decided to make peace with food, and come face to face with "official permission," she found that she did not care for most bakery birthday cakes. She had always eaten them so fast, often on the sly, that she had not truly experienced the taste and texture of the cake! With her newfound permission, Molly took the time to *taste* the cake (whether in the privacy of her home or at a party). She found more often than not that the cakes were stale or bland, and would not finish a single piece, let alone go for more pieces. Eventually, Molly would not settle for cakes that were less than superb. She now often turns down cake at parties—because she wants to, not because she is a diet martyr.

Annie had a similar "taste experience." Her commitment to making peace with food sparked an enthusiasm for taste sensations that had been buried by her restrained eating. Annie gave herself unconditional permission to experience forbidden foods one at a time, day after day, often in preference to all other foods. Annie went through her red licorice phase, her Pop-Tart phase, and her mashed potato phase. While in the midst of each phase, she ate the favored food with relish and delight. For some foods, she found that it took a few weeks for the desire to peak and then slowly taper off. For other foods it took longer, and for a few, she found that they didn't taste half as good as she had imagined.

To Annie's surprise (and delight), she discovered that once she completed a particular food-freeing phase, she found that *she stopped craving that food, hardly ever thought of it, and sometimes she never wanted it again*! Removing deprivation from Annie's eating diminished the alluring quality of foods, and instead put them in a rational perspective.

Fears That Hold You Back

Even clients who come ready to give up dieting have a strong resistance to eating whatever they *really* want. They are terrified. While they feel comfortable learning to *honor their hunger,* they are ready to bolt out the door when we talk about giving unconditional permission to eat what they like.

If people are so afraid to advance to this part of the Intuitive Eating process, why do we insist that this must be explored? Legalizing food is the critical step in changing your relationship with food. It frees you to respond to inner eating signals that have been smothered by negative thoughts and feelings of guilt about eating. When you don't truly believe that you can eat whatever food you like, you will continue to feel deprived, ultimately overeat, and be blocked from feeling satisfied with your eating. And when you are not satisfied, you will be on the prowl for more food! When you know the food will be there and allowed, day after day, it doesn't become so important to have it. Food loses its power.

In spite of the knowledge that deprivation leads to backlash eating, many people are apprehensive about making this peace pact with food, in part due to the following perceived obstacles.

I won't stop eating

At first you may experience an overpowering fear that you won't stop eating a favorite forbidden food. Just remember that when you know that previously forbidden foods will always be allowed, the urgency to have large quantities of them eventually dissipates. Also, research shows that people will tire of eating the same kind of food—it's called habituation. Habituation studies have shown that the more a person is exposed to a particular food the less appealing it becomes. (See the sidebar "Habituation Response Explains Why Foods Become Less Enticing with Exposure.") In fact, you may have already witnessed this type of eating in other people. For example, observe the all-you-can-eat buffet dining that is popular in vacation spots such as Las Vegas. On the first day, people typically load up their plates and grab three or four desserts. By the last day, however, they are choosing their food selectively. The novelty has worn off, and they know there is plenty of food.

My entire family (ET) encountered the habituation effect when I was working on a two-hundred-recipe cookbook. Whether I was testing salads, appetizers, or casseroles, we eventually tired of eating the same kind of food. This was especially evident while creating the dessert chapter. Not only did we tire of eating sweets, but one family member to this day cannot bear to take a bite of pineapple upside-down cake, which was once his favorite! I made that cake at least eight times before I decided to give up on that particular recipe.

The only way that *you* will come to believe that you will be able to stop eating is *to go through the food experience, to actually eat.* That's why we are fond of the word "process." This is not about knowledge of food, but rather rebuilding experiences with eating. You cannot have an experience through knowledge; rather, you need to go through it, bite by bite. Otherwise it would be like trying to learn how to play the guitar by reading a book on music theory. You may understand the components, but only after you practice and struggle with the strings personally will you truly know how to play. And the more you practice, the more confidence you will have.

Sometimes people express a fear about being addicted to food—there are many reasons, other than addiction, that can explain the reward aspect of eating. (For more information, see the sidebar "Can You Really Be Addicted to Food?" p. 122.)

Pseudo-permission: I've tried it before

Many of our clients will recount that when they "allowed" themselves to eat certain forbidden foods, they still overate and felt out of control. But for most people, these foods were never really *unconditionally* allowed; rather, they were only given pseudo-permission. These forbidden foods were actually being eaten with a sense of temporarily breaking the rules, or with a little voice saying, "You really shouldn't eat that." The moment that food touched the tongue, feelings of guilt and remorse flooded in. And with these feelings came a conviction to limit these foods in the future and counter this indulgence by "eating right" tomorrow. Although physically eating the food, they were emotionally depriving themselves in the future. And, so, the cycle perpetuates. Pseudo-permission does not work—it's only an illusion. Your mouth may be chewing, but your mind is saying, "I shouldn't." Your mind is still on a diet.

Self-fulfilling prophecy

Sometimes just the thought that you will overeat is enough to actually make you overeat. Carolyn initially had held the strong conviction that white flour would cause her to overeat. She believed that even one bite of a bagel would trigger a binge. And it did. Carolyn had created a self-fulfilling prophecy. Because of diet culture, she "knew" these foods were "fattening," she "knew" she would binge, and she feared that she would gain weight. Every time she gave in to her craving for white bread, she sincerely told herself that this would be the last time. Of course, the depriving thoughts and feelings, along with her sense of being bad, sent her out of control.

It took a long time before Carolyn was truly able to permit herself to eat foods with white flour, but now she rarely binges on these foods. Every now and then a fleeting, archaic thought of restriction occurs and drags her back to the world of deprivation. And with that thought comes her occasional sense of loss of control. Now, though, she only has a few cookies instead of the whole bag, and this happens once every six months instead of every week. Because Carolyn has had so many positive experiences with foods containing white flour, it has become much easier for her to let go of her restrictive thinking and make peace with these foods.

I won't eat healthfully

In case after case, when people are given free choice and access to all varieties of food, after going through the peace process, they end up balancing their intake to include mostly nutritious foods with a smattering of "play foods." As nutritionists, we continue to honor and respect nutrition, but at this point in the Intuitive Eating process, nutrition is not the driving force. If nutrition were the overriding priority now, it would only perpetuate your restrictive thoughts. (It took us years to come to terms with this factor, and it is why nutrition issues are reserved for later in this book.) As you go further along in the process and all foods are completely allowed, your intuitive signals will give you good advice. But even right now, if you think about eating a hot fudge sundae for every meal, how soon do you think you will be craving something completely opposite, such as a salad or a piece of grilled chicken?

Lack of self-trust

A mighty obstacle to making peace with food is a strong lack of self-trust. Most clients say that they intellectually trust us and our philosophy. They truly believe that it has worked for "other" clients, but they distrust themselves and are frightened that it won't work for them.

Ironically, the process of giving yourself permission to eat is actually the stepping-stone to rebuilding your trust with food and with yourself. In the beginning, each positive food experience is like a tiny thread. They may be few and far between and seem insignificant, but eventually the threads form a strand. The strands converge into strong ropes, and finally the ropes become the bridge to a foundation of trust in food and in yourself.

Betsy was feeling desperate when she first came in. She had been on several very restricted diets and was now rebound eating in an out-of-control fashion. After a short time of giving herself permission to eat, she began to find herself eating only *one* candy bar instead of three, which was a major breakthrough. At first these experiences were sporadic, and her successes were interspersed with large periods of bingeing behavior. But Betsy was gradually able to see her successes build upon each other and watch her loss of control eating gradually disappear. Soon she began to redevelop that sense of self-trust that had been eroded by her history of dieting.

For some, the trust issue goes even deeper. Several studies have shown that the regulation of food intake has its foundation in early eating experiences. If as a child your parents took control over most of your eating without respecting your preferences or hunger levels, you easily got the message that you couldn't be trusted with food.

Sarah described this as the push-or-pull-away effect. Her mom was either pushing her to eat, while exerting pressure about Sarah's weight, or pulling food away. At dinnertime, for example, Sarah's mom forced her to clean her plate, even though she was full. Sarah remembers coming home from school on several occasions feeling famished and heading for the fridge for a snack. Her mom would chastise her, "You can't be hungry," and forbid her to eat. Consequently, Sarah would sneak food when her mom wasn't looking. By that time, however, hunger was no longer mild, but intense. Sarah would overeat in response to hunger, but she felt guilty from overeating and shame from sneaking the food. And she grew to believe that her mother was right—she couldn't be trusted with food. Wrong!

Don't underestimate the profound impact self-trust can have. Psycho-analyst Erik Erikson, a noted pioneer in human development, explains how critical trust is. According to Erikson, all people must go through a series of psychosocial stages throughout their lives. The first developmental stage deals with basic trust. During each stage there is a significant issue or crisis that presents itself and must be resolved. If this task is not handled well, a person will continue to struggle with it into adulthood. If food becomes a battleground during this stage, the ability to trust yourself with food becomes tarnished. The "you-can't-be-trusted-around-food" message becomes compounded if you were put on diets by your parents or your doctor. As an adult, try as you may, you still don't trust yourself. That child can still reside within you, making you fearful about giving yourself permission to eat unconditionally.

Fortunately, Erikson had an optimistic belief that childhood crises can be resolved at any time later in life. If you take back ownership of your eating signals by making peace with food, you can heal one of the most basic trust issues and go on to a healthier relationship with food.

Five Steps to Make Peace with Food

Keep in mind as you read through these steps that it's okay to proceed at a pace with which *you* are comfortable. There is no need to feel over-whelmed by going to the grocery store and buying every single forbidden food—we find that is too big of a step and not necessary. It takes time to build up trust in yourself. Before you proceed, please be sure that you are consistently *honoring your hunger*. A ravenous person is bound to engage in rebound eating, regardless of their intention.

1. Pay attention to the foods that are appealing to you, and make a list of them.
2. Put a check by the foods you actually do eat, then circle remaining foods that you've been restricting.
3. Give yourself permission to eat one forbidden food from your list, then go to the market and buy this food, or order it at a restaurant.
4. Check in with yourself to see if the food tastes as good as you imagined. If you find that you really like it, continue to give yourself permission to buy or order it.
5. Make sure that you keep enough of the food in your kitchen so that

you know that it will be there if you want it. Or if that seems too scary, go to a restaurant and order the particular food as often as you like.

Once you've made peace with one food, continue on with your list until all the foods are tried, evaluated, and freed. If your list is quite large, which is possible, we have found that you don't have to experience each and every food listed. Rather, what is important is that you continue this process until you *truly know* you can eat what you want. You will get to a point where you don't have to experience the "proof" by eating.

If these steps seem like too much to handle right now, don't worry. Maybe you can call a ceasefire; that's okay—it's progress. The next chapter will give you some tools to help you loosen up with your food. Just as many peace treaties require a team of negotiators—and time. The next chapter will help you discover powerful allies to help keep the peace with food.

Beware the "I Can Eat Whatever I Want, as Much as I Want, Whenever I Feel like It" Trap

This perception, or trap, actually distorts the premise of Intuitive Eating. Yes, make peace with food, and eat what pleases your palate. Yes, give yourself the freedom to eat unconditionally, and eat as much as you need to satisfy your body. But eating whenever you feel like it, without regard to hunger and fullness, might not be a very satisfying experience and might also cause physical discomfort. Attunement with your body's satiety cues is an important part of this process.

HABITUATION RESPONSE EXPLAINS WHY FOODS BECOME LESS ENTICING WITH EXPOSURE

One reason that having unconditional permission to eat is important is because of the habituation response. Habituation explains why we quickly adapt to a repeated experience—and subsequently experience less pleasure each time. It's a universal phenomenon that applies in many situations—such as when you buy a new car. At first, it's super exciting, but then the novelty wears off. Or when you hear a special person say "I love you" for the first time. It's magical, but then it becomes routine, and even expected. Psychologist and author Daniel Gilbert aptly describes habituation this way: "Wonderful things are especially wonderful the first time they happen, but their wonderfulness wanes with repetition" (Gilbert 2006).

Habituation is also one of the reasons why leftovers are less appealing, especially on days two and three. When you eat a food over and over, it simply loses its appeal. There is a lot of research on food habituation, which shows that people habituate to a variety of foods, like pizza, chocolate, and potato chips (Ernst 2002). Scientists describe food habituation as a form of neurobiological learning, in which repeated eating of the same food causes a decrease in behavioral and physiologic responses (Epstein 2009).

Studies also show that the habituation response is delayed by eating novel foods and by stress and distraction. This works against chronic dieters, in particular. Dieting heightens the novelty and desirability of the forbidden foods. When they go off the diet, dieters often eat those forbidden foods in excess, in part because of the lack of habituation. When you combine low habituation with the fear of never being able to eat a particular food, it can become a powerful force in overeating, which we call Last Supper eating. It's difficult to tire of eating a food you think you may never eat again!

The purpose behind having unconditional permission to eat is not to "get sick of" or burn out on a particular food—it's partly to experience habituation, in which the heightened novelty of eating a particular food wanes.

A recent study provided the first promising evidence of long-term food habituation (Epstein 2011). Two groups of women were given the same food with their meals, daily, over a five-week period. This resulted in an increase in the rate of habituation.

CAN YOU REALLY BE ADDICTED TO FOOD?

There has been a lot of research speculation and media attention on "food addiction." Scientists are curious, because the brain region (and neurochemicals) involved with substance abuse are also implicated in loss of control. But there are many reasons, other than addiction, that can explain the reward aspect of eating.

Survival of the species. This brain-reward system is believed to be necessary in order to ensure human survival. This involves the brain chemical dopamine,

cont.

Cont.

which triggers both a pleasurable feeling and motivation behavior. Engaging in activities necessary to survival (such as eating and procreating) triggers a rewarding feel-good experience.

Hunger enhances reward value. Hunger by itself enhances the reward value of food, through triggering more dopamine-related activity. For example, if you discover you are hungry, you might find yourself suddenly interested and motivated to cook a meal. Dieting (which can be a form of chronic hunger) also has this effect.

Pavlovian conditioning. The dopamine effect could be attributed to Pavlovian conditioning. (Recall the classic study in which Pavlov's dogs salivated at the mere ringing of a bell. This anticipatory salivation occurred because the dogs were conditioned to receiving a treat each time, after a bell rang.) This is not addiction; it is a learned response.

Dopamine deprivation. Many pleasurable activities trigger dopamine, including socializing, hiking, and playing games. The great majority of people we see in our practices who binge eat are often leading very unbalanced lives. These unbalanced lives "deprive" them of the dopamine benefits. When needs are not being met, food becomes even more enticing, more rewarding.

Music lights up dopamine brain centers. A clever study showed that when people listen to music, it lights up the same region of the brain (nucleus accumbens) that has been implicated in the euphoric component of psychostimulants, such as cocaine (Salimpoor 2011). Just the anticipation of hearing the music lit up the dopamine brain centers. (Yet we really don't think you can make the case for "music addiction"!)

Food addiction studies are limited and flawed. The research on "food addiction" is too limited to be drawing any conclusions from it. The great majority of studies have been on animals, mainly rats. Fascinating studies on food-restricted rats show that they will consistently overeat sugar. Yet in the same studies, the control rats that have regular access to food do not overeat sugar. This might suggest that food restriction is the gateway to making food more rewarding, but we wouldn't call that addiction (Westwater et al. 2016). No such studies have been done in humans. The limited research on humans has only been focused on brain-imaging studies with a very small number of people and not much exclusion criteria, such as dieting history (Benson 2010).

Yale Food Addiction Scale (YFAS) questionnaire. When you combine a prestigious university (Yale) and add "Food Addiction" to the title of questionnaire, it might give you the impression that food addiction is a bona fide diagnosis. But it's not! (If it were, it would be in the most recent *Diagnostic and Statistical Manual of Mental Disorders,* fifth edition, also known as the DSM-5.) While the concept of food addiction has generated a lot of headline news, it has been criticized by researchers. One scientific review in 2015 by Long and colleagues concluded, "At the present time, the concept of so-called FA [food addiction] at the individual level as putative biological cause of overeating is controversial and lacks convincing support." Some scientists believe that the YFAS is a proxy for other maladies, such as trauma, PTSD, or eating disorders. And we'd like to add one other possibility—that the YFAS is a proxy for chronic dieting.

Upon a closer look, the YFAS questionnaire seems to actually be measuring compulsive eating or rebound eating from chronic dieting. Here is a sampling of the questions from the updated questionnaire YFAS 2.0 (Penzenstadler et al. 2018):

- I tried and failed to cut down on or stop eating certain foods. (*Chronic dieting and overeating can cause this.*)

- When I started to eat certain foods, I ate much more than I planned. (*Chronic dieting and overeating can cause this.*)

- I had such strong urges to eat certain foods that I couldn't think of anything else. (*Chronic food restriction for the purpose of losing weight can cause this.*)

Studies show eating "forbidden food" decreases binge eating. Finally, there are five studies, to date, in which binge eaters eat their "forbidden foods" as part of the treatment process. (Kristeller 2011; Smitham 2008). Binge eating decreased significantly in all of these studies. If food addiction were an issue, you would not expect these types of results. Food addiction theory would predict increased binge eating, triggered by eating "addicting food." Yet the opposite happened.

cont.

Cont.

The problem with the food addiction concept is that it is fear-mongering, demonizes food, and labels people, which is very disempowering. Also, the language we use to name symptoms (overeating) makes a significant difference in how you treat them.

Chapter 9

PRINCIPLE 4:

Challenge the Food Police

Scream a loud NO to thoughts in your head that declare you're "good" for eating minimal calories or "bad" because you ate a piece of chocolate cake. The food police monitor the unreasonable rules that diet culture has created. The police station is housed deep in your psyche, and its loudspeaker shouts negative barbs, hopeless phrases, and guilt-provoking indictments. Chasing the food police away is a critical step in returning to Intuitive Eating.

> *I felt so guilty eating an extra piece of birthday cake that when I felt nauseous for three days, I thought that I had earned and deserved this misery. To my surprise, I found out one week later that nausea was not my penance for my eating indulgence—I was pregnant!*
> —A chronic dieter

We have become a nation riddled with guilt based on how we eat. Even non-dieters experience eating angst. In a random survey of 2,075 adults, 45 percent said they feel guilty after eating foods they like! And nearly all of our clients also feel that way—guilty, guilty, guilty.

The thought of stealing or lying would instill a sense of guilt in most people. Yet most dieters are able to create an equivalent level of guilt when they've eaten French fries or a hot fudge sundae. The quantity of any of these "bad" foods has almost nothing to do with the level of despair that is felt when they are eaten. The first bite often evokes a sense of having failed or being bad. Eating a "bad" or "illegal" food then becomes a morality issue. The subsequent guilt that builds is enough to initiate a period of overeating that can destroy any feeling of perceived "diet success."

Foods are often described in moralistic terms, independent of dieting: decadent, sinful, tempting—all the words of food fundamentalism and eating morality. Historian Roberta Pollack Seid concluded in her book *Never Too Thin* that our beliefs about food resemble dietary laws of a false religion—we pay homage to dieting, and its rules, but it doesn't work.

Since we are a culture that worships the lean body, it easily becomes virtuous to eat foods associated with slimness and guiltlessness. It is no wonder that dieters have been found to think of food in terms of *absence* of guilt.

Food companies, magazines, social media, and commercials are capitalizing on consumer eating morality with absolving themes:

- Oreo Thins ad depicts a regular size Oreo cookie with "minus the guilt"
- Pop Chips ad promotes "Less guilty, more pleasure"
- *5 Surprisingly Healthy Sin Foods*, title of a magazine article

With these daily reminders it becomes difficult to view eating as simply a normal pleasurable activity; rather, it becomes good or bad, with the societal food police chastising each blasphemous bite of food. The food police are alive and well—both as a collective cultural voice, and at the individual level, in the thoughts of our clients.

As you embark on your journey to Intuitive Eating you may encounter your fair share of societal food police—from the well-meaning yet naïve friend who comments, "How can you eat *that*?" to unsolicited commentary on your eating habits from a stranger. Just because someone makes an inappropriate comment does not make it true! Yet it can shed seeds of doubt as you begin to explore a new eating world that runs counter to the doctrine of fatphobia.

Some years ago on a vacation, I (ET) experienced an unwelcome food police barb. I placed my order at the customized omelet bar and requested an egg white omelet with mushrooms and *cheese*. The chef nearly gave me hell for my order; he reprimanded, "How can you order an egg white omelet with that fatty cheese, it's loaded with cholesterol." That unsolicited remark would have devastated most of our patients. I was on vacation and did not feel like defending my consciously placed order. I knew full well what I was doing—I don't really like egg yolks. I'm not crazy about cheese, but since I was pregnant during this vacation, it was one way I was able to get my calcium in, since I'm not fond of the taste of milk. It was our clients' worst fear personified.

We have found that regardless of the level of inappropriate comments from the collective food police—the inner food police that reside in the minds of our clients are even harsher. If our nation is being possessed by a food fundamentalism, then certainly no less than a food police exorcism will do.

FOOD TALK

In the world of diet culture, we develop a whole retinue of thoughts that can work against us. These thoughts can come from sneaky diet culture books and programs masquerading as a "lifestyle," "detox," "cleanse," or wellness diet, and a generalized pervasive diet mentality in society itself. Self-awareness, or having the ability to think about our thoughts, distinguishes us from animals. It's also human, however, to let our busy lives lead us from one routine activity to the next without stopping to be aware of or examine our thoughts. Food thoughts and judgments run rampant through our minds, but how often do we take a moment to examine them? We're not born with these thoughts. We hear the ideas behind them as we grow up, take them in, and sometimes then adopt them as "well-known" rules, which must not be defied.

Here is some of the "knowledge" and thoughts that prevail in the minds of our clients when they first come to see us:

- Sweets are bad for you.
- I shouldn't eat anything after 6 P.M.
- You should take in zero grams of fat.
- You should avoid carbs.
- If I eat breakfast, it will just make me eat more throughout the day.
- Dairy products are bad for you.
- I shouldn't have any salt.
- Beans will make me gain weight.
- Bread will make me gain weight.

Even when these thoughts are evaluated, they stick like glue in the consciousness of the people who think them. Although there has been a great deal of evidence to refute these thoughts, they've become so well entrenched that it often takes years to loosen their hold and replace them with reality. The thoughts themselves can be very damaging and can affect subsequent behavior. These thoughts are called cognitive distortions, and we call the voices that speak these distortions the Food Police.

WHO'S TALKING

There are many psychological ways of looking at personality structure. Psychotherapist and MD Eric Berne tells us that the way we feel and the ways in which we act make up what are called "ego states." If you watch the way a person is standing and listen to their voice, the words they use, and the views they're stating, you'll be able to detect which ego state they are in. Dr. Berne simply labels these ego states as the Parent, the Adult, and the Child. He believes that at any particular time, you may be in any one of these three ego states and can shift quite easily from one to another. Each ego state can direct the thoughts floating around in your head. You can begin to identify just which one of them is speaking by listening carefully to what is being said.

We have found that in the world of diet culture, specific voices crop up from moment to moment, which influence how we feel and how we behave. We have extrapolated from Berne's theory of ego structure and identified the following eating voices. There are three that can be primarily destructive: the Food Police, the Nutrition Informant, and the Diet Rebel. But we also can develop powerful allies; these voices are: the Food Anthropologist, the Nurturer, and the Nutrition Ally.

Let's look at each food voice—how each can help or harm our thinking process in the world of eating. The diagrams on the next two pages give an overview of how they interrelate:

The Food Police

The Food Police is a strong voice that's developed through dieting and diet culture. It's your inner judge and jury that determine if you are doing "good" or "bad." The Food Police is the sum of all your dieting and food rules and gets stronger with each food plan. It also gets strengthened through new food rules that you may read about in magazines, social media, or messages you hear from friends and family. The Food Police is

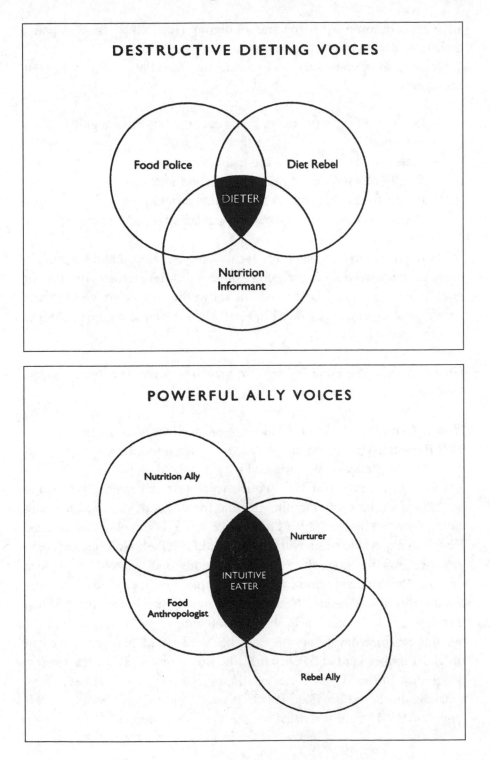

DESTRUCTIVE DIETING VOICES

Food Police

Diet Rebel

DIETER

Nutrition
Informant

POWERFUL ALLY VOICES

Nutrition Ally

Nurturer

INTUITIVE
EATER

Food
Anthropologist

Rebel Ally

alive and well even when you are not dieting (like a lobbyist positioning their issue during an election year).

Here are some common rules by which the Food Police may judge your eating actions:

- Don't eat at night (therefore if you eat at night, you are guilty of a violation).
- Better not eat that bagel—too many carbohydrates.
- You didn't exercise today, better not eat dinner.
- It's not time to eat yet—don't have that snack.
- You ate too much (even though it was based on being hungry).

It's important to remember that even when you reject dieting and begin to make peace with food, the Food Police will often surface. But it's not always obvious—just like a weed cut above the surface. A weed that is strongly rooted can easily flourish, even when there are no green tendrils peeking through the soil.

How It Hurts. The Food Police scrutinizes every eating action. It keeps food and your body at war.

How It Can Help. *It doesn't!* This is one voice that does not turn into an ally. By identifying its strong presence in your mind, however, you will learn how to challenge its power and loosen its hold on you.

Cyndi had a powerful Food Police voice that criticized every eating act. She woke up every morning praying for a "good" day, which meant eating only diet foods. But her Food Police voice set impossible standards. Her good day would begin with a light breakfast of a boiled egg. On some days her growling stomach would beg for more food—just adding a piece of toast. Cyndi would "cave in" and have a piece of dry rye toast, and her Food Police would shout, "Now you have to skip lunch or dinner." When Cyndi was able to skip lunch, she'd get too hungry and find herself at the vending machine devouring whatever she could afford. Now, once she had officially broken her Food Police rule, she would reactively overeat the rest of the day. In fact, Cyndi's vicious disconnected cycle would begin any-time she disobeyed her Food Police. It wasn't until Cyndi began to challenge the Food Police voice that her reactive eating stopped.

The Nutrition Informant

The Nutrition Informant provides nutrition evidence to keep you in line with dieting and diet culture. The Nutrition Informant voice may tell you to fastidiously count macros or eat only carb-free foods, often in the name of health (pretty sneaky!). While this may seem innocuous or even healthy, it's a facade.

The Nutrition Informant makes statements like:

- Check those macros, any deviation is unacceptable.
- Don't eat foods with added sweeteners.

It's not unusual for someone to say, "I've rejected dieting, I truly believe I can eat what I want—I *want* to start eating healthfully." It's therefore possible to consciously reject dieting, but instead unknowingly continue to diet as a politically correct regimen for shrinking the body (it's subtle diet culture, which has co-opted terms like "healthy," "lifestyle," and "wellness").

How It Hurts. This voice colludes with the Food Police. It operates under the guise of health, but it's promoting an unconscious diet. It can be a little difficult to identify, because its messages can mimic the "sound" advice of health authorities or social media influencers.

For example, Kelly declared, "I've made peace with food; I'm never going to diet again, but I'm ready to start eating healthfully." She was actually burned out on exploring "junk foods," which in and of itself was something she never thought she would accomplish!

Here's what happened. One afternoon at work, Kelly got hungry, so she honored her hunger and ate an apple, in the name of "healthy eating." But one hour later, she was hungry. Her Nutrition Informant voice chimed in with the Food Police telling her, "You shouldn't be hungry—you just had a healthy apple. Wait until you get home to eat." She waited until she arrived at home and proceeded to devour her pantry out of ravenous hunger. Later, we talked about satisfying snacks, including a bagel or bean soup. "But aren't those . . . unhealthy?" she asked. "The only snacks I thought I should eat were either fresh fruit or cut-up vegetables." Kelly's description sounded like the diet culture dogma of snacking, yet she did not see it as such, because she was focused on health and had sincerely rejected dieting. Yet one of Kelly's Food Police rules had surfaced: "If you snack, you can't possibly be hungry later."

This rule merged with the Nutrition Informant voice, which declared, "If you snack, it should only be raw veggies or fruit because they're good for you and healthy." While Kelly chose the apple in the name of health and nutrition, she had difficulty honoring her true hunger that surfaced only one hour later, because her Food Police and Nutrition Informant voices were overpowering (yet subtle, because she did not recognize them).

How It Can Help. The Nutrition Informant becomes the Nutrition Ally when the Food Police are exiled. The newly emerged Nutrition Ally is interested in healthy eating with *no hidden agenda*. For example, if you were choosing between two brands of cheese that you like equally and that have saturated fat, the Nutrition Ally would advise choosing the brand with lower saturated fat. It's a choice based on health and satisfaction, *not* deprivation, or dieting. We have found that the helpful version of this voice is one of the last to truly appear without being tied into the Food Police. (We will address nutrition later in the book. Remember, however, that focusing initially on nutrition can undermine your attempts to be truly free from the influence of diet culture. It's not that nutrition is not important, but rather that it can be self-defeating in the beginning stages of Intuitive Eating. Remember, we *are* nutritionists, and we honor health!)

One distinguishing factor between the Nutrition Ally and the Nutrition Informant is how you *feel* when you respond. If you make, or reject, a food choice in the name of health, but feel acquiescent or guilty, then you know the Food Police still have a stranglehold on your Nutrition Informant, who's guiding your decision.

The Diet Rebel

The voice of the Diet Rebel often bellows loudly in your head. It sounds angry and determined. Here are some typical statements of your internal Diet Rebel:

- You're not going to get me to eat that plain broiled chicken!
- Let's see how many cookies I can stuff in before Mom comes home.
- I can't wait until my partner goes out of town so I can eat whatever I want, without their chastising glares.

How It Hurts. Unfortunately, these rebellious comments reside in your head, because you're usually too scared to confront your "space invaders" and tell them to bug off. Feeling powerless over their messages, you feel resigned to merely possessing the thoughts you wish you could say out loud, and then end up carrying out the "threats" just to spite them. Ultimately, this is a form of acting out.

Janie had a strong Diet Rebel voice. Every time her mother put her on a diet as a child, Janie's sneak-eating would escalate. The Diet Rebel voice was Janie's primary guiding force as a child and as an adult. Janie would hang out at her friends' homes so she could eat as much of their treats as she could. A large child, Janie became larger as an adult. When her ex-husband carried on with the parental diet admonishment messages, Janie's silent Diet Rebel became loud and angry. It was her "forget you" inner voice that directed her to go against any rules imposed upon her, which resulted in reactive eating. Janie's boundaries were being invaded everywhere she turned. In order to protect her autonomy, Janie's Diet Rebel was overpowering all other voices to help keep her independent. Yet it only ended up in private food riots of overeating.

Unfortunately, when the Diet Rebel rules the roost, self-destruction always ensues. Rebellious behavior often has no limits, and severe reactive eating may be the result. How often does the diet rebel break forth in your thoughts? How often do you feel compelled to follow its directions, because you're so angry at the Food Police (and diet culture) in your life imposing their dieting rules on you?

How It Can Help. You can turn your Diet Rebel into the Rebel Ally. Use the energy of the Rebel Ally to help you protect your boundaries against anyone who invades your eating space. *Use your mouth for words instead of acting out with food* in a direct but polite way—it's surprising how powerful it can make you feel, while giving you a tremendous release.

- Ask your family members to not comment on your food choices or amounts. For example: "Aunt Carolyn, please don't push that second portion on me. I'm full, thank you." Or: "No thanks, Mom, I don't like macaroni and cheese. You know I've never liked macaroni and cheese."

- Tell your family and your friends and people on the street that they may not make comments about your body. For example: "Dad—my body is *my* business!" Or: "Joey, you have no right to comment about my body." Simply put, it's your body, your rules.

The Food Anthropologist

The Food Anthropologist is simply the neutral observer. This is the voice that makes observations *without* making judgment. It's a neutral voice that takes note of your thoughts and actions with respect to your food world, without an indictment—just like an anthropologist would observe an individual or culture. It's the voice that will let you explore and discover. The Food Anthropologist will help pave the way to the world of Intuitive Eating. For example, noticing when you're hungry or full, what you ate, the time of day, and what you're thinking are the actions of the Food Anthropologist. This voice simply observes and shows you how to interact with food both behaviorally and inwardly. The advantage to developing this voice is that only *you* know what you feel and think. No outside observer could possibly know this.

The statements of the Food Anthropologist are purely observational, such as:

- I skipped breakfast and was ravenous at 11 a.m.
- I ate ten cookies. (No judgment here, just the facts.)
- I experienced guilt after eating dessert with dinner. (No condescending statements, just an observation of how you felt.)

One easy way to call your inner Food Anthropologist into action is to keep a food journal. Sometimes simply noting the time of day and what you ate can give you some interesting clues about what drives your eating. Or note your thoughts before and after you eat. Do they affect how you *feel*? Does your feeling state affect how you behave or eat? If so, how? Consider this as one big experiment, *not a tool for judgment*.

Many of our clients have had negative experiences with food journals because it was a requirement of past diets. But in those cases, the food journal was used as evidence to convict "bad" eating! When we use the Intuitive Eating journal, we use it as only a learning and discovery tool. Yet in spite of the fact that we emphasize this, our first-time clients still expect to get verbally beat up upon their return visit for any perceived "eating indiscretion" or violation. Remember, this is not a tool of the Food Police, but a tool to help you access the Food Anthropologist.

How It Helps. The Food Anthropologist can help you sort through the facts rather than get caught up in the emotionally labile experience of eating. It keeps you in touch with your inner signals—biologically and psychologically. We often play the role of the Food Anthropologist with our clients until they can build their own voice. (It can be hard to be just neutral when you've had a critical voice harping on every food choice.) The Food Anthropologist can help find the loopholes in your thinking, similar to the way a sharp attorney can find the loopholes in a contract. But using this voice does take practice—it's the practice of neutrality, rather than judgment.

The Nurturer

The Nurturer's voice is compassionate and gentle. It has the soothing quality that might be associated with the voice of a loving grandparent or best friend. It has the ability to reassure you that you're okay and that everything will turn out fine. It never scolds or pressures. It's not critical or judgmental. Instead it is (or can be cultivated as) the vehicle for most of the positive self-talk in your head.

Here are some of the messages you might hear from the Nurturer in your head:

- It's okay to have cookies. Eating cookies is normal.
- I really overate to the point of feeling very uncomfortable. I wonder what I was feeling that could have made me need more food to comfort myself?
- When I take care of myself, I feel great.
- I'm doing so well this week. There were only a few times that I didn't honor my hunger signals.
- I'm getting more in touch with myself every day.

Alice is a mother who usually knows just the right thing to say to her children to make them feel safe and secure. But for many years, Alice had not learned to speak to herself kindly about her body. The voice of the Food Police punished her severely through all of her diets. On her journey to becoming an Intuitive Eater, Alice learned to counter the messages of the Food Police with the supportive messages of the Nurturer. She listened to herself speak to her family and realized that the voice she used when speaking to them was the same voice that she needed to comfort herself.

Alice learned to be understanding of the stumbling blocks in her path and to patiently reassure herself that she was in the midst of a process. When she would have difficulty honoring her hunger, she'd gently ask herself what was bothering her and what she really needed instead of food. When she found herself craving a food she had restricted on one of her many diets, the Nurturer gave her permission to eat that food.

How It Helps. When you get in touch with the Nurturer inside your head, you will experience one of the most significant tools necessary to becoming an Intuitive Eater. The Nurturer will be there for you to help you to challenge the Food Police and support you compassionately through this process. The Nurturer provides coping statements for the harsh zingers that the Food Police and the Diet Rebel can throw.

The Intuitive Eater

The Intuitive Eater speaks your gut reactions. You were born an Intuitive Eater, but this wisdom has probably been suppressed for most of your life by diet culture and the voices of the Food Police (prevailing in your family and in society), the Diet Rebel, and the Nutrition Informant.

The Intuitive Eater is a compilation of the positive voices of the Food Anthropologist, who is able to observe your eating behavior neutrally, and the Nurturer, who holds you with supportive statements to get you through the tough times, as well as the Rebel Ally and the Nutrition Ally. The Intuitive Eater knows how to quell or reframe the negative voices out of your head. For example, it knows how to challenge the distorted messages of the Food Police and how to get the Rebel Ally to speak out loud to fend off the boundary invaders.

The Intuitive Eater voice might say some of the following things:

- That little rumble in my stomach means I'm hungry and need to eat.
- What do I feel like eating for dinner tonight? What sounds good to me?
- It feels so good to be out of that dieting prison.

These statements all tell you about your gut reactions. They're instinctual and hit you out of nowhere, without your having to think about them. You'll find that you'll be in the midst of a meal and the Intuitive Eater voice knows that you're satisfied. Or you'll be doing some writing and a hunger pang will emerge. Or maybe your eyes lock on to the food on the menu that connects with your craving. When you have reached the last stages of your path to Intuitive Eating, the Intuitive Eater, rather than the dieter, will prevail most of the time. But there will be times when you find that you'll need to evoke one or all of the positive eating voices to help you get centered and in touch with your Intuitive Eater once again. There are no rigid rules in this process. Diets are rigid—Intuitive Eating is fluid and adapts to the many changes in your life. Go with the flow without trying to control it.

The integrated Intuitive Eater honors gut reactions, whether they are biological, satisfaction-based, or self-protective. *The Intuitive Eater is a team player* and can draw from the voices of the Nurturer, the Food Anthropologist, and the positive traits of both the Diet Rebel (the Rebel Ally) and the Nutrition Informant (the Nutrition Ally).

EATING VOICES: HOW THEY EMERGE AND EVOLVE

Each of the voices may prevail at different times. Some of the voices were there at birth but may have become buried. Others were instilled by family and society. And some need to be learned and developed so you can become an Intuitive Eater.

You're born with the innate ability to sense when you're hungry and full. These are primitive signals and are the basis for the emerging voice of the Intuitive Eater, which is operating in the toddler as they start eating solid food. The Intuitive Eater tells you what you like and what you don't like. If your parents are not sensitive to your signals, you may learn to mistrust them and ultimately lose touch with them.

If you happen to live in a family that is weight-focused with an array of eating issues, you might have had your first experience with the voice of the Food Police when you were very young. You might have been told to stop eating so much or been restricted from eating certain foods. It doesn't take long before you internalize those negative messages and create your own powerful Food Police. If, on the other hand, you're lucky enough to have a family that is not invasive, making no food or body

SUMMARY: HOW VOICES HELP OR HARM		
Voice	How It Harms	How It Helps
Food Police	Causes guilt and food worry. Full of judgment. Keeps you in diet culture, and out of touch with inner cues of eating.	It doesn't.
Nutrition Informant	Uses nutrition as a vehicle to keep you dieting.	Once uncoupled from the Food Police, it becomes the *Nutrition Ally* and can help you make healthy food choices without guilt or deprivation.
Diet Rebel	Usually results in loss of control eating and self-sabotage.	When the Diet Rebel becomes the *Rebel Ally,* it can help you guard your food turf/ boundaries.
Food Anthropologist	It doesn't.	A neutral observer that can give you a distant perspective into your eating world. Nonjudgmental. Keeps you in touch with your inner signals—biologically and psychologically.
Nurturer	It doesn't.	Helps to compassionately disarm the verbal assault from the Food Police. Gets you through the tough times.

judgments, you may not encounter the Food Police until you start school or until you become a teen scrolling social media and listening to your friends talk. If diet culture is strong in your community, you are at risk of making the Food Police messages your own at any time in your life. And the Nutrition Informant constantly feeds nutrition information about food to the Food Police.

The voice of the Diet Rebel will crop up soon after you've encountered the Food Police. It usually goes hand in hand. The Food Police come in and invade your boundaries by interfering with your intuitive biological and food preference signals. In order to protect your private space, the Diet Rebel feeds you "forget you" messages that not only counter the Food Police but often send you off into a one-person food riot.

The Food Anthropologist will help give you a neutral perspective. For some individuals, interaction with this voice is often the first nonjudgmental, non-negative encounter they have with food.

The Nurturer can get you through outside abuse and your own self-defeating behavior if you have access to its positive voice. If your family has given you a sense that you are competent and adequate and has modeled positive ways of coping, you may easily find the voice of your nurturer to combat the societal voices of the Food Police. If, however, your family has colluded with diet culture and you have grown up with criticism and judgment, the Nurturer will have to be found elsewhere. Sometimes a grandparent, aunt or uncle, or dear friend may teach you how to speak kindly to yourself. For some, seeking help from a psychotherapist or dietitian may be their first experience with learning compassionate, positive self-talk. However you learn to bring forth the voice of the Nurturer, this is a critical step in becoming an Intuitive Eater. You must make it available to yourself so you can buffer the negative voices that bombard you without notice and cause a barrier to your progress.

And finally, you find yourself back at that place where the Intuitive Eater is running the show. The Intuitive Eater integrates the voices of the Nurturer and the Food Anthropologist, the Nutrition Ally, and the Rebel Ally. The Intuitive Eater knows when your biological signals are calling; it tells you what you need and want, and with guidance from the other positive voices helps you make adult, neutral decisions about how you will take care of yourself.

Let's now take an eating situation and listen for the dialogue of voices that can affect its outcome.

You've been invited to dinner at the home of a gourmet cook. Many appetizers will be served during the cocktail hour, and later a spectacular dinner will be placed before you. Unfortunately, you arrive at the party in an overly hungry state.

THE FOOD POLICE: You'd better be careful of what you eat. Everything is bad for you. Don't touch the appetizers. If you even taste that little quiche, you're a goner. And you can be sure you'll be tempted with lots of rich desserts. Watch out!

THE NUTRITION INFORMANT: You shouldn't have any cheese because there's too much fat in it, and the salt will make you feel bloated. You can only eat the raw veggies.

THE DIET REBEL: Nobody is going to tell me what I can eat at this party. I hate that stupid diet. I've had to succumb to cardboard crackers and diet cottage cheese. Well, not tonight. I'm going to get my fill of these amazing foods. I don't care what happens to my diet. I'll show my partner what they can do with comments about my body.

THE FOOD ANTHROPOLOGIST: Look at the interesting array of appetizers. A lot of them look great. You're overly hungry—better eat something, or you'll probably eat past comfortable fullness at dinner.

THE NUTRITION ALLY: I don't think I'll have any cheese or fried appetizers tonight. They will make me feel too full for dinner. I'd rather have some crab and veggies now, so I still have some hunger for dinner.

THE NURTURER: This food looks terrific. I want to taste *everything*. It's scary to feel such an overwhelming desire to devour these appetizers. That's okay, it's normal to feel this way when you're ravenous. This isn't the usual situation, and I'm human.

THE INTUITIVE EATER: I'm starving. But I think I'll pace myself, so I won't feel too full to enjoy the dinner later. Let's see, of all the appetizers, which look the best? Oh, I haven't had pizza in a long time—that looks good, and so does the baked brie. I think I'll try them both. The brie is great, but the pizza is kind of soggy—think I'll *throw it out* and taste the stuffed mushrooms.

(*Halfway through dinner.*) This is delicious, but I'm starting to feel full. Probably just a few more bites, and I'll feel satisfied. I feel great getting to eat anything I like and leaving some of it (without feeling deprived).

THE REBEL ALLY (*to the hostess, who is pushing seconds*): The dinner is delicious, but I'm quite full and couldn't eat another helping. Thanks anyway.

SELF-TALK: SPECIAL ARSENAL FOR CHALLENGING THE FOOD POLICE

Identifying the inner voices is useful for challenging the Food Police. But this powerfully negative voice requires more ammunition. The Food Police can throw many tricks that require special attention—especially in the thought process department.

When working with dieters in our offices, we have seen over and over that there is actually a middle step between the initial dieting thought and the subsequent eating behavior. We have found that the inner dieting myths (which are cognitive distortions) lead to feeling bad when the self-imposed dieting rules are broken. This concept is widely accepted and well explained by Dr. Albert Ellis and Dr. Robert A. Harper, highly respected pioneers in the field of rational-emotive psychotherapy, a system of psychotherapy that deals with the effect of our thoughts on our feelings and then our behaviors. (An offshoot of this therapy is called cognitive-behavioral therapy, or CBT.)

According to Ellis and Harper, we routinely flood our heads with unrealistic and sometimes absurd notions as well as sane and rational messages. These thought processes are called internalized sentences, or *self-talk*. Negative self-talk often makes us feel despair. The feeling of despair can trigger sabotaging behaviors. Ellis and Harper believe that if we challenge the "nonsense" in our heads, we'll end up feeling better. When we feel better, we'll act better. In a review of hundreds of research studies of this type of therapy, it has been shown that if we can first change our *beliefs,* our feelings and behaviors will also change in a chainlike reaction. Therefore, it makes sense to examine our food or diet beliefs and the influence they can have.

Here's a favorite story that illustrates this principle. Let's say that you've been a dieter who has been carefully following your food plan for several weeks. Your diet is low carb and prohibits any kind of fatty desserts. You decide that you're going to visit your grandmother, whom you haven't seen for a while. You walk into Grandma's house and the first thing that strikes you is the enticing aroma of brownies hot out of the oven. Here are the *food beliefs* and *thoughts* that might fill your head:

- I've been so good on my diet the last few weeks.
- I haven't had any ice cream or candy or cookies.

- I'd sure love to have one of those brownies, but I can't—I shouldn't—I won't!
- If I have a brownie, I'll blow my diet.
- I won't be able to stop eating the brownies.
- Oh, maybe just one will be okay.

You eat the brownie.

- Oh, no—I shouldn't have done that.
- That was really stupid.
- I have no willpower.
- I'm going to be out of control.
- Will I ever be at peace with my body?

Now, let's sense what you are *feeling*:

- Disappointment
- Fear of future deprivation
- Sadness
- Fear of being out of control
- Despair

Typical eating *behavior* that follows will be something like this:

- You slowly take a second brownie.
- . . . and a third brownie.
- Before you know it, you've gobbled up the whole plateful.
- You collapse on the couch, stuffed and miserable, and fall right to sleep.

Now, let's see how challenging your basic food beliefs can change your feelings and your behavior. The *beliefs* and *thoughts*:

- I'm so glad I gave up diet culture.
- I can eat anything I want, any time I want.
- I'd sure love to have one of those brownies.

You eat the brownie.

- Boy, was that delicious.
- I'm satisfied with just this one, although I could have a second if I wanted.
- There's nothing like Grandma's home-baked brownies.

And now the *feelings*:

- Satisfaction
- Pleasure
- Contentment (no worry about future deprivation)

And the *behavior*:

- You leave the rest of the brownies on the plate.
- You put the plate of brownies on the kitchen counter.
- You're free to enjoy the afternoon with Grandma without another thought about the brownies.

Andrea is a college student who had been suffering from years of bouts of low self-esteem associated with her so-called dieting failures. For a short time, she actually became bulimic when she saw no other way to control the bingeing that inevitably followed her dieting "falls from grace." Andrea was an expert at telling herself that carbohydrates were bad and that even a few grams of fat in a day would mar her "good" eating behavior (*belief*). As soon as these *thoughts* formed in her head, she *felt* bad the moment she would eat carbohydrates. The conflict between her restrictive thoughts and her craving for the forbidden food always created angry and hateful feelings. When she *felt* bad in her mode of shaky "willpower," she was off and running to her latest eating disaster (*behavior*).

As soon as Andrea succumbed to her natural desires to eat that food, the system of negative thinking led to negative feelings, which led to negative behavior.

Andrea has learned to check her food thoughts as soon as they arise. Old diet rules and thoughts get challenged immediately. Because she is free from distorted dieting thoughts, she feels better about herself and eating. Instead of feeling bad about wanting French fries or ice cream, she feels great about her new relationship with food. And you guessed it—her bingeing days are over.

NEGATIVE SELF-TALK (AND HOW TO CHANGE IT)

> *. . . for there is nothing either good or bad but thinking makes it so. To me it is a prison.*
>
> —Hamlet

When eating thoughts are irrational or distorted, negative feelings escalate exponentially. As a result, eating behavior can end up extreme and destructive. It's the classic case of perception becomes reality. Therefore, to change our "food reality," we need to replace the irrational thinking with rational thoughts. This in turn helps to moderate our feelings and then behavior.

To get rid of distorted diet thoughts, you first need to identify irrational thinking. Ask yourself:

- Am I having *repetitive* and *intense* feelings? (This is a clue that you need to challenge your thoughts.)
- What am I *thinking* that's leading me to feel this way? (What are you saying to yourself?)
- What is true or correct about this belief? What is false? (Examine and confront the *distorted* beliefs that support this thinking. Your Food Anthropologist voice can be very helpful here.)

Once you have uncovered your distorted beliefs, you need to replace them with thoughts and beliefs that are more rational and reasonable. Here's one example, but the remainder of this chapter will show you how to do this in various ways:

Replace this disorted thought	With a more rational thought
Every time I eat pizza, I feel unhappy with my body the next day. I shouldn't be eating pizza.	I am salt sensitive. Since pizza is pretty salty, I'm most likely bloated; it's just water retention. While it's uncomfortable, it's temporary.

Irrational beliefs often present themselves to us through negative self-talk. Let's examine the various types of negative thinking and how you can recognize their signs before they drag you into the ditches of overeating.

Dichotomous or Binary Thinking

When I (ER) furnished my first office, I purposely chose gray fabric for the couches. I decided that it was a symbolic gesture to help my patients get away from the "black and white" thinking that usually coexists with the diet mentality. Here are some typical examples of dichotomous thinking: If you get on the scale in the morning and it drops a pound, you say that you've been "good." If it goes up a pound, you're "bad." When you're dieting, you think in terms of "all or none." You're not allowed to have any cookies, and if you eat one, you think and feel that you must finish them all. With dichotomous thinking comes all-or-nothing behaviors. Here are some typical eating examples:

- On a food plan or off a food plan
- Never eating snacks or always eating snacks
- Always eating alone or only eating with others

Dichotomous or binary thinking can be dangerous and is often based on the premise of achieving perfection. It gives you only two alternatives, one of which is usually neither attainable nor maintainable. The other then tends to be the black hole into which you inevitably fall after failing to get to the first. You set your sights so high, constantly chasing an ideal that you can grasp only moments at a time. When the standard for being okay is this lofty, you're destined to feel lousy most of the time.

For example, Hillary is a client who set herself up for failure by thinking in an all-or-nothing manner. She would give herself permission to eat only when she felt ravenous. If she ate when just moderately hungry, she would consider it overeating. As a result of thinking that she had "blown it" when she didn't meet her "starving standard," she would feel awful and then go into a binge.

When you think in terms of how good or bad your eating is or how large or small your body is, you can end up judging your self-worth based on these thoughts. If you begin to feel that you're a bad person, you're likely to create self-punishing behaviors.

Rae is a young woman who set up perfectionistic standards in her eating style throughout her high school days. She never allowed herself to eat anything with sugar, artificial sweeteners, salt, or fat in it. When Rae got to college and was away from the familiarity of home, she found that her standards were becoming impossible to keep up. As soon as she began to expand her food choices as a result of availability and peer pressure, things began to fall apart for Rae. As a dichotomous thinker, her thoughts began to run like this:

- The only correct way to eat is the way I ate in high school.
- This new kind of eating is bad.
- I've lost my willpower to eat in the right way.
- The only way I can eat now is wrong.
- That's bad, I'm bad, and I deserve to feel bad.

Rae ultimately began to binge as a result of her dichotomous thinking and was willing to acknowledge that much of her bingeing behavior was done as a way to punish herself for her "bad" acts. The bingeing made her feel increasingly worse, but, ironically, this was okay with her, as she felt that she deserved the punishment. Rae is only now learning to change her thinking. She's stopped talking to herself negatively, has stopped punishing herself with bingeing, and is slowly feeling comfortable in her body.

How do you get out of the dichotomous thinking trap?
Go for the gray. Gray may seem to be a dull color, while black and white are dramatic extremes. In the world of eating, however, going for the gray can give you a rainbow of choices. Give up the notion that you must eat in an all-or-nothing fashion. Let go of your old all-or-nothing dieting rules. Allow yourself to eat the foods that were *always* restricted, while checking your thoughts to be sure that they support your choices.

You'll find that the thrill of being in the extreme area of diet restriction is gone, but so is the misery of being in the other extreme of out-of-control behavior.

Absolutist Thinking

When you think in this way, you believe that one behavior will absolutely, irrevocably result in a second behavior. This is considered magical thinking, because in reality, you can't and don't control life in this way. It leads you to believe that you "must" act in a certain way or else something "awful" will happen.

In the world of eating, absolutist thinking will lead you to statements like the following: "I *must* eat perfectly these next two months or else I won't look good for my daughter's wedding, and that would be *awful*." You don't really have any proof that eating "perfectly" will actually cause you to "look good." You're not even sure what "looking good" actually means. And you really can't define this "awful" state that you imagine. You end up feeling frantic trying to eat perfectly, and then, of course, eat "imperfectly." Fearing that your body won't look good enough makes you more anxious and believing that the outcome will be awful turns you into a wreck. The result, of course, of all of these absolute thoughts and anxious feelings is destructive behavior.

How do you get out of this kind of thinking?
Banish the absolutes and replace them with permissive, flexible statements. Carefully listen for the "absolute" words that you use. Get rid of the *musts, oughts, shoulds, need to's, supposed to's,* and *have to's.* Every time you think that you *must* go on a diet, or you *ought* to have a light lunch like a salad and tea, or you *shouldn't* eat before you go to bed, stop yourself and replace those thoughts. Those kinds of words and thoughts will only cause you anxiety about not being able to carry out the command. Thinking in this absolute way has no guarantee of resulting in the behavior you desire and is likely to create self-sabotaging behavior. In fact, it's fairly sure to make the result *awful,* which is just what you're trying to avoid.

Use words such as *can, is okay,* and *may.* Give yourself permissive statements such as:

- I can eat whenever I feel like it.
- If I want, I can eat whatever foods I like.
- I may have anything that looks good to me.

Catastrophic Thinking

Each time that you think in exaggerated ways, you create miserable feelings for yourself and, once again, compensate with extreme behaviors. The following are examples of catastrophic thoughts:

- I'll never like my body.
- It's hopeless.
- I'll never get a significant other or a job in this body.
- My life is ruined, because of my body.
- If I let myself eat candy bars and fries, I'll never stop.

This kind of thinking is a real setup. It makes a bad situation worse and ties all of your future successes in life to your ability to eat in a particular way or to changing your body. You tell yourself that all your happiness hinges on your eating and your body. If that is your premise, then you're bound to feel all the more unhappy than you are at the moment. You may be desperately unhappy right now, but you may become despairing by catastrophizing your bleak future.

Marion is a highly successful screenwriter who owns her own home and has many devoted friends and two loving dogs. But Marion feeds herself a daily litany of catastrophic thoughts. Because she doesn't think her body is good enough, she tells herself that she'll never get married, never have children, and never be happy. Looking forward to this negative self-created future only makes her feel miserable.

How do you get away from catastrophic thinking?
Climb out of the abyss. Replace your exaggerated thoughts with thinking that is more positive and accurate. Treat yourself to hopeful, coping statements. Marion is learning to nurture herself by telling herself that many people of diverse sizes find partners who love them as they are. She's practicing positive self-talk that confirms her current as well as her future happiness. As a result, Marion is becoming body-accepting. She knows that she won't return to her episodes of negative self-talk.

Pessimistic Thinking, or "The Cup Is Half-Empty"

People who view the world in this way tend to see every situation in its worst-case scenario. They usually think that life is terrible, that they don't have enough of what they want, and that everything they do is wrong. They're highly critical and blameful, not only of themselves but of others.

Bonnie walks into the office each week with a scowl. She complains about her husband and her job and says that her children are stressing her out. She begins each session with accounts of how terrible her week has been and how badly she has "blown" her eating. Bonnie would evaluate the cup as half-empty. This kind of negative thinking is insidious and often goes unnoticed by the participant. It needs to be pointed out on a regular basis, so the person can reevaluate their thought process and see that it only leads to a pervasive sense of unhappiness. It also perpetuates self-destructive behaviors. A person who thinks this way has great difficulty appreciating their small successes. They often even miss them and tend to condemn their progress.

How do you get out of this kind of thinking?

Half-Empty	Half-Full
1. I had a terrible week.	1. I had some progress this week.
2. I overate so many times.	2. I had many times when I ate to satisfaction.
3. All I ate was sweets.	3. I had sweets more than I wished, but I had lots of other foods, too.
4. I feel so fat.	4. Fat is not a feeling, but it is a form of body shaming, rooted in diet culture and weight stigma. I am appreciating all the things my body can do.
5. I'm such a failure.	5. I'm doing better little by little.

Make the cup half-full. The most obvious way to heal cup-is-half-empty thinking is to consciously catch each of your negative statements and re-place the words with more positive ones.

After you have done this consciously for a while, you'll find that you hear your own negative thoughts transform into more positive words. You will also become sensitive to how hard you've been on yourself. Once you begin to see the world in terms of the cup being half-full, you'll find that your daily dose of happy moments increases regularly. Soon you'll see much of your negative eating habits disappear along with the negative thoughts.

Linear Thinking

If you've been on even one diet, you'll know that diet thinking goes in one straight line. You follow a very specific plan that allows for no deviations. It's like trying to walk along the white line in the middle of the highway to get to your destination. If you put one foot in front of the other in perfect style, you'll successfully make it to the end. If you accidentally step off the line for even a moment, you're likely to be a highway disaster. We tend to be a society of linear thinkers. We want to get to the goal without appre-ciating the means. We're success-oriented and rarely stop long enough to just be and check out the scenery along the way.

Here are some examples of linear thinking that can set you up:

- The faster I do it, the more successful I am.
- To be successful, I must reach my goal by the specified target date.

How do you get out of this kind of thinking?

Switch to process thinking. The solution for linear thinking is *process thinking,* which focuses on continual change and learning, rather than just the end result. If you start thinking in terms of what you can learn along the way and accept that there will be ups and downs, you will go forward. By becoming a process-thinker you will enjoy the opportunity to enrich many aspects of your life, while re-creating your relationship with food. Process thinking will help you become more sensitive to your Intuitive Eating signals, rather than endpoints, such as how much you ate today.

Here are some examples of process thinking:

- This was a rough week. But I learned some new things about myself that will help me make changes in the future.
- I ate more than I wanted to at the restaurant tonight. But I learned that by giving myself permission to eat dessert, it took away the urgency to have sweets again. Usually I would have binged when I got home, alone.

COMPASSIONATE SELF-AWARENESS: THE ULTIMATE WEAPON AGAINST THE FOOD POLICE

The next time you see yourself eating in a way that feels uncomfortable, unsatisfying, or even out of control, give yourself the gift of remembering what you were thinking before you even took the first bite of food. Get curious. Examine that thought and challenge it. As you get more adept at the Intuitive Eating process, you'll be able to catch these thoughts before they make you feel bad or cause undesirable behavior.

Become self-aware. Pay attention to the food talk that inevitably arises when you approach any eating situation. Listen for the different voices that can serve as either your support or your saboteur.

Banish the Food Police that keep you from making your peace with food. Challenge the pseudo-nutrition thoughts that come from the Nutrition Informant. Observe your eating through the eyes and voice of your Food Anthropologist and allow it to guide you sensibly. Speak out loud the thoughts of your Rebel Ally, so you find coping mechanisms other than using food to take care of you. The real protection will come from your Nurturer, who knows just how to soothe you and get you through tough situations. And, finally, become acutely sensitive to the positive voices that comprise your Intuitive Eater. It was there when you were born. Discard the layers of negative voices that have buried it so deeply that it seemed lost forever. By listening to its instinctual signals, you'll have the opportunity to form a healthy relationship with food.

Chapter 10

PRINCIPLE 5:

Discover the Satisfaction Factor

The Japanese have the wisdom to promote pleasure as one of their goals of healthy living. In our fury to comply with diet culture, we often overlook one of the most basic gifts of existence—the pleasure and satisfaction that can be found in the eating experience. When you eat what you really want, in an environment that is inviting, the pleasure you derive will be a powerful force in helping you feel satisfied and content.

So, what is it about satisfaction that is so powerful? Abraham Maslow has taught us that we are driven by our unmet needs. We want what we can't have and will do whatever it takes to calm down the sense of deprivation that inevitably arises when our needs are not satisfied. Whether it is food or relationships or career—if we're not satisfied, we're not happy. In the twenty-five years since *Intuitive Eating* was first published, it has become more evident that finding satisfaction in eating is the driving force of this process. We explain this to our clients by describing the following visual:

Imagine a wheel with many spokes. At the hub is satisfaction, surrounded by ten spokes. Each spoke represents an Intuitive Eating principle that influences satisfaction.

To be satisfying, a meal includes foods that you enjoy and that "hit the spot." Eating a salad when you want a steak will not lead to satisfaction. If you are served an appealing food or whole meal when you're not very hungry, your satisfaction will be diminished. You may eat anyway, but food tastes much better when you're moderately hungry. Conversely, if you eat when you're ravenous, your taste buds will barely have a chance to register the exquisite tastes before you've bolted down the entire meal. Definitely not a satisfying experience! But when you begin to eat a deli-

SATISFACTION: The Hub of Intuitive Eating

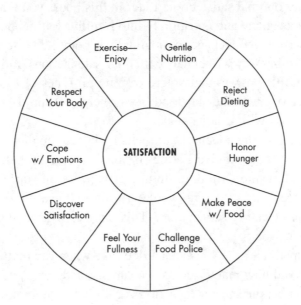

cious meal when you are moderately hungry, you are likely to find that you're comfortably full before the meal is finished. If you finish eating the whole meal, there will be diminished taste to the food, because your taste buds become desensitized to the nuances of the food, especially if you become overfull.

Now think about eating when you're in the middle of a fight with a family member. How delicious is the food you eat during that meal? You may not even notice that you've eaten! Or think about an experience you've had when you've eaten to push down feelings. Again, not a very satisfying eating experience!

Honoring your hunger, making peace with food, feeling your fullness, and coping with your emotions with kindness are four of the spokes on our imaginary wheel. Another spoke on the wheel involves *rejecting the diet mentality*. If you're still in diet mentality when you eat, it's likely that you're not choosing the most satisfying food, or, if you do choose it, you are judging yourself for eating it.

Respecting your body is yet another spoke on the wheel. Eating while you're wearing comfortable clothes and eating without body bashing will free you to have more satisfaction in your meal. *Challenging the Food*

Police, who chastise you for what you eat or for even eating at all, will also allow for optimal satisfaction. Later in this book, you will learn more about how movement and nutrition fit into Intuitive Eating, but suffice it to say that a person who feels good moving their body will also find that eating in a satisfying way will enhance this self-satisfaction. And when you're at a point in this process that you're craving all types of food—nutrient-dense food, along with the play food (see principles 9 and 10)—your eating satisfaction level will be at its peak.

You may be taking a leap of faith when you give up diet mentality and jump headfirst into Intuitive Eating. If you're looking for the motivation to make this transition, think of finding satisfaction in your everyday eating experiences. After all, who wouldn't want to live a life that is built on a foundation of eating satisfaction? This chapter will crystallize finding satisfaction for you.

How many times have you eaten a rice cake when you really wanted potato chips? And how many rice cakes, carrots, and apples have you eaten attempting to get the same satisfaction you would have found with a handful of chips? If you are unsatisfied, you will likely eat more and be on the prowl, regardless of your satiety level.

For example, one client, Fran, wanted a piece of cornbread with lunch, but she fastidiously refrained from eating it. Fran thought about having cornbread with dinner, but again stopped herself. That night, she ate six Weight Watchers desserts, and realized that what she was really seeking was cornbread—no amount of diet desserts would satisfy her cornbread craving. When Fran was eating the diet desserts, she was chasing her *phantom food*—trying to fill the void created by denying the satisfaction factor from the food she originally wanted to eat.

THE WISDOM OF PLEASURE

Americans have gotten so focused on the alchemy of foods—whether as an adjunct to shrinking their body or seeking health, that we have neglected a very important role that eating plays in our lives—provision of pleasure. The Japanese promote pleasure as one of their goals of healthy eating. "Make all activities pertaining to food and eating pleasurable ones" is one of their dietary guidelines for health promotion. How ironic this advice is for dieters, who have come to see food as the enemy and the eating experience as the battleground between "tempting" foods and the willpower to avoid them. Most dieters with whom we work have lost sight of how important it is to have a satisfying, let alone pleasurable, eating experience. For some, any experience that smacks of pleasure triggers feelings of guilt and wrongdoing. It's not too surprising, since we live in a society with strong puritanical roots and a tradition of self-denial. Dieting and rigid food plans play right into the puritanical ethic—make sacrifices, settle for less. Yet if you settle for food that doesn't match what you desire, it will often leave you wanting.

Jill is an example of a young woman who let the fear of eating pleasurable foods turn her into a restrictive eater. Her food choices were based primarily on trying to shrink her body. She was convinced that if she even tasted a pleasurable food, she would never again be able to control herself. Every time that Jill was in a dieting phase, she would find herself having strong cravings for forbidden foods. She chased her "phantom food," searching for a food that would quell her cravings. If she craved a chocolate cookie, she would spread sugar-free jam on fat-free saltines. When that didn't satisfy her, she'd move on to cinnamon-flavored rice cakes, then to fat-free "healthy" cookies (which she disliked since they "tasted like sweetened cardboard"), and lots of dried fruit. By the end of an evening, *Jill had eaten ten times more diet foods than she would have eaten had she just allowed herself to have the chocolate cookie.* And, not surprisingly, she would usually "succumb" to the chocolate cookie anyway at the end of her frustrating food chase.

After learning the Intuitive Eating process, Jill quit the phantom food searches and allowed herself to eat what she really wanted. She can now even order a hamburger *with fries* and finds that she ends up leaving some of her food when she feels comfortably full, because she's so *satisfied*. She's also found that she eats plenty of nutritious food along with enough play food to satisfy her whole spectrum of taste cravings!

DON'T BE AFRAID TO ENJOY YOUR FOOD

Like Jill, our clients are initially afraid that if they let the pleasure of eating into their lives, they might continue to seek food in an uncontrollable fashion. Yet letting yourself enjoy food will actually result in self-limiting, rather than out-of-control eating. Remember, as we explained in chapter 8, deprivation is a key factor that leads to backlash eating.

Satisfied Now, Content Later

For many of our clients, feeling a sense of satisfaction in a meal actually decreases their yearning for foods at a later time. We have had our clients compare having a full-course meal for dinner with just "picking" or scrounging. When they take the time to prepare a meal that attracts their sense of smell, taste, sight, and so forth, they invariably report a feeling of satisfaction and a decreased need for more food later in the evening. Those who come home and drop on the sofa with cheese and crackers find themselves getting up at each commercial break for yet another snack. They feel that they haven't really eaten and never seem to get satisfied. By the end of the evening, they feel overfull and frustrated.

Kelly is a busy person who often neglects her own needs. Sometimes, she'll be so busy with work and her child that she doesn't stop to prepare an entire meal for herself. On the days when she takes the time to figure out what she really wants to eat and ends up eating exactly what she wants for lunch or dinner, she finds that she rarely has desire for more food. On the days when she restricted her eating, she never felt satisfied, and her dessert cravings at night were insatiable.

When you allow yourself pleasure and satisfaction from most eating experiences, your contentment will increase.

HOW TO REGAIN YOUR PLEASURE IN EATING

As a result of dieting and the fear of giving it up, dieters have lost their pleasure in eating, and they don't know how to get it back. Here are the steps we use with our clients to help them achieve pleasure and satisfaction in their eating.

STEP 1:
ASK YOURSELF WHAT YOU *REALLY* WANT TO EAT

Satisfaction is derived when you take the time to figure out what you really want to eat, give yourself unconditional permission to eat, and then eat in a relaxing, enjoyable atmosphere.

The problem for most people with whom we've worked is that they have been engaged with diet culture for so long and have figured out many "tricks" to avoid eating that they no longer know what they like to eat! When you're about to begin a new diet, have you ever asked yourself what you *feel like* eating? That thought rarely enters a dieter's mind. After all, the basic premise of dieting is to be told what to eat—why would you begin to question your own needs?

Such was the case with a forty-year-old woman, Jennifer, who had lived in a large body and been on some sort of food plan all of her life. As a child, she was put on diets by her mother and her doctors. When Jennifer first visited my (ER) office, she rebelliously stated that she didn't want to hear another word about dieting. She had only come because her doctor had insisted, and she insisted that she knew all there was to know about dieting. I told her that I didn't believe in dieting, but all I really wanted to know was what she liked to eat. Astonishment crossed her face. She could hardly respond, but when she did, she told me that no one in her entire life had ever asked her what *she* wanted to eat. She had been on diets since she was a child and had always been told what she *should* eat. She went deeply into thought for a few moments and then said that she had no idea what she liked. In fact, Jennifer wasn't even sure if she liked food at all.

At the end of the session, I suggested that she spend the next week experimenting with food so that she could learn more about her taste preferences. During that week, Jennifer could only find ten foods that she actually liked and discovered that she could do without the rest! The following week, Jennifer's task was to eat only those ten foods and see how much she actually consumed. Again, she was surprised by the results. When she ate what she liked, she found that she was satisfied by much less and that her total food intake that week was more attuned to her fullness signals than it had been in years. One night, all she had for dinner was a scoop of chocolate ice cream. In the past she would down a huge dinner of foods she thought she *should* eat, even though she wasn't very hungry, and would then finish the half gallon of ice cream, because she felt guilty about having any of it.

Jennifer was on her way to becoming an Intuitive Eater. In addition to appreciating that she could have exactly what she wanted any time that she ate, she realized that eating when she was hungry would give her the most satisfaction. As a result of this revelation, she found herself eating only when she was hungry, for the most part. She also found that eating past comfortable fullness was pointless, as the food no longer tasted good, her body felt miserable, and she could eat the same food again at her next meal if she liked. As time went on, Jennifer felt continually satisfied by her meals, without feeling deprived. Also, she had had a history of chronic knee problems, which led to virtual inactivity. Since she felt good for the first time in her life, she was motivated to begin a program of regular swimming—not because she *had* to but because she worked on accepting living in a larger body and *wanted* to feel even better physically!

If you also have trouble figuring out what you truly like to eat, the next step will give you clarification.

STEP 2:
DISCOVER THE PLEASURE OF THE PALATE

Our clients are focused on every aspect of food except the here and now. They lament the past and worry about the future (what will I eat, how will I work off these calories), but very rarely do they focus on the actual experience of eating. Therefore, they are not tasting—not experiencing or savoring food. It's almost as if the art of eating needs to be relearned without bias.

The Sensual Qualities of Food

To discover what foods you really like and how to increase satisfaction in your eating, explore the sensual qualities of foods. For most people, this means a conscious period of experimentation. Take your taste buds and palate for a sensory joy ride. As you eat, consider:

- *Taste.* Put a particular food in your mouth to see which of your taste sensations gets stimulated. Roll the food on your tongue to see if it's predominantly sweet, salty, sour, or bitter. Is that taste pleasant, neutral, or maybe even offensive? Try this experiment at various times during the day to see if certain tastes are more pleasurable at different times. Some people are drawn to the sweet taste at breakfast and want waffles or pancakes. Something spicy, such as eggs with salsa, might be a turn-off early in the morning. Others can't think of something sweet until later in the afternoon.
- *Texture.* As you roll the food on your tongue and begin to chew

on it, experience the various types of textures that foods can provide. How does crunchy feel to you? Is it abrasive to have to break into a crunchy food, or is it a satisfying experience? What reaction do you have to a food that is smooth or creamy? Does it remind you of baby food, and is that appealing or annoying? Some foods are chewy and require a lot of work from your teeth and tongue. What is that like for you? Sometimes you might just want the flow of a liquid through your mouth and down your throat. Certain food textures might be appealing at different times of the day or even on different days.

• *Aroma*. Sometimes the aroma of a food will have more of an effect on your desire for it than does its taste or texture. Appreciate the various aromas that foods can emit. Walk by the bakery and smell the yeasty bread coming out of the oven or inhale the coffee vapors as the coffee is dripping through the filter. If the aroma of a food is not appealing, you probably won't get your optimal satisfaction from it. If it smells great to you as it is cooking or served to you, however, it will probably increase your satisfaction.

• *Appearance*. Food artists who design commercial food sets or menus for restaurants know that foods that look appealing are alluring and make a person want to try them. Take a look at the food you're about to eat. Is it attractive to your eye? Is it fresh looking? Is its color interesting to you? Imagine a plate with a poached chicken breast, a boiled potato, and cauliflower—not too thrilling. You'll probably get less satisfaction from that meal than one that's more exciting to look at.

• *Temperature*. A steamy bowl of soup might just be the order of the day if it's cold and rainy outside. But chilly frozen yogurt is not usually desirable when you're shivering under an umbrella. Ask yourself what the most appealing temperature of your food is. Do you like your hot foods boiling hot or temperate? Do you like your cold drinks with lots of ice or very little? Or is room temperature just fine for you for everything?

• *Volume or filling capacity*. Some foods are light and airy, while others are heavy and filling. The filling capacity of your food choices can make a difference in how much food you need to satisfy you or how you feel after you're finished eating. Some days you might only be satisfied by a plate of pasta, which fills your stomach, while at other times, a lighter salad is more appealing. Even if something tastes and feels great on your tongue and in your mouth, if it makes your stomach feel queasy or too full, it will diminish the satisfying experience.

Respect your individual taste buds. Keep in mind that everyone has a different experience with taste and texture sensations. Not all foods will be desirable to you. People may rave about the best sushi in town, but the thought of eating raw fish might be intolerable to you. If you have gotten sick after eating corn, regardless of the cause, corn might never seem appealing again. Your preferences may be lifelong or may change from time to time. Keep in touch with what is appetizing to you so that you can choose what is most satisfying.

Think about what you really feel like eating

Once you've gone through this hyperconscious experimentation with the sensory qualities of foods, the next time you feel like a meal or a snack, take a few moments to decide what you *really* want for a meal or snack. If you have trouble deciding what to eat, or need a little clarity, ask yourself:

- What do I feel like eating?
- What food aroma might appeal to me?
- How will the food look to my eye?
- How will the food taste and feel in my mouth?
- Do I want something sweet, salty, savory, sour, or even slightly bitter?
- Do I want something crunchy, smooth, creamy, soft, lumpy, or fluid?
- Do I want something hot, cold, or moderate?
- Do I want something light, airy, heavy, filling, or in between?
- How will my stomach feel when I'm finished eating?

If you have a general knowledge of your taste preferences, it will lead you to the right place on the menu or in the supermarket. Checking in with yourself before a meal will give you the specifics of the moment.

A further critical key to finding satisfaction in your eating is to take a time-out *after* you've had a few bites of your food. Is the taste and texture consistent with your desire? Is the food satisfying enough to eat? If you continue to eat a food just because it's there, despite the fact that it's unappealing, you'll only end up feeling unsatisfied when you're finished and find yourself on the prowl for something else that will satisfy you.

Step 3:
Make Your Eating Experience more Enjoyable

Savor Your Food

Europeans seem to have a market on slow, sensual eating experiences. Businesses often shut down temporarily to allow for a long lingering lunch, so the meal can be savored and appreciated. Friends tend to gather together to enjoy the conversation and the food. Americans, on the other hand, often engage in desktop dining (fifteen minutes if you're lucky) while going over notes for a meeting or zipping through the fast-food drive-through while racing to pick up the kids from school. Who do you think has the most satisfying meal experience?

Alice is an executive in a company that stresses high productivity. Taking time to sit down for lunch is unheard of, and she's so anxious to get into the office in the morning to begin her calls to the East Coast that she never allows herself to eat breakfast at home before she leaves. By the time Alice gets home in the evening, the frenetic pace of her day has become a part of her—she ends up gulping down her entire dinner before her husband and daughter get through their salads.

When you race through your meals as Alice does, you don't give yourself the opportunity to experience the sensual aspects of your food. You don't have time to appreciate the attractiveness of the different colors and shapes of the food. You can barely take in their aromas or feel their textures on your tongue and teeth—let alone their tastes.

To help you savor your food and get more satisfaction from your meals:

- *Make time to appreciate your food.* Give yourself some time to allow for a meal. Even fifteen minutes is better than nothing. If even that seems impossible, try and savor a few bites.
- *Try sitting down at the table or your desk.* Standing at the refrigerator or walking around decreases attention and satisfaction.

- *Take several deep breaths before you begin to eat.* Deep breathing helps to calm and center you, so you can be focused on eating slowly.
- *Pay attention to the sensations of eating.* Remember that your taste buds are on your tongue, not in your stomach. If you rush through your meal, and gobble your food, it takes away your chance to really savor it.
- *Taste each bite of food that you put in your mouth.* Experience the different taste and texture sensations that the food can provide.
- *Feel your fullness.* Take a time-out in the midst of the meal to check your fullness level (see chapter 11). Food won't taste as good or be as satisfying after you've reached the last-bite threshold.
- Finally, remember the three S's of **satisfying** eating:
  - Eat **slowly.**
  - Eat **sensually.**
  - **Savor** every bite.

Eat When Pleasantly Hungry Rather Than When Over-hungry

If you sit down for a meal when you're over-hungry, your biological need for energy supersedes your ability to eat slowly and taste what's before you. Likewise, if you begin to eat when you aren't really hungry, it can be difficult to decide whether what you're eating is really what you want and whether it's satisfying. When you're not very hungry, food is not as compelling. If you find this is true for you, this may be a sign that you're not ready to eat just yet. Wait a little while, until your hunger is somewhat more obvious, and you'll find that you'll have an easier time getting in touch with what you really want to eat.

Eat in a Pleasant Environment (When Possible)

Most people find that they get the greatest satisfaction from their meals by eating them in a pleasing setting. Restaurants spend a great deal of time and money creating an environment that is appealing and will draw people back again and again. The aesthetics of a restaurant can be as important as the taste of the food. At home, the same thing goes. If you set your table in a pleasing manner (a placemat or tablecloth, attractive dishes, and so forth), your food enjoyment will increase. But eating while standing or driving can diminish satisfaction. If you eat in the car, you are distracted by the traffic and by balancing food on your lap.

Avoid Tension

Keep heated fights off-limits at the table. One of the surest ways to decrease your satisfaction in eating is to try to eat when you're having an argument with a family member or friend. You'll probably end up eating faster and might even use your chewing as a way to show your anger. You definitely won't have your focus on the food and might eat everything before you without even noticing it—not a satisfying experience!

Provide Variety

Eating a variety of foods is not only nutritionally wise, but it will give you a much broader and more satisfying eating experience. Many clients take pride in keeping empty refrigerators and barren cupboards. They believe that if certain foods aren't around, they'll be less tempted to overeat. The reality is that a lack of appealing food choices creates a sense of deprivation and promotes a creative food foraging experience that never seems to produce a satisfying result. Give yourself the gift of keeping a variety of foods around, from soups to pastas to cookies to fruits and vegetables. You never know what you might feel like eating. Finding satisfaction in your eating will be a futile attempt if what you want isn't there.

STEP 4:
DON'T SETTLE

You are not obligated to finish eating a food just because you took a bite of it. How often have you tasted what appeared to be a mouthwatering dessert, only to discover it was mediocre—and yet you kept on eating? One of the biggest assets of being an Intuitive Eater is the ability to toss aside food that isn't to your liking. This can easily be done when you are truly tasting and experiencing food, combined with the knowledge that you can eat whatever you want again. (One caveat—bear in mind that if you have food insecurity, tossing food may not be something you're able to do.)

For the most part, adopt the motto "If you don't love it, don't eat it, and if you love it, savor it." Order something else, find something different in the refrigerator, or eat the parts of the meal that you like, and leave the rest. For example, Barbara spoke of a meal served to her at a banquet that was comprised of salad, chicken, vegetables, and pasta. She took just one taste of the salad and left the rest when she found that the lettuce was soggy under a sea of dressing that she didn't like. The chicken and pasta were delicious, so she ate most of them. The vegetables were so buttery that they overwhelmed her taste buds, so she left them on the plate. In her old diet days, she would have eaten only the salad and vegetables, thinking that was the "diet" way to do it and would have left her meal unsatisfied, only to go home to search for something else to eat.

Melody is another client who is learning to discard what she doesn't find satisfying. One of Melody's favorite foods is a trademark muffin at a local restaurant. Every time she goes to the restaurant, she savors her muffin and feels satisfied. One day, Melody got the inspired notion to bake the trademark muffins from the restaurant's prepared mix. And bake she did. When she took a bite of the freshly baked muffin, she was sadly disappointed. It didn't taste anything like what she had eaten in the restaurant. Melody's connection with her Intuitive Eating allowed her to throw out the muffins, with the conviction that she would only eat them when she could get the "real thing."

STEP 5:
CHECK IN: DOES IT STILL TASTE GOOD?

Have you ever eaten a whole bag of cookies or a whole carton of Häagen-Dazs? If so, you can probably attest to the fact that the first couple of cookies or spoonfuls of ice cream tasted much better than those at the bottom of the barrel. Even the taste satisfaction of a large apple dwindles by the time you get down to the core. In studies of hedonics to food cues (hedonics is the branch of psychology dealing with pleasurable and unpleasurable feelings), researchers find that as you're eating a particular food, a decrease of desire for that food emerges. Researchers call this concept *sensory-specific satiety* (Epstein 2009). Relatedly, it does not take many bites of food to reach "taste satisfaction." Sensory-specific satiety is defined as a decrease in the subjective liking for a food that is eaten. This decline occurs within minutes of eating a particular food, which is highly influenced by the sensory aspects of food, such as flavor, texture, or aroma. We also see that in our clients.

Try your own hedonic experiment. Rate the taste pleasure you get from the first few bites of a food from ten to one—ten being the most pleasurable and one being the least pleasurable. Then stop halfway through the food and check your taste buds. Finally, rate the food when you're down to the last bite. You're likely to find that the numbers diminish along with the food.

Routinely, check in with yourself to see if the food tastes as good as it did when you started. If it doesn't, consider stopping, as your satisfaction level is diminishing by the bite. Wait until you're hungry again. Food will taste better, and you'll be more satisfied. And, remember, no one is going to take that food away from your eating repertoire. You can have it for the rest of your life. So why waste your time and your food on a less-than-satisfying experience?

IT DOESN'T HAVE TO BE PERFECT

We've discussed how taking the time to figure out what you really want to eat and eating in a favorable environment can lead you to more pleasurable, satisfying eating experiences. But what if this isn't always possible? There will be times when you don't have the option to get exactly what you want. You might be served a meal at a friend's or relative's house that offers little to say for it. Many a client has bemoaned meals made by a relative or an old friend who might boil the vegetables until unrecognizable or cook the chicken until it's the texture of an old shoe. At those times, remember the concept of *thinking in the gray* rather than in all-or-nothing terms (see chapter 9). Intuitive Eating is not a process that seeks perfection, but one that offers guidelines to a comfortable relationship with food. Remember, most of your eating experiences will be more satisfying and pleasurable than you've experienced in years of diets. After all, it's only one meal—you will survive! It's how you jump back into taking care of yourself afterward that makes the difference.

Sometimes *honoring your hunger* is the best you can do. And for many of our patients, that alone is significant progress. But if survival eating occupies most of your experiences with food, your satisfaction factor will most likely be low.

RECLAIM YOUR RIGHT TO PLEASURABLE, SATISFYING EATING

If dieting has been a significant part of your life for many years, you may need to make a serious commitment to reclaim your right to enjoy your food. You may have been so programmed to eat what you were told, especially foods that have little taste pleasure, that you hardly know where to begin to find satisfaction. *Knowing what you like to eat and believing that you have the right to enjoy food are key factors in a lifetime of enjoyable eating without dieting.* If it takes you some time to accomplish all of this, be patient. After all, it's taken you many years to lose your ability to truly enjoy eating.

DISTRACTED VERSUS MINDLESS EATING

There seems to be a common perception that mindless eating is a condition in which you have no idea that you just ate, akin to "eating amnesia." Many of our clients eat while distracted—but don't consider themselves mindless eaters, because they are aware that they are eating while engaging in another activity, such as watching television.

Similarly, most car drivers would not readily identify themselves as mindless drivers, because they are aware that they are driving. However, if you describe someone as a *distracted driver,* it conjures up a clearer image—such as driving while talking on the cell phone or while applying makeup. The problem, we believe, is a terminology issue. Unless you are trained in mindfulness, the description of "distracted," rather than "mindless," seems to resonate with more people. One recent study makes a good case about the effect of distraction on eating (Oldham-Cooper et al. 2011).

DISTRACTED EATING STUDY

Scientists divided people into one of two groups. The distracted group ate lunch while playing a computer game of solitaire. The non-distracted group ate the same type of lunch, but without the same distraction condition. The study's findings showed that distraction made a significant impact on the eating experience, both qualitatively and quantitatively. When compared to the non-distracted group, the distracted people:

- Ate faster.
- Couldn't remember what they ate.
- Ate more snacks.
- Reported feeling significantly less full.

The research also showed that distraction during a meal influenced meal size later in the day.

SATISFACTION AND SATIETY AFFECTED BY DISTRACTION

We are living in such a multitasking, high-urgency era that even when not pressed for time, it seems that many people are in the routine of eating while distracted. The distracted conditions in the study are similar to how our clients eat, such as eating while checking email, scanning social media feeds, texting, surfing the internet, tweeting—you get the idea.

The irony of eating while distracted is that you end up missing out on the eating experience, which often means that eating needs to be repeated. This is akin to having a phone conversation with a friend while you are checking email. You might respond to the conversation at the right times, but something is missing, there is a disconnect—and usually the person on the other line can tell you are not 100 percent there. In the case of distracted eating—it is your body that knows.

ARTIFICIAL SWEETENERS

Artificial sweetener consumption has steadily risen over the past few decades. Currently, there are thousands of foods that contain one or more artificial sweeteners, ranging from baby food to frozen foods and beverages.

People often assume that using artificially sweetened foods and drinks is a healthier choice because it usually has fewer calories, and it will help shrink their body. Yet research suggests that the opposite may occur. A scientific

cont.

Cont.

review describes how consuming artificial sweeteners may have unintended consequences. (Yang 2010):

- Artificial sweeteners may increase appetite, because they result in less satisfaction in eating.
- Calorie-free sweeteners offer only partial, but not complete, activation of the food reward pathways in the brain. This incomplete activation of the reward may contribute to increased food-seeking behavior.
- Artificially sweetened foods may encourage sugar cravings. The more someone is exposed to a flavor, the more this flavor becomes a preference. For example, people who are used to very salty foods often find unsalted foods to be bland and unfavorable. Similarly, people who use artificial sweeteners become accustomed to the intensely sweet taste of artificially sweetened foods and beverages. This repeated exposure can lead to an increased preference for an unnaturally sweet taste.
- People tend to see artificially sweetened foods as lower in calories than foods that are naturally sweet or foods sweetened with sugar, leading them to disconnected eating.

Chapter 11

PRINCIPLE 6:

Feel Your Fullness

In order to honor your fullness, you need to trust that you will give yourself the foods that you desire. Listen for the body signals that tell you that you are no longer hungry and observe the signs that show that you're comfortably full. Pause in the middle of eating and ask yourself how the food tastes, and what your current hunger level is.

The vast majority of chronic dieters we have worked with belong to the clean-plate club. And most of them say that they've tried not to clean their plates. It may seem that an obvious step to healing your relationship with food is to respect your fullness, rather than to habitually clean your plate. Yet leaving food on the plate can be difficult to achieve, especially for the chronic dieter.

Dieting instills a license to eat at mealtime—when it is "legal." Ironically, this sense of entitlement reinforces a clean-your-plate mentality. This is particularly true for our clients who have sipped on over-the-counter liquid diets, such as SlimFast. (Liquid diet programs typically have you drink a "beverage meal" for breakfast and lunch, and then "allow you to eat a sensible dinner" of "real" food.) Naturally, most of our patients practically licked their plates clean when given the opportunity to eat their one real meal. It's not that they overate; rather they ate *all* of their precise and "entitled" portions. We have also seen this with our clients who were engaged in intermittent fasting—entitled eating during the "allowed" timeframe of eating.

Other diet plans using regular food typically offer small portions at meals. This, too, encourages you to eat while you can. Who would leave any morsel of food when quantities are meager? For example, even frozen diet meals are low in calories, and more suitable as a snack! Consequently, the meager food amounts leave you less than satisfied. This type of eating hardly fosters getting in touch with your inner eating signals, especially signals of satiety. Instead you eat it all.

Perhaps you've tossed your diet plans out years ago, but now carefully count macros. You may find, however, that you clean your plate when it comes to eating whatever food is deemed acceptable to diet culture. Years ago, fat-free foods were all the rage. We've had several clients eat an entire package of *fat-free* chocolate cake (or other fat-free goodies) with carefree abandonment because of the entitlement factor. They would rationalize, "I can eat as much as I want." Diet and food trends are like fashion, they come and go. And whatever food is considered "safe" or "clean" or "acceptable" is eaten with a similar abandonment and disconnection. One patient, Brittany, went on a very-low-carbohydrate diet. The only allowable food that she liked was peanut butter. She got to the point where she was eating entire jars of peanut butter because it was legal, and she got totally disconnected from the fullness sensations in her body.

Of course, other factors can easily condition you to polish off every crumb on your plate, including:

- Having been taught to finish everything on your plate by well-meaning parents.
- Respecting economics and the value of food—thou shall not waste. Remember, however, that eating more than your body needs may be respecting economics but is not necessarily respecting your body.
- Having an ingrained habit of eating to completion. Out of sheer habit you finish an entire plate of food, or a *whole* hamburger, or a *whole* bag of chips, regardless of how hungry or full you are. This is a reliance on external cues. You stop eating when the food is *gone,* regardless of the size of the initial portion.
- Beginning a meal (or snack) in an overly ravenous state. In this state, eating intensity is revved up, and it's all too easy to bypass normal satiety cues.
- Food insecurity. This is when a person truly does not know when their next meal is going to be. They often go hungry and may be living paycheck to paycheck. This is a survival response. The challenge is that even when there is no longer food insecurity the traumatizing effect lingers.

Even if you don't clean your plate, it's still possible that you may be bypassing your comfortable satiety level. With our clients who don't clean their plates, we have often discovered that while there may still be food left on the plate, it took an *uncomfortable* level of fullness to get them to stop eating. The problem is the inability to recognize comfortable satiety or the sadness that arises when realizing you're full and need to stop eating.

THE KEY TO RESPECTING FULLNESS

Respecting fullness, or the ability to stop eating because you have had enough to eat biologically, hinges critically on giving yourself unconditional permission to eat (principle 3: *make peace with food*). How can you or any dieter expect to leave food on your plate, if you believe that you won't be able to eat that particular food or meal again? Unless you truly give yourself permission to eat again when you are hungry, or have access to that particular food, respecting fullness simply becomes a dogmatic exercise without roots. It won't take hold. The Intuitive Eater in training learns to stop eating when they have enough to fill the stomach comfortably without being overfull. It's easier to stop eating at this point and leave food behind, when you *know* you can eat it again later. We also want to emphasize how important it is not to turn this (or any) principle of Intuitive Eating into a rigid rule!

RECOGNIZING COMFORTABLE SATIETY

We are surprised at how often our clients do not know what comfortable satiety feels like. Oh yes, they can usually describe with great detail how overeating or overstuffed feels. But knowledge of what comfortable satiety feels like is often elusive, especially to the chronic dieter. Yet if you do not know what comfortable satiety feels like, how can you expect to achieve it? It's like trying to shoot at a target without ever seeing it, or even knowing where it resides. When respecting fullness is the target, it could easily be missed if you are not looking for it, especially when you have been conditioned to clean your plate. Also, if you start eating when you are not hungry, it's harder to know when to stop out of fullness.

Can you *imagine* how comfortable satiety feels? Here are some common descriptions offered by our clients:

- A substantive feeling of stomach contentedness
- Feeling satisfied
- Pleasant completeness

The sensation is highly individual. And while we can describe it endlessly, it's akin to trying to tell someone what snow feels like. We can give you a good idea, but it's something that needs to be experienced at the personal level, so that *you* know what it feels like, in *your* body.

HOW TO RESPECT YOUR FULLNESS

When you habitually clean your plate, your eating style easily evolves into autopilot—you eat until completion, until the food is gone. To break this pattern of eating, we have found it helpful to be keenly aware or hyper-conscious of your eating. This means being conscious or mindful of your eating experience. While you may certainly be aware that you are engaged in the act of eating, we find that somewhere between bites one and one hundred, there is a significant level of unawareness. Quite often the food is not even being tasted! Likewise, it's all too easy to bypass comfortable satiety. Here are some examples:

- I wasn't aware of how much candy I would eat at the movies until, suddenly, my hands were scratching at the bottom of an empty box.
- I wouldn't even consider splitting a meal when eating out until my boss asked if I would split an entrée at her favorite restaurant. Begrudgingly I agreed. To my surprise I was thoroughly satisfied with half an entrée, *knowing all too well that had I ordered the full portion I would have eaten it all, out of sheer habit.*
- Once I opened up a package of *any* food, I had to eat it all. God forbid I'd leave a few tidbits. I know I'm not even tasting the food most of the time.

Conscious-Awareness Eating

This initial step away from the blind autopilot eating mode is *conscious-awareness eating*. It's a phase where you neutrally observe your eating as if under a microscope. (Your Food Anthropologist voice will be very helpful here.) We have broken this stage into a series of steps, which begins with taking a mini time-out from eating. This will help you regroup and assess where you're at in your eating. It's like a time-out that athletes and coaches take during a game to help improve their play or strategy. Here's what to do.

• *Pause in the middle of a meal or snack for a time-out.* Keep in mind that this time-out or pause is not a commitment to stop eating. Rather, it's a commitment to check in with your body and taste buds. (If you thought that by pausing you were obligated to leave food on your plate, you'd be reluctant to go through this step. In fact, many of our clients who initially appeared resistant to this step later admitted that they were afraid that they would have to stop eating from that point on.) During this time-out, perform these checks:

TASTE CHECK: We find that this check is usually pleasurable, which is why we like to begin with it. Ask yourself how the food tastes. Is it worthy of your taste buds? Or are you continuing to eat just because it's there?

SATIETY CHECK: Ask yourself what your hunger or fullness level is. Are you still hungry, do you feel unsatisfied, or is your hunger going away, and are you beginning to feel emerging fullness? In the beginning, this may seem like a hit-or-miss process. Be patient, and remember, you are getting to know yourself from the inside out. Just as you would not expect to get to know a person over one meal, how could you expect to understand your satiety levels in one meal or snack? It will take time. However, the more in tune you are with your hunger level, and the more you honor your hunger, the easier this step will be. Remember to be open to any answer. There can be considerable fluctuation in your fullness level depending upon the last time you ate and what you ate. If you find you're still hungry, then resume eating.

• *When you finish eating* (whatever the amount), *ask yourself where your fullness level is now.* How would you describe fullness—pleasant, unpleasant, or neutral? Did you reach comfortable satiety? Did you surpass it? By how much? If you reached an unpleasant fullness, would you choose to feel that way again? If not, what would you do differently next time? Use the Fullness Discovery Scale to help you get in touch. (Note: This is the same scale as the Hunger Discovery Scale on page 99—only now we're focusing on fullness.)

• *Discovering your fullness level will help you identify your last few bites threshold.* This is the endpoint(-ish). You have a growing realization that you are just a few bites away from fullness—eventually knowing that the bite of food *in* your mouth is your last—finis! It may take you a long time to get to this point. (It's really okay, please be kind and patient with yourself.) The longer you have been disconnected from your body's sense of fullness, the longer it will take to identify this point. If you *honor your hunger* (principle 2), it is much easier to know fullness. If, however, you do not eat from biological hunger, how could you expect to stop from biological fullness (or to even know what it feels like)? Please be patient with yourself.

• *Don't feel obligated to leave food on your plate.* If you find that you have a level of resistance to this activity, it may be from past dieting experience. You may be feeling obligated to leave food on your plate—which is a remnant of the diet mentality. Remember, there is no commitment to leaving food on your plate. The commitment, instead, is to getting to know your satiety level and your taste buds. It's perfectly normal, even when you discover your specific satiety level, to opt to eat past fullness. That's okay. We have found that many clients continue to opt for more food—they are still testing the "unconditional permission" to eat. After a while, when the newness wears off and the deprivation feelings subside, you will find that it's quite easy to leave food on your plate. It does require, however, a degree of consciousness and staying present—checking in with yourself. But, if most of the time you can recognize your fullness, and respect it, it will make a considerable difference in your physical comfort level and peace of mind.

How to Increase Awareness

The mind can only place its awareness on one thing at time. While you certainly may juggle a zillion activities, your mind places its awareness on only one. That's why, for example, so many people accidently lock their keys in their car. Their minds are somewhere else, such as getting into the office on time, or unloading the groceries. We find that to get the most out of eating, it needs to be a conscious activity, whenever possible.

• *Eat without distraction.* Value and enjoy the eating experience when possible. For example, Adelle, a fast-paced, hard-driven lawyer, always made the best use of her time and would usually eat while doing something else. Adelle would read briefs while eating lunch at work and dine with a magazine at home. She took a step forward when she decided to try eating without distraction when at home (she was too busy at work to even consider "just" eating lunch). Adelle discovered that if she ate a meal or snack at home without engaging in reading, she would feel more satisfied. To her surprise she detected her fullness level much sooner; consequently, she ate less food. She was thrilled that "without trying" she was eating in a way that left her feeling satisfied without deprivation, and not dieting. Up until now she would feel lethargic after meals. Adelle was willing to eat this way at home but did not view it as realistic for work—and this was progress!

Many clients have taken the suggestion to eat without distraction as a hard and fast rule and feel guilty if they happen to read the newspaper with breakfast or have a snack watching TV. Remember, Intuitive Eating is not another diet with rules to be broken. As in every other aspect of Intuitive Eating, you are the only one who has the internal wisdom about what works for you. You also know what doesn't work. Whatever the "other" activity may be, be honest with yourself about whether you are able to get the most satisfaction in your eating, while engaging in this activity or whether you're being distracted by it.

• *Reinforce your conscious decision to stop.* Many of our clients have found that when *they* decide to stop eating, because they've reached the last-bite threshold, it's helpful to *do* something to make it a conscious act, such as gently nudging the plate forward half an inch or putting their utensils or napkin on their plate. This simply reminds them of their decision. Otherwise it may be all too easy to innocently nibble on the remaining food, even though you had no intention of doing so. (If you have trouble with the idea of wasting food, try putting your leftovers away for tomorrow's lunch or dinner or giving them to a homeless person. If you're going to a restaurant, try bringing a small cooler to keep the food safe until you get home.)

• *Defend yourself from obligatory eating.* This usually means practicing saying "No, thank you!" I (ET) never realized the significance of this act until I attended a very elegant cocktail party in which there seemed to be one server for each guest. The moment my hand was empty of food or drink, an all-too-eager server was there to offer more food or beverage. I found it was so much easier to say yes, especially if I was in the middle of a conversation. It took much more energy, however, to say no. The same is true if you attend any function in which there are well-meaning "food-pushers," from the gracious host to the obnoxious relative. A special caution to those of you who enjoy wine by the bottle at a good restaurant: a good server will often keep your glass full. Unless you are conscious of that, you may drink more than you intend. Remember, *you* are in charge of how much to eat or drink.

THE FULLNESS FACTORS

"I just ate two hours ago—I honored my hunger *and* respected my fullness, so how could I be hungry again so soon?" While the ebb and flow of satiety signals may seem puzzling, it's quite normal to have different degrees of hunger and fullness, especially when you begin listening to your body's eating cues. There are also several factors that affect fullness. These factors are both biological and learned. When you have a general understanding of some of these satiety factors, it makes it easier to trust your body and *feel your fullness.*

The ability to recognize comfortable satiety or fullness can ultimately determine how much food will be consumed in a meal. And the amount of food eaten in a meal is influenced by these fullness factors:

• *The amount of time that has passed since the last time you ate.* The more often you eat, the less hungry you will be. This has been found to be true in nibbling studies. These are studies in which people are given several snacks or mini-meals throughout the day. The nibblers are consistently *less* hungry than those fed identical calories divided into three meals. While the purpose of these studies was to examine the metabolic effects of snacking compared to traditional meals, the researchers have consistently noted that the nibblers were less hungry, even though calories and fat were identical in both groups.

• *The kind of food you eat.* The macronutrients, protein, carbohydrates, and fat influence subsequent food intake by their contribution to the total amount of food energy in the stomach. Other food factors such as fiber will also affect the fullness factor because of its bulk and water-retention properties. Protein in particular seems to have a suppressive effect on intake beyond its contribution to total calories, according to several studies.

• *The amount of food still remaining in the stomach at the time of eating.* If your stomach is empty you will eat more than if some food is still present (from a prior snack or meal).

• *Initial hunger level.* If you begin a meal or snack in a famished state, you are more likely to override satiety mechanisms.

• *Social influence.* Eating with other people can influence how much *you* eat. Studies have shown that:

—The more people gathered at a meal, the more people tend to eat.

—Eating with others increases the duration of the meal.

—Eating more on weekends is usually due to being around people.

—Dieters, however, have been shown to eat less when they know someone is "watching" them. The same can be true for non-dieters, when they dine with a "model" eater. In one study, when the model eater refrained from eating, so too did the non-dieter.

There is a tendency to ignore or be distracted from biological signals in social settings. However, we believe that social connection is a very important part of quality living. We have found that the key to the social dilemma is to continue making eating a *conscious* activity with purposeful food choices.

Clearly, there are many factors that influence how full you feel from eating. With so many variables that exert influence on your eating, it should be no surprise, then, that the amount of food that you desire to eat can and will fluctuate. A big key is to stay tuned in and remember conscious eating.

Beware of Air Food: Fake Fullness

Simply shoving some food in your mouth like a pacifier to ease hunger pangs may backfire, and the comforting effect may not be long-lasting. This is especially true for "air food"—food that fills up the stomach but offers little sustenance. Air food includes such low-energy foods as air-popped popcorn, rice cakes, puffed rice cereal, fat-free crackers, celery sticks, and calorie-free beverages. There's nothing inherently wrong with these foods. But if you eat them expecting to get full, it will often take massive quantities—and you might also find yourself on the prowl for something more substantial to "top off the meal." It also may be a lingering effect from diet culture, trying to trick your body into feeling full. We call that fake fullness, because while your stomach might feel full, there's something amiss, there's still a wanting of sorts. (Your body is smart and knows that this is not enough food, which can feel confusing!) That's where having a balanced snack or meal, which includes a substantial carbohydrate, some protein, or some fat, is especially helpful if you're looking for a little "staying power" or the stick-to-your-ribs kind of feeling from eating.

If, on the other hand, you know you will be going out for a fabulous dinner or to a party and want just a little something to take the edge off your hunger, lighter foods may serve your purpose just fine.

Foods with Staying Power

Snacks or meals with a little fiber, complex carbohydrates, some protein, and some fat will help increase satiety. Ironically, many of our chronic food restrictors shy away from the very foods that could help them feel more satisfied at meals—complex carbohydrates and fat. Here are some common unsatisfying food choices and suggestions for how you can round them out to be more satisfying. (There's nothing inherently wrong with these light foods; they just may not provide staying power.)

Less-Filling Foods	Staying Power Boost Add these types of foods to perk up your satiety
Salad (no carbohydrates; little protein unless it's an entrée)	Protein: tuna, chicken, garbanzo or kidney beans Carbs: crackers or whole grain roll Fat: salad dressing
Fresh fruit (no protein, can be low on carbs depending on quantity)	Protein/carb/fat: cheese and whole grain crackers; half sandwich; yogurt
Turkey breast (no fiber, no carbs)	Carb/fat: whole grain pita; whole grain bagel; whole grain crackers; mayonnaise

WHAT IF YOU CAN'T STOP EATING?

If you discover, after time, that you still are eating even though you are not hungry, there's a good chance that you might be using food as a coping mechanism. This is not always as obvious and dramatic as some magazines suggest. Chapter 12 is devoted to this issue. A history of food insecurity, which is a form of trauma, is also related to binge eating. It could be helpful to work with a specialist trained in both eating disorders and Intuitive Eating.

TABLE 5. FULLNESS DISCOVERY SCALE JOURNAL

After you eat your meal or snack: Check the quality of your fullness as pleasant, unpleasant, or neutral. Place an X in the box that applies to you. Next, circle the number that best reflects your fullness level, where 0 = unpleasant/painful hunger and 10 = unpleasant/painful fullness.

Time	Quality of Fullness			Fullness Rating											Meal/Food Eaten
	Pleasant	Unpleasant	Neutral												
				0	1	2	3	4	5	6	7	8	9	10	
				0	1	2	3	4	5	6	7	8	9	10	
				0	1	2	3	4	5	6	7	8	9	10	
				0	1	2	3	4	5	6	7	8	9	10	
				0	1	2	3	4	5	6	7	8	9	10	

Adapted with permission from The Intuitive Eating Workbook *(New Harbinger, 2017).*

Chapter 12

PRINCIPLE 7:
Cope with Your Emotions with Kindness

First, recognize that food restriction, both physically and mentally, can, in and of itself, trigger loss of control, which can feel like emotional eating. Find kind ways to comfort, nurture, distract, and resolve your issues. Anxiety, loneliness, boredom, and anger are emotions we all experience throughout life. Each has its own trigger, and each has its own appeasement. Food won't fix any of these feelings. It may comfort for the short term, distract from the pain, or even numb you. But food won't solve the problem. You'll ultimately have to deal with the source of the emotion.

Becoming an Intuitive Eater means learning to be gentle and compassionate with yourself about how you use food to cope and letting go of the guilt. As odd as this may sound, eating may have been the only tool you had to get through difficult times in your life. It may also have been an inevitable result of years of dieting and feelings of deprivation and despair that arose from dieting. *Dieting itself can trigger emotions, which ultimately leads to using food as your primary coping mechanism for dealing with these feelings*—chalk another vicious cycle up to dieting.

Indeed, a study of more than 35,000 men and women found that former or current dieters have more emotional eating than those with no history of dieting (Peneau et al. 2013). What many folks have labeled as emotional eating is merely a psychological and biological consequence of food restriction. It's important to heal the deprivation effects of food, which have both psychological and biological consequences. To make matters worse, diet culture villainizes emotional eating, which reinforces another round of food restriction to compensate for emotional eating.

Eating doesn't occur in a void. Regardless of your size or shape, food usually has emotional associations. If you have any doubt, catch a glimpse of food commercials. They push our eating buttons—not through our stomachs but through the emotional connection. They imply that in sixty seconds or less you can:

- Capture romance with an intimate cup of coffee.
- Bake someone happy.
- Reward yourself with a rich dessert.

Eating can be one of the most emotionally laden experiences that we have in our lives. The emotional rhythm to eating is set from the first day that the infant is offered the breast or the bottle to quell their crying. It's then reinforced each time a cookie is offered to soothe a scraped knee, or ice cream is eaten to celebrate a Little League victory. Nearly every culture and religion use food as an important symbolic custom, from the wedding cake to the Jewish Passover Seder. Each time a significant life experience is celebrated with food, the emotional connection deepens, from the I-got-the-promotion dinner celebration to the annual birthday cake. Likewise, each time food is used for a little wound-licking or comfort, the emotional bond strengthens.

Food is love, food is comfort, food is reward, food is a reliable friend. And, sometimes, food becomes your *only* friend in moments of pain and loneliness.

Our patients are embarrassed that food has become so important to them—that food is their best friend. But if you consider how emotionally charged food is, it's no surprise that food can evolve into a special salve. When a dieter eats during rough emotional times (whether periodically or chronically), it is usually obvious that food is used as a coping mechanism. For others, it is not so clear.

Some of our clients are emotionally unaware—they have not yet learned to identify their feelings. It may not be obvious to them that they are using food to cope. Sometimes, these clients don't know why they are eating. Often the "why" is an uncomfortable feeling that has not been discovered. Or they may be engaged in a subtle form of emotional eating, such as boredom eating. Nibbling to kill time between classes or appointments is not emotionally charged, but the results can be the same as using food to numb strong feelings—*disconnected eating*.

The eating experience itself, especially perceived overeating, evokes feelings, and those feelings can affect your ability to eat with attunement. One of the most detrimental feelings that overeating can stir up is guilt and shame. When our clients say, "I feel guilty because I ate _____," we ask these questions: Did you steal that food? Or did you steal money to get that food? They look aghast, and emphatically declare, "Of course not!" Feelings of guilt imply that a crime or moral code was violated. Guilt is an appropriate emotion if you killed the chef or the farmer, but guilt and morality have no place in your eating world. Studies have shown that although you might have immediate emotional comfort from eating, the negative rush of guilt that bursts forth is powerful enough to completely wipe out the relief. If you replace the guilt with feelings of self-compassion, you'll be freed to get curious about your underlying issues and find ways to understand and deal with them.

THE CONTINUUM OF EMOTIONAL EATING

Food can be used to cope with feelings in myriad ways. Using food in this way is not a component of biological hunger, but of emotional hunger. Emotional eating is triggered by feelings, such as boredom or anger, not by biological hunger. These feelings can trigger anything from a benign nibble to an out-of-control binge.

It's important to understand that this coping mechanism lies on a continuum of intensity that begins at one end with mild, almost universal sensory eating to the opposite end with numbing, often anesthetizing eating. The following diagram illustrates this spectrum:

•sensory gratification •comfort •distraction •sedation •punishment

←———→

Sensory Gratification

The mildest and most common feeling that food can call forth is pleasure. The significance of receiving pleasure from eating is emphasized in principle 5: *discover the satisfaction factor.* This concept is not only critical to

Intuitive Eating, but is a normal, natural part of living. Don't underestimate the importance of pleasing your palate. As we explained in chapter 10, by letting yourself enjoy and appreciate eating, you will be able to tune into the amount of food you need to feel satisfied when biologically hungry. For example, allowing yourself to truly taste all of the special foods that appeal to you at Thanksgiving or any holiday, without restriction, will usually offset disconnected eating.

Comfort

Just the thought of certain foods has the ability to evoke feelings from a comfortable time or place. For example, do you ever crave chicken noodle soup when you are sick, or macaroni and cheese on dreary days—because that's what your mom fixed on these occasions? Those are examples of comfort foods. If you want to curl up with a blanket in front of a fireplace and sip hot cocoa with your dinner, that's fine. Eating comfort foods can be part of a healthy relationship with food, if you do it while staying present and without guilt. If, however, food is the first and only thing that comes to mind to take care of you when you are feeling sad, lonely, or uncomfortable, it can keep you from getting to the core of your feelings.

Distraction

If you go a little further on the continuum of emotional eating, food can be used to distract you from feelings you choose not to experience. Using food to cope in this way can become troublesome, as it can be a seductive behavior that blocks your ability to detect your intuitive signals. It can also inhibit you from discovering the source of the feelings and taking care of your true needs. Whether you're the teenager who sits in front of the TV with a bag of chips to distract you from the feelings of boredom while doing your homework, or you're the executive who goes through a whole bowl of peanuts on your desk to distract you from the anxiety of an arduous meeting, this kind of eating needs to be explored. There is nothing wrong with occasionally wanting to distract yourself from feelings. Experiencing your feelings twenty-four hours a day can be tedious and overwhelming. But if you find that you're using food as a way to distract yourself from your feelings on a regular basis, this might

be a cue to seek some help, in order to deal with them in a more beneficial way.

Sedation

A more serious form of using food to cope is eating for the purpose of
numbing or anesthetizing. One client calls this form of eating a "food
coma." Another suggests that this kind of eating results in a "food hangover." In either case, it's eating to sedate yourself. It keeps you from experiencing any feeling for extended periods of time. It becomes impossible
to sense your intuitive signals of hunger and satiety, and it deprives you of
the satisfying experience that food can bring to your life. Most clients who
use food in this way talk about feeling out of control, out of touch with life,
and generally zoned out.

Connie is a young woman who had an abusive childhood. She learned
to use food at a very early age as a numbing agent to escape her pain.
She continues to sedate herself through the anxiety, fear, and sadness of
her present life. What she finds most frightening is the complete detach-
ment from life that she experiences each time. She isolates herself from
her friends, calls in sick to work, and feels completely hopeless about life
itself. Connie has sought counseling treatment so that she can improve the
quality of her life.

When eating to numb and sedate is occasional and short-term, it tends
to have little detrimental effect. But this kind of eating can escalate into a
habitual behavior before you notice it.

Punishment

Sometimes, eating for the purpose of sedation becomes so frequent and
intense that self-blame ensues and ultimately triggers punishing behaviors.
Clients find themselves eating large quantities of food in an angry, forceful
manner that allows them to feel beaten up. This is a severe form of emotional eating and can lead to loss of self-esteem and self-hatred. Clients
who use food to punish themselves report no pleasure in their eating and
actually begin to hate food. Fortunately, this type of eating behavior disappears when the Nurturer voice can be cultivated to give understanding
and compassion.

Note: Seeking eating disorder counseling from a psychotherapist and registered dietitian nutritionist who are trained in Intuitive Eating is highly advised when there is frequent and severe emotional eating.

EMOTIONAL TRIGGERS

We've looked at general emotional reasons for eating; now, let's examine the specific feelings involved. A craving for certain foods, or simply a desire to eat, can be triggered by a variety of feelings and situations.

Some people use food to cope when they have no idea that's what they're doing. They think that they're overeating "just because it tastes good" and deny or minimize that they're eating emotionally. If you find that you're doing quite a bit of eating when you're not biologically hungry, then there's a good chance that you are using food to cope. You may not have deep-seated emotional reasons to eat, but just getting through life's hassles with some of its irksome tasks and boredom might trigger you to seek food to make it all easier, or you just might not want to feel the sadness that emerges when you need to stop eating because you've reached comfortable fullness. The best way to gauge whether you're using food in this way is to ask yourself the following question: "If my body only needs a certain amount of food to feel satisfied, but I continue to eat after I'm clearly full, then what other need am I trying to fill with food?" You may discover that the food is taking care of some of the feelings mentioned below.

Boredom and Procrastination

One of the most common reasons that our clients eat when they're not hungry is boredom. In fact, studies have shown that boredom is one of the most common triggers of emotional eating. One particular study divided college students into two groups. One group had the monotonous task of writing the same letters over and over again for nearly half an hour. The other group was engaged in a stimulating writing project. Students in each group were given a bowl of crackers to nibble on. Guess which group ate more? The "bored" group ate the most crackers.

In boredom eating, food is used as a way to fill time, or to make a boring task more tolerable, as well as a way to put off doing mundane work. For some people, the thought of the food and the actual experience of going for it and eating it breaks the tedium. Here are some situations that trigger boredom eating:

- Lying around the house on a Sunday afternoon when you've made no plans for the day.
- Having to get through an afternoon of studying, paperwork, or a writing project.
- Watching a boring night of television with nothing else to do but take food breaks.
- Killing time: waiting for a meeting to get started, waiting for a phone call, and so forth.

We also see this type of eating in our overworked clients—they feel they must always be *doing* something, being productive. The moment a tiny hole opens up in their schedule, they feel the need to fill it—often with food. (In their mind, it's acceptable to eat, but not to rest!)

Bribery and Reward

Have you ever promised yourself that you could have a treat once you finished writing a term paper or a contract, or cleaning the house? If so, you have experienced reward eating. It's not unusual to use food as a motivation to accomplish undesirable tasks. For example:

- Children are bribed with treats such as candy or ice cream if they behave—at the shopping center, at the doctor, for a babysitter, and so on.
- People often reward themselves for working hard: at work, at home, or at school—with an extra bagel or a muffin, for example.

Using food as a reward can be self-perpetuating, as there will always be ongoing tasks and challenges that can be made more tolerable if they're mitigated by food gifts. Remember, you can always eat whatever you like—you don't need to make it conditional on accomplishing a task.

Excitement

Food and the eating experience itself can serve as a way to add excitement when life begins to feel dull. At a subtle level, planning a special meal or making a reservation at a favorite restaurant can create a sense of excitement. (And there's nothing wrong with that!)

The notion of going on a diet can trigger excited feelings of hope. This is one of the reasons that dieting is so alluring. Our clients talk of how even contemplating a new diet gives them a rush of adrenaline—just imagining a new body and new life. When the diet fails, the excitement is replaced with despair. At this point, the experience of going to the store to buy large quantities of forbidden foods can be one way to re-create the excitement. And then the cycle continues—diet/compensatory eating, diet/compensatory eating. This may be exciting, but at what cost?

Soothing

It's not hard to understand the soothing power that food can provide. It can be more appealing to go to the kitchen for cookies and milk than to sit on the couch and experience uncomfortable feelings. This is especially true if those cookies and milk remind you of a time that was pleasant, and life felt less complicated. Habitually eating to soothe what ails you can evolve into disconnected eating.

Food can have other symbolic meanings of comfort. Ellen is a sixteen-year-old who has battled with her father since she was a small child. She describes him as mean and nasty with a bitter personality. It was not surprising to hear Ellen talk about her obsession with eating large amounts of candy every day as a way to bring "sweetness" into her life. To her, the sweets countered the bitterness of her daily experiences with her father.

Love

Food can become connected to the feeling of being loved. There is certainly a romantic link with food—chocolate on Valentine's Day is a classic example. When dating, there's an unspoken ground rule, that your relationship is elevated to a more intimate level when you have experienced a home-cooked meal for two.

Clients frequently describe how their parents' only way to show love was through food. Their parents may not have been able to show physical attention or speak to them in loving ways, but food was always plentiful.

Frustration, Anger, and Rage

If you find yourself going through a bag of hard and crunchy pretzels when you're not hungry, it's a good bet that you may be feeling frustrated or angry. The physical act of biting and crunching can serve as a way to release these feelings for some people. One client, Nancy, a lawyer, discovered that she had a habit of subduing her anger at some of her clients by grabbing some crunchy food, whether it was carrots or crackers, and munching away.

Stress

Many of our clients say they head for the nearest candy bar under stressful times. Yet, in most individuals, biological mechanisms associated with stress *turn off* the desire to eat.

The rush of adrenaline during stressful times sets in motion a cascade of biological events to provide immediate energy. As a result, blood sugar is elevated, and digestion is slowed. These two elements alone tend to suppress hunger and heighten the sense of satiety when eating. The biological reactions are a form of self-preservation—to ready our bodies for "fight, freeze, or flight." While this was quite useful for survival in an acute situation—*fighting off* a ravenous tiger or *fleeing* from danger required immediate energy—a growing body of research suggests that in our modern day, this mechanism can actually become chronic and may lead to chronic diseases. It may be stressful to *fight off* rush-hour traffic or to *flee* from a deadline, but you don't need the extra blood sugar that the stress reaction provides. Chronic stress also raises cortisol, which is a steroid hormone produced by the adrenal gland and secreted into the bloodstream. Prolonged higher levels of cortisol alter its effectiveness to regulate inflammatory and immune responses. For these reasons, seeking help to find ways to reduce stress can improve your overall health. These biological problems are compounded if you cope with stress by eating. Studies show that people who have been dieting are especially vulnerable to overeating during stressful times. Stress becomes one more reason to "blow" the diet. Furthermore, dieting itself can be a source of stress.

Anxiety

Worries, of any magnitude, from an upcoming final to waiting to hear if you got the job, can trigger an urgent need to eat to relieve anxiety. Sometimes generalized anxiety can be described as that uncomfortable feeling that you are unable to put a finger on; our clients say it feels like butterflies in your stomach. With the focus on the stomach, so goes the food.

Mild Depression

It's not uncommon for many people to turn to food when they are mildly depressed. In one particular study, 62 percent of the dieters and 52 percent of non-dieters stated they ate more when feeling depressed.

Being Connected

The need to feel part of a group or to feel a connection to others can be very powerful for some people, which can affect how and what they eat. This experience was poignantly described by Matthew, when he was talking about the dinner he had eaten one night with some friends. Although he didn't like the food served, he ate it anyway. He made the choice to feel connected but dissatisfied with the food, rather than feeling different. How many times have you eaten to be part of the crowd—from running out to get ice cream to sharing a pizza? Participating in this type of eating can be emotionally healthy. Although you may not be able to honor your taste buds, you can still honor your body, while also honoring your connections.

Loosening the Reins

Frequently, clients who are highly successful in every aspect of their lives, except in their eating, discount their accomplishments. They feel as if their food problems indicate they are truly failures in life. We have found that in most cases, out-of-control eating is the only mechanism that such a person has for letting go and letting loose of the tight reins of control in their life. A good example is Larry, a wealthy businessman who was the chief executive officer of a large business. He dresses impeccably, keeps his car perfectly washed and waxed, and lives in a beautifully decorated house in an affluent neighborhood. He maintains rigid discipline with his children and has high expectations for his partner as well. He never drinks or uses drugs; he keeps perfect records of his household finances; and he has an immaculate calendar that maintains his punctuality. Larry's only outlet from his self-imposed militaristic control is overeating—it is his way of letting off some steam.

COPING WITH EMOTIONAL EATING

Whether your response to emotional hunger is mild emotional eating or out-of-control bingeing, there are four key steps to making food less important in your life. Ask yourself:

1. *Am I biologically hungry?* If the answer is yes, your next step is to honor your hunger and eat! If you are not hungry, explore the following questions.

2. *What am I feeling?* When you find yourself reaching for food when there is no biological hunger, take a time-out to find out what you are feeling. This is not such an easy question to answer, especially if you are not in touch with your feelings. Try the following:

- Write out your feelings.
- Call a friend and talk about the feelings.
- Talk about the feelings and record them into your phone.
- Just sit with the feelings and experience them if you can.
- Talk to a counselor or a psychotherapist.

3. *What do I need?* Many people eat to fulfill some unmet need, which is related to the emotional or physical feeling being experienced. If you are a chronic dieter, or chronically on some food plan, you can be particularly vulnerable. Eating to assuage an unmet need can be at play.

For example: Molly is a freelance writer who was working into the wee hours to meet her deadline. Around three o'clock in the morning she found herself walking downstairs into the kitchen. She realized that she was not hungry, yet she was about to devour a bowl of ice cream. When Molly asked herself what she was feeling, she discovered frustration, exhaustion, and an unfocused mind. She realized that she was trying to feed both her fatigue and her frustration. But what she really *needed* was rest—no amount of food would replace sleep. She decided to call it a night and go to bed. But before Molly made that decision, she told herself she could have the ice cream tomorrow if she still wanted it. She also realized the ice cream would taste better if she experienced it fully awake rather than half-asleep.

4. *Would you please . . . ?* It's not unusual to find that when you ask the question "What do I need?"—the answer can be simply speaking up and asking for help. Laurel Mellin, a health psychologist, has found that kids often have trouble speaking up for their needs. We also find this to be true for many of our clients. The "Would you please" step originated from Laurel Mellin's work, and we find it extremely helpful for our clients.

Danielle, a full-time stay-at-home mom, learned that she was using food as a momentary time-out. Eating was her only retreat between baby cries. Danielle discovered that what she needed was not food, but time just for herself. To obtain this she used the "Would you please" step. She asked her partner to give her thirty minutes of uninterrupted quiet time after they came home from work. Having gained this, food for this need was no longer important.

MEETING YOUR NEEDS WITH KINDNESS

There are various ways in which we learn to handle the unending emotions that life can trigger. Some people learn early on that it's okay to express their feelings or to ask for a hug. Others aren't lucky enough to be taught how to take care of themselves in productive, nurturing ways. The first task in learning how to cope with kindness is to acknowledge that you are entitled to having your needs met. But basic needs are often discounted, including:

- Getting rest
- Getting sensual pleasure
- Expressing feelings
- Being heard, understood, and accepted
- Being intellectually and creatively stimulated
- Receiving comfort and warmth

Seek Nurturance

Feeling nurtured can allow you to feel comfort and warmth so that food loses its number-one position in this role. There are many routes and avenues available for nurturing yourself and receiving nurturance from others. For example:

- Rest and relax.
- Watch a sunset.
- Take a relaxing walk.
- Spend some time in a sauna or a jacuzzi.
- Listen to soothing music.
- Take time to breathe deeply.
- Learn to meditate.
- Play games with friends.
- Take a bubble bath in candlelight.
- Take a yoga class.
- Get a massage.
- Play with your dog or cat.
- Develop a network of friends.
- Ask friends for hugs.
- Put fresh flowers in your house.
- Spend time gardening.
- Give yourself a manicure or pedicure.
- Hug a teddy bear.

Deal with Your Feelings

If you receive a steady flow of comfort and nurturing, you'll be better prepared to face the emotions that feel so frightening. Acknowledge what is troubling you—allow your feelings to come up. This will reduce your need to push them down with food. Here are some suggestions for how to deal with your feelings:

- Write your feelings in a journal.
- Call a friend (or several).
- Record your feelings in your phone.
- Confront the person who is triggering your feelings.

- Let yourself cry.
- Sit with your feelings and discover how the intensity will diminish with time.
- If you have trouble identifying your feelings or coping with them, it may be helpful to talk with a therapist, especially if it is a persistent issue.
- Get curious about the *physical sensation* of an emotional feeling. Where do you feel it in your body? Is the physical sensation pleasant, unpleasant, or neutral? Notice that when you get really curious, it tends to stop ruminating thoughts. Every time you connect with the physical sensation in your body from emotion, it's an opportunity to really get to know your body. The ability to feel the felt sense of emotion is a component of interoceptive awareness, which is the basis of operation for Intuitive Eating.

Find a Different Distractor

Many people use food as their primary distraction from their feelings. It's okay to get away from the feelings from time to time, *but you don't need to rely on food as your primary coping tool.* Many teens tell us that they come home from school every afternoon and plop in front of the TV with a bag of chips and a soda. When asked why they do this, they say that they're avoiding the boredom feelings of having to do their homework. When it's suggested that they first have a snack to take care of their biological hunger and *then* watch some TV to distract themselves for a while before settling down to homework—they exclaim that their parents would never let them. *As long as they're eating, they can legitimately procrastinate from homework, but having other distractors is not allowed!* This is also true for many workaholic clients. It's socially acceptable to take a time-out to eat (coffee break), but to just sit at their desk, even while entitled to a break, is not allowed. They fear that it will appear as if they are doing nothing. Others use food to distract themselves from loneliness, fear, and anxiety. Since it would be overwhelming to try to feel your feelings twenty-four hours a day, give yourself permission to take a break from them for a while. Take the assertive stance of distracting yourself in an emotionally satisfying way. Try the following:

- Read an absorbing book.
- Rent a movie.
- Talk on the telephone.
- Go to the movies.
- Take a drive.
- Clean out your closet.
- Put on some music and dance.
- Peruse a magazine.
- Take a stroll around the block.
- Work in the garden.
- Listen to an audio novel.
- Do a Sudoku or a crossword puzzle.
- Work on a jigsaw puzzle.
- Play a game on the computer.
- Take a nap.
- Curate amusing videos on social media.

One last note about distraction: if you spend a good deal of time on social media as a distractor, be aware of the images that come up, and the people you follow. If they are posting before and after pictures showing off their bodies or any references to dieting or food plans, please unfollow them. There are many non-diet, Intuitive Eating accounts that give positive, affirming messages for you to follow. On Instagram you can follow the hashtag #IntuitiveEatingOfficial.

HOW EMOTIONAL EATING HAS HURT *AND* HELPED

As you begin to examine your use of food as a coping mechanism, it's helpful to take a look at how food has actually helped you. The notion that overeating or undereating can have benefits may sound absurd to you, especially if you're feeling distressed by this behavior. *But if there were no upside to this, you probably wouldn't continue it.* Take a piece of paper and divide it in half. On one half, make a list titled "How Coping with Food Serves Me," citing all the benefits you receive. Title the other side "How Coping with Food Disserves Me," and examine the ways in which food has become harmful or destructive to you. A list might look like the following:

How Coping with Food Serves Me	How Coping with Food Disserves Me
• It tastes good.	• It's not a satisfying eating experience.
• It's reliable—it's always there.	• It disconnects me from my body.
• It keeps me from feeling bored.	• It disconnects me from relationships.
• It soothes me.	• I feel overfull and uncomfortable.
• It numbs my bad feelings.	• I'm numbed to the joys of life.
• It gives me something to control.	• I feel too hungry and grouchy.

As you look over your lists, you might be surprised to learn that the use of food is not just a negative experience for you. In fact, it may give you some valuable perks. But if you're feeling bad and guilty about using food to cope, it will be hard for you to recognize its benefits in relation to its burdens. By recognizing that there are indeed some benefits to using food, you'll begin to own your eating experience, rather than feeling out of control.

WHEN FOOD IS NO LONGER IMPORTANT

Many clients have talked about having strange, uncomfortable feelings when they're no longer using food to cope as their primary way to deal with their emotions. At the same time, they're feeling happy and secure in their new Intuitive Eating style and have stopped struggling with food. There are a couple of reasons for the conflicting feelings.

• You no longer have the "benefits" of using food. While coping with food can be problematic, one client noted that on tough days she knew she could always go home to her chocolate. Now, instead, she's "stuck" with experiencing her feelings. You might even need to go through a grieving period for the loss of this coping mechanism as comforter and companion.

• You may also notice that you're experiencing your feelings in a deeper, stronger way. Since you're no longer covering them up with food, they may have a profound effect on you. This is a point at which some people decide that it would be helpful to get counseling as a way to process these long-buried feelings.

Sandy is a client who experienced the loss of using food as a coping mechanism. By acknowledging what food used to do *for* her as well as *against* her, Sandy was able to understand that her uncomfortable feelings were normal and appropriate. Sandy had either dieted or used food to cope all her life. She talked about feeling very frustrated when she would stop eating after finding the threshold bite and truly not wanting any more food. She knew that she'd had enough, didn't want to feel uncomfortable by eating more, yet felt unhappy that she wouldn't be able to continue to have the taste sensations that the food provided. She also talked about feeling angry that she no longer had food or the next diet to turn to when she was feeling bad. Eating isn't as exciting as it used to be when Sandy would restrict and then overeat. Soon, however, after mourning the loss of being able to *use* food or diets, she was able to leave these feelings behind and feel mainly the exhilaration of being an Intuitive Eater who copes with kindness.

A STRANGE GIFT

You may go for a long time without using food to cope, when all of a sudden emotional eating catches you by surprise. If this occurs, it's not a sign of failure or that you've lost ground; instead, it's a strange gift. Overeating or undereating is simply a sign that stressors in your life at that moment surpass the coping mechanisms that you have developed. Some of these stressors are divorce, a job change, a move to a new city, the death of someone close, marriage, or the birth of a child. These may be new or unexpected experiences for you. As a result, you haven't had the opportunity to develop coping skills to deal with them. So, you revert back to eating as the familiar way to take care of yourself.

Coping with food can also occur when your lifestyle becomes unbalanced with too many responsibilities and obligations, with too little time for pleasure and relaxation. Consequently, food is used to indulge, escape, and relax (albeit so briefly). When you find this happening, it may be a signal for you to reevaluate your life and find ways to put more balance into it. If you don't make these necessary changes, food remains important by filling an unmet need.

In both of these situations, turning to food as a coping mechanism becomes a red flag to let you know that something isn't right in your life. Once you truly appreciate this, you'll realize that this is an early-warning system. Recognize how lucky you are to have this mechanism to alert you that something is off-kilter in your life! (At first, our clients think this notion is a bit absurd, until they realize the truth behind it in their own lives.) Those people who have never had an emotional eating problem often have no ostensible warning of excess stress in their lives. If you can see that your eating problem can have benefits as well as negative effects, you won't get into a pattern of self-defeating behaviors that become destructive and difficult to reverse.

APPROACHING FOOD KINDLY

Once you learn new ways of coping, think about how food can continue to nurture you in a constructive way. You have a right to feel good—and that means just not feeling stuffed or ravenous, but also feeling satisfied with your food choices. Your relationship with food will become more positive as you begin to let go of food as a coping mechanism and bring it into your life as a nonthreatening, pleasurable experience. In chapter 15, we discuss how you can eat healthfully without falling back into the diet mentality. But first you need to learn how to respect your body and appreciate how it feels when you include movement in your life.

Chapter 13

PRINCIPLE 8:

Respect Your Body

Accept your genetic blueprint. Just as a person with a shoe size of eight would not expect to realistically squeeze into a size six, it is equally futile (and uncomfortable) to have the same expectation about body size. But mostly, respect your body so you can feel better about who you are. It's hard to reject the diet mentality if you are unrealistic and critical about your body size or shape. All bodies deserve dignity.

Body vigilance begets body worry, which begets food worry, which fuels the cycle of dieting. As long as you are at war with your body, it will be difficult to be at peace with yourself and food. For every disparaging glimpse in the mirror, the Food Police gain power, and with that comes vows of just one more diet, one more food plan.

We blame our bodies by dwelling on the parts that we see as imperfect or criticize ourselves every time we step on the scale. Has this thinking helped you in any way? Or has it merely made you feel worse? We have yet to find one client who says that focusing on their body in such negative ways is helpful. Studies have shown that the more you focus on your body, the worse you feel about yourself. Moreover, this type of body criticism is a form of personal gaslighting, perpetuated by diet culture and weight stigma. Sadly, we:

- Blame our bodies for the meanness of other people.
- Police our bodies to avoid the judgments of weight-stigmatizing people.
- Engage in performative eating for the expectations of others.

The problem isn't your body, it's our fatphobic culture, which is everywhere, including healthcare, schools, places of worship, media, social media, grocery stores, the beauty industry, the fitness industry, family, and friends.

It's hard to escape the self-induced body torture game when the whole culture is playing it. In the name of fitness, a lean and hard shape has become the body icon for modern times. Self-proclaimed fitness gurus insist that you can "sculpt" your body as if it were a lump of clay, that you can change your genetic shape with an aerobic huff and puff. We are ardent advocates of being strong and recognize the health benefits of movement, but we feel we must point out where unrealistic expectations are being painted. It is widely accepted in the research community that you cannot change fat into muscle or spot-reduce (lose fat in just one specified place). For example, no amount of abdominal crunches are going to directly remove abdominal fat. So how could it be that you can simply sculpt your body by working on certain body parts? Yes, you can build specific muscles through strength and resistance training. Yes, you can make your heart healthier through exercise. But you cannot personally select where that fat will be lost (or even if it will be lost). It's possible to build muscle, but this is not the concept of body sculpting that most have in mind. Many clients we speak with take body-sculpting classes in hopes of shrinking their body.

The fashion world has also shaped the "ideal look" for women into various versions of thin—from the Twiggy figure of over fifty years ago to the waif look first embodied by supermodel Kate Moss. Fortunately, things are beginning to change with larger-body folks: fashion models like Ashley Graham and Tess Holiday; fat activists like Sonya Renee Taylor and Sonalee Rashatwar; performers and actors, such as Lizzo and Aidy Bryant; and fat athlete activists Latoya Shantay Snell and @Fatgirlshiking. They are challenging society's skewed body-shape expectations.

If the culturally ideal body type for women is sandwiched between the spandex-fitness look and fashion-runway waifness, most bodies don't stand a chance. No wonder body dissatisfaction has become the norm. Repeatedly, we seem to be sold the message: If they can do it, you can do it; just try harder. With such standards, it's no wonder that people are at war with their bodies. For all genders, fat is considered the enemy.

There is no doubt that there are unrealistic pressures to be thin with contributions from social media, advertisers, fashion industry, beauty industry, and on and on. We could groan and point fingers at the causes leading to increasing body dissatisfaction. Yes, there are myriad cultural factors that lead to unrealistic body expectations. We will address some of these important factors later in the chapter. Let's first focus on how you can get past body vigilance. Besides, plenty of good books have been written on this topic, especially *The Body Is Not an Apology* by Sonya Renee Taylor.

BODY IMAGE

Most of our clients are adept at being overly critical or hating their bodies. And putting an end to body worry and self-loathing is no easy task. Most of us have trouble accepting a compliment, let alone accepting our bodies. We have found that the notion of accepting your body was too far of a stretch for our clients as a beginning point, because we live in a culture that stigmatizes body sizes. They feared that if they accepted their current body size, it would mean complacency, giving up on changing their relationship with food, and simply accepting the weight stigma that comes with their current body size, without a fight. They talked themselves into the belief that there's honor and dignity in continuing the fight. Our clients also argued that embracing the notion of body acceptance felt hypocritical. After all, the reason they sought our help is because they did *not* accept their current body—they wanted a change.

What a paradox. Science has shown us that DNA programs each body's size and shape. Rather than focusing on changing your body, now is the time to treat your here-and-now body with the respect it deserves. At some point, we hope that you will embrace Mother Nature's plan for your unique body.

Remember, repeated diets and a disparaging attitude toward your body have not helped. When you are caught in the I-hate-my-body mindset, it's all too easy to keep delaying good things for yourself, waiting until you have a body that you think is more deserving. But that day never comes (especially when your standards are unreachable). So, you put off treating yourself better. Many aspects of your life get put on hold. "I'll go on a special vacation after I reach my goal weight"; "I'll start going out with my friends when I just get some of this weight off"—and so the empty promises go. And life gets a little emptier during these times. The irony is that waiting to feel "deserving" of care will reinforce the feeling that you don't deserve it! Conversely, *doing* the things that a person would do who felt deserving is a way to actually *feel* deserving. Shifting your focus to appreciating the body you have, rather than wishing for a different body, will help you fill this emptiness with meaningful and satisfying life experiences.

Taking weight loss out of the picture opens the door to the freedom that can come with respecting your body. *We are not saying disregard your body—we are urging you instead to respect and appreciate your here-and-now body.* Respecting your body means taking care of your health, which includes your mental health. There is a growing movement that shifts the focus to all forms of well-being, rather than weight—it's called Health at Every Size (HAES). Instead of focusing on numbers (weight), the emphasis is on forms of well-being and behaviors that are sustainable for people in all bodies, as well as the practices, environments, and policies that maximize access to well-being for all the people in all the bodies. Weight is not a behavior! For example, physical activity is vital for health, and it's a sustainable behavior. (To learn more, see the sidebar "Health at Every Size," on page 214.)

Respecting and appreciating your body is a key aspect of making peace with your body and your genetics. It is probably the most difficult thing that you will do. It's a powerful practice of resistance to diet culture and weight stigma. You really can't make peace with food when you are at war with your body. (This is especially difficult if you have chronic illness, disability, or are in a trans body.) If you can place your priorities on making peace with your food and body (becoming an Intuitive Eater), it will allow you to loosen up. Otherwise, it will be a constant tug of war.

It's normal to feel panicky when thinking about respecting your body, because it feels so foreign, even wrong. But doing so will allow you to go through the Intuitive Eating steps much more easily. Ironically, we observe a marked difference in our clients who are able to move away from specific weight goals and get to a place of respect for their bodies, versus those who are not. Those who are able to find respect for their bodies have more patience for the Intuitive Eating process. This patience allows them to explore further and move forward more quickly.

Those who have trouble respecting their bodies often find themselves in conflict. When they feel loathsome toward their bodies, they struggle with an intense desire to diet and "just get the weight off." Then they vacillate with intermittent feelings of peace when working through the Intuitive Eating process. It is those moments of peace that give them hope, however, to continue Intuitive Eating.

WHY "RESPECT"

We chose the word "respect" as a launching point for working through your body issues. It's a tough place to begin for most of our clients. Just keep in mind these points, which will ease you into the idea of body-respect: You don't have to like every part of your body to respect it. In fact, you don't have to immediately accept where your body is now to respect it. *Respecting your body means treating it with dignity, while holding the intention of meeting its basic needs.* Many of our clients treat their pets with more respect than their own bodies—they feed them, take them out for a walk, and are kind to them. Using this metaphor can be helpful in your journey: What would you do for your beloved pet? How would you take care of it?

Respecting your body is a critical turning point in becoming an Intuitive Eater. It's not easy. Our culture has a built-in bias against larger body sizes, while placing a premium on appearance, including granting social power based on the culturally thin ideal. It's important to recognize that these biases exist, because it may seem like you are a salmon swimming upstream against the cultural norm. After all, it's all around us in both subtle and blatant forms, from the thin actresses in diet soft drink ads to glaring magazine covers, such as the issue of *People* magazine's "Diet Winners and Sinners of the Year: Here's the skinny on who got fat, who got fit and how they did it." It takes a conscious effort to move away from this diet culture norm. Just because seeking a smaller body is the societal norm does not make it right. Moreover, this toxic norm is pervasive, so it takes an active practice of resistance to fight body oppression. Most people will benefit from joining a supportive community, because body discrimination is rampant.

How to Respect Your Body

Think of respecting your body in two ways: first, by making it comfortable, and second, by being responsive to its basic needs. You deserve to be comfortable. You deserve to get your basic needs met.

Consider these basic premises of body respect:

- My body deserves to be fed.
- My body deserves to be treated with dignity.
- My body deserves to be dressed comfortably and in a style I like.
- My body deserves to be touched affectionately, with my consent and with respect.
- My body deserves to move comfortably, to the extent it is possible.

Let's explore how you can offer more respect to your body (and to yourself). It's an easy concept to understand, but far more difficult to implement. The following ideas and tools have helped our clients begin a new relationship with their bodies.

Getting comfortable. Let's get personal here. When is the last time you bought new underwear? Don't laugh. All too often we have clients who feel that they don't deserve new underwear (let alone new clothes) until they reach a certain weight or clothing size. Think about what that means at a basic level. Wearing panties, a bra, or briefs that are constantly pinching or riding up is highly uncomfortable. How can you be comfortable in your body when you have an unpleasant reminder constantly binding your body? How can you be at ease when your body is constantly pinched and squeezed by poorly fitting garments? This is especially challenging for folks in large bodies who can't find clothing and underwear in their size. For decades, major clothing stores and fashion designers generally catered to one type: the white, thin customer. The majority of American women (67 percent) wear sizes 16 and up, yet the majority of clothes available for purchase only go up to size 14, which is completely discriminatory for those who don't fit the clothing company's idea of "ideal" size.

While initially you may snicker at the simplicity of changing your underwear, it's had a significant impact on many of our clients. "I just had a baby a few months ago. My maternity underwear was laughably big, but my regular panties fit too snugly. They were a constant reminder that I was "too big." I felt miserable, until I invested in underwear that fit. The funny thing is that I didn't want to spend the money—even though I had shelled out plenty on a weight loss program that did not work. I was amazed at how a simple act made such a difference in feeling better about myself."

Cassandra was in her fifties and hadn't bought new bras in years. (The ones she had were of very high quality and quite expensive, so they lasted.) Sadly, the underwires in her bras were jabbing and scarring her, but she didn't feel she deserved to buy new bras until she lost weight. Every day, she was miserable. Her first step toward respecting her body was buying new bras and tights. She learned that wearing a tortuously tight undergarment would hinder the process of listening to her body's signals. When she was more comfortable in her underwear, she was able to be more relaxed about her eating.

The comfort principle goes beyond undergarments. How you dress can be a step toward a newfound respect for your body. We are not saying to be subservient to the fashion industry, however. Rather, dress in the manner to which you are accustomed. If you are used to dressing in a particular way, why should you stop just because you're not happy with your shape? You should not have to settle for leftovers or clothes that you don't enjoy. There's nothing wrong with dressing in worn-out jeans and an oversized shirt, *if that is what you are used to and are comfortable in*. If, however, you prefer wearing stylish jeans and a casual blazer and settle for leggings, it may affect how you feel about yourself and your body. It's an issue of being consistent. Once again, this can be challenging if you are in a larger body because of the lack of availability of clothing that fits *and* is stylish. Retailers are starting to get the message and trying to be more size inclusive, but they still have a long way to go!

All too often, weight loss programs have urged you to "get rid of your fat clothes"; otherwise, they warn, you are issuing an invitation to failure. Not to mention that the fashion industry has a vested interest in influencing you to buy new clothes, urging you to shell out money for them. This is another diet culture message telling you your body is wrong. It is the job of the clothes to fit your body, not the other way around! It's important to dress for your here-and-now body and be comfortable.

Get rid of body-assessment tools. We have found that most of our clients who weigh themselves frequently have difficulty living in their present body—they get too worried about the numbers. Our advice: stop weighing yourself. Remember, the scale is the tool of diet culture's oppression.

Also, beware of substituting a tight pair of jeans as a pseudo-scale or body assessment tool. Hanging on to a small piece of clothing and trying it on daily or weekly can equally undermine how you feel about yourself and your body. It's important that you don't organize your life around an arbitrary size. Rather, build a life that works day to day in your here-and-now body.

Jamie, a young account executive for a public relations firm, was doing quite well with Intuitive Eating. She quit dieting, honored her hunger, respected her fullness, and so forth. Jamie had also gotten rid of the scale. But she began to assess her progress by trying on a tight pencil skirt. Every time she tried the skirt on, she felt bad about herself. It conveyed the message "You haven't made enough progress. You need to lose weight." Jamie eventually got rid of the skirt and her bad feelings about her body. *Regardless of body size, anyone will feel uncomfortable in a piece of clothing that feels too tight.*

Quit the body-check game. Most of our clients are embarrassed to admit this, but when they enter a room with other people, they play the silent game of body-checking. The game of body-checking revolves around the theme "How does my body compare to the rest of the crowd?" Perhaps you've played this game (and maybe are not even quite aware of it).

For people who face more weight stigma, they may ask themselves, "Am I the biggest one here, or is there danger here for me?" as a strategy to manage their fear of stigma. For those with thin privilege, their questions might be, "Who's got the best body? How does my body rate, compared to the others?" This body comparison can be a dangerous game. It can lead to a fleeting sense of superiority, only to result in more envy and insecurity. Either way, they end up feeling bad.

We've had clients admire and envy a stranger's body shape. They're not only feeling bad about themselves but may hold the fantasy that if they were thin, it would fix everything in their lives that is distressing for them (which is easier and less threatening than doing the work on the distressing things, such as marital difficulties or changing jobs). "Oh, if I only had their body. They must work out daily. Look at them eat—they must not eat carbs. I should be able to do that. Something is wrong with me. I need to try harder." These are big assumptions. You don't know if the person is truly eating! The person may have had surgery (such as liposuction), is suffering from an eating disorder, or even have cancer. You can't judge the shape of someone's body and assume they "earned" it. This person could just be genetically programmed for a smaller body.

In one session, Kate described a party that she had attended and how good a particular woman's body looked. Kate thought that she should be able to get those kinds of "results" too, if she just tried harder. Little did Kate know, however, that the acquaintance at the party was a client of mine (ET), who happened to have cancer. (Of course, Kate would never know this from me because of strict patient confidentiality.) Kate had been admiring a woman who was fighting for remission with chemotherapy. The bottom line is, you never know. Even if it was a friend or relative, you still don't know. We have worked with clients whose own spouses and roommates did not know that they had an eating disorder or some illness. It's normal to want more safety, to envy someone who seems to have more body safety and privilege.

Playing the body-comparison game may lead to more disconnected eating and more body dissatisfaction. The process of Intuitive Eating, however, redirects our attention to our own needs, our own agenda—rather than basing our decisions on the perceptions of other people's bodies and food choices, which is illustrated in the next case.

Both Sheila and Cassie had been on their share of diets, and they silently compared their bodies and eating decisions. (This is another unfortunate by-product of diet culture—constant body and food vigilance.) When Sheila became an Intuitive Eater, this dynamic began to change. Sheila had made substantial progress over six months. Fortunately, Sheila accepted this process and was feeling good. Meanwhile, her neighbor, Cassie, had just finished another crash diet and was rather proud of her weight loss.

That night, Sheila and Cassie went out together for dinner with their husbands. Sheila ate what she wanted, enjoyed a good meal, and, overall, felt satisfied. Meanwhile, Cassie proudly nibbled like a bird, and boasted how easy her current diet was. (Another phenomenon of diet culture is loud evangelizing of the latest, greatest diet, lifestyle, food plan, and so on.) Sheila got sucked into the comparison trap, and next to Cassie, she felt as if she were overeating. Fortunately, she kept listening to her Intuitive

Eater voice that told her to respect her body and that her body deserved to be fed. Her voice gently reminded her that Cassie was on a path to diet destruction—the euphoria wouldn't last long. Sheila knew this all too well from her old dieting days.

Sheila's private body competition with Cassie made her feel inferior about her own body and progress. Nonetheless, Sheila continued to focus on her journey of Intuitive Eating. Predictably, one month later, Cassie "failed" yet another diet and was binge eating in spurts. One year later, Sheila was continuing her Intuitive Eating and was at peace with food and her body. Meanwhile, Cassie continued to be stuck in diet culture. Rather than being triggered back into diet culture and body comparison, Sheila felt compassion for Cassie and hoped one day she would be as free and healed as she was.

Doing what's best for you for "big events." Whether it's a class reunion or a wedding, it's natural to want to look your best at important occasions. If this involves shrinking your body to squeeze into that special outfit, it will only backfire. You'll only add another notch on the belt of yo-yo dieting— this time, however, it's yo-yo dieting with a cause.

Remember, there will always be important occasions in your life. One particular client was attending the Grammy Awards, because her husband was up for an award. Of course, she wanted to look not just good, but great. It became clear, however, that she would not be at what she believed was her ideal body size for this prestigious event. Her thinking was steeped in diet culture, believing that looking great would mean looking thinner. She was feeling desperate and considered a quick fast to shrink her body. She was asked, "When will the dieting stop?" There will always be an important award or event, always a "legitimate" reason to diet. At that moment she saw the future futility of crash diets triggered by competitive body-checking, as well as how the pursuit of weight loss perpetuated weight stigma. She decided to respect her current body. She kept her usual standards of dress and wore a custom-made outfit. This time, however, the outfit was designed for her here-and-now body. She did not have to squeeze into a gown and worry about every move she made. She still maintained her other routine standards—stylish hair, glittery accessories, and so forth. The only thing different was that this time she felt comfortable, rather than self-conscious.

It's all too easy to cross over into the dieting mentality if you rationalize that the specialness of an event makes it okay to diet. The more you exert pressure on yourself to be a certain body size, the more you are bound to create problems. Jesse would always panic when a special occasion arose, whether it was a wedding or her company's annual awards banquet when she had to give a keynote speech. First, she would worry about what to wear, which would lead her on an intense shopping foray. Eventually, she would buy a stunning dress that was just a little too small. Jesse always shopped for her "future body," rather than her present body. But she knew she could "make weight" for the big day, just like a boxer weighing in for the big fight. As the big day drew near, Jesse would feel more pressure. She'd try her dress on daily and chastise herself for not fitting into it. Then the meal skipping would begin. On the big day itself, Jesse would allow herself a light breakfast. She would forgo eating the rest of the day to make sure she fit into her dress. Yes, the dress would fit. But by the time Jesse reached her destination, she would invariably rebound eat (discreetly, of course) at the special function. Her body was famished, and she'd rationalize that she earned it. But by the end of the night, the combination of her overfull stomach and her tight dress amplified her body discomfort. She'd spend the event worrying about her body rather than having a good time.

Alarmingly, one of the most profound arenas where we see this played out is the cultural phenomenon of dieting for a wedding dress, to be memorialized in photos. Sadly, this sets you up to be a lifelong repeat customer for the weight loss industry. Each time you look at the wedding pictures, the focus is on your body, rather than remembering the feelings on your special day.

How much time and energy have you spent getting your body ready for a big event? What if the energy was directed on recognizing your inner qualities, such as wit, intelligence, or listening ability? What if you came prepared for a function by spending your time thinking of ways to engage in meaningful conversation, or getting to know someone new? You'd probably have a better time! Jimmy almost skipped his twenty-year class reunion because he thought he was too big and didn't have a suit that fit. He could not bear the thought of shopping for a larger suit size. Eventually, Jimmy decided to put his body worries aside and attend his reunion. Instead of worrying about his body, Jimmy focused on finding out what his old buddies had been doing over the years. He even danced the night away with old friends. (He had not danced in years!) Jimmy's reunion experience had far exceeded his expectations. He found his "old self"—the witty and charming person who loved to have fun and dance. Over the years, Jimmy's private body war had only served to isolate him and keep him from doing the activities he enjoyed. The sad irony is that Jimmy came so close to avoiding his reunion, because his body was not ready for the big event.

Stop body bashing. Every time you focus on your "imperfect" body parts it creates more self-consciousness and body worry. It's difficult to respect your body when you are constantly chastising yourself for looking the wrong way.

Many of our clients are surprised at how often they degrade their bodies in one day. How many times a day do you chide yourself about your body? Try keeping count for a day or a few hours. It is surprising how often we can be triggered to worry about our body, whether it's a quick glimpse in a store window reflection or passing a mirror. Each disparaging thought lands another nail in the coffin of body dissatisfaction. Surrounding yourself with these body thoughts will only make you more unhappy and frustrated. It can also bleed over into how you feel about yourself in general.

Instead of focusing on what you don't like about your body, focus on your relationship with your body and how you can improve it by speaking kindly of yourself. Start simply. Perhaps one of these appreciative statements resonates with you:

- I love that my hand can hold the hand of my lover or child.
- I'm grateful that my feet allow me to walk.
- I've noticed that my smile connects me to other people.
- How lucky I am that my skin allows me to feel the sensation of touch.

When you participate in conversations disparaging your own body, or the bodies of others, it perpetuates weight stigma. Studies show that refraining from this type of discussion is helpful in reducing body dissatisfaction, dieting, and eating disorder symptoms.

Respect body diversity, especially yours. We come in all shapes and sizes, yet we somehow expect that we should all be "one size fits all," as long as it's thin. As long as we feed into this cultural stigma, it will be a long time before societal norms will change into a healthy acceptance of body diversity.

There are many factors that contribute to one's weight, especially genetics. You cannot assume, for example, that just because someone is in a larger body, they are overeating. Several studies have documented that people in larger bodies do not necessarily eat more than their smaller counterparts. Humans are supposed to come in a diverse range of sizes, not just one body. Yes, there are compulsive eaters. Yes, there are those who are not active. You cannot assume that someone with a large body overeats and does not move. Conversely, you cannot assume someone in a thin body is healthy and engages in physical activity. Many classic studies on twins have shown that genetics plays a powerful role in determining our body build.

Beware of stereotyping large people. Try beginning with a place of neutrality and compassion. Check your body bias at the door.

It's important to recognize that some people are naturally born with a leaner body type, although they are in the minority. Similarly, we cannot assume that because someone is unusually thin, that they have an eating disorder or are obsessed with dieting.

Be realistic. If maintaining or obtaining your weight requires living on rice cakes and water, while exercising for hours, that's a glaring red flag that your goal is not realistic. If your parents are higher-weight people, chances are you will never be model-thin. Remember, genetics is a strong determinant of body size.

Do nice things for your body. Your body deserves to be pampered and touched with the resources you have. If you are able, schedule massages as often as you can, even if it's just a fifteen-minute neck rub by a loving friend. Try a sauna or a whirlpool, if you have access to them. Buy lotions and creams to rub on your body. Take bubble baths with bath oils and salts. (Try this in candlelight with classical music!) Doing these things for your body shows that you respect it and want to make yourself feel good.

View your body as an instrument, not an ornament. This is a powerful mantra from the creators of Beauty Redefined, a nonprofit created by Lexie Kite, PhD, and Lindsay Kite, PhD, experts in body image resilience. It's important to empower yourself by realizing what your body can do, rather than how it appears. When you focus on appearance, it's a form of objectification, which undermines your self-worth.

YOUR NATURAL BODY WEIGHT

One of the first questions that we are invariably asked is, Can you help me lose weight? Or how much should I weigh? As we've said before, we have compassion for those who hold the hope of weight loss, which is understandable because of diet culture. But our sincere hope is that we can help people shift their focus to enjoying eating and treating their bodies with respect and kindness. No one can really say what a specific ideal weight is. In fact, the 1990 edition of U.S. Dietary Guidelines threw out the recommendation that Americans reach or maintain an *ideal weight,* because no one knows exactly what that number is! Unfortunately, the 2015–2020 Dietary Guidelines urge Americans to "maintain a healthy body weight," which is based on the incredibly flawed body mass index (BMI) metric, which is a ratio of weight to height, to determine weight categories.

Initially, scientists used the BMI as a screening tool for large populations. Ironically, the BMI was created by a mathematician more than two hundred years ago and was *never* intended to be used on individuals, let alone as an indicator of health!

Several large studies have shown the profound problems with using BMI:

- Wildman and colleagues (2008) found that using BMI as a proxy for health resulted in the misdiagnosing of over half the people (51 percent) as unhealthy.
- A research team from UCLA found that 54 million Americans were labeled "obese or overweight" but were in fact healthy according to metabolic indicators (Tomiyama et al. 2016).
- In a seminal book, *The Obesity Paradox: When Thinner Means Sicker and Heavier Means Healthier* (2014), cardiologist and researcher Carl J. Lavie describes the numerous problems with the BMI and focusing on weight, rather than behavior, to predict health outcomes.

The BMI has also been criticized because it does not take into account muscle composition. Notably, muscle weighs more than fat. That's why many professional athletes have high BMI values that would classify them as overweight

when, in fact, they are actually lean. Much more important than a number is
the issue of how to improve the health of the nation. If the factors necessary
to improve health can be changed, everyone benefits, no matter their BMI.

We agree. That's why, in part, we use the concept of *genetically determined weight*. This is the weight your body will maintain with *normal/
intuitive* eating and *normal* movement.

The problem with most of the people we see is that their eating relationship is *not normal,* due to years of dieting.

Your genetically determined weight may not match what you have in
mind. The weight that many people wish to achieve or maintain often has
more to do with aesthetics than the unproven pursuit of health. According
to the National Institutes of Health, many people in this country who are at
the weight they are born to be continue to try to lose weight—and it may be
in part from chasing an unrealistic body size, healthcare demands, public
health policy, and ongoing weight stigma.

A seminal study reviewed the weights of Miss America contestants
and Playboy models from 1959 to 1988 and found that their weights and
body sizes got *thinner* as the years went on. That level of thinness over-
lapped with one of the criteria for anorexia nervosa. If the cultural ideal
for women overlaps with eating disorder criteria, American women are
not only chasing an unrealistic body goal but are engaged in a potentially
dangerous pursuit. (Note that eating disorders come in a variety of body
sizes.) In 2011, the Succeed Foundation commissioned a body image survey, the findings of which prompted a scientifically supported campaign in
the United Kingdom, aiming to improve body image and prevent the onset
of eating disorders. Their survey revealed the following:

- 30 percent of women say they would trade at least one year of
  their life to achieve their ideal weight and shape.
- 46 percent of the women have been ridiculed or bullied because
  of their appearance.

If you have a weight aspiration in mind that comes from a time when
you were dieting, this sheds information on how low your body weight was
able to go under duress—which is *not* realistic. Remember that research
shows that the actual process of dieting itself, losing or recycling the same
amount of weight lost and gained, is harmful to your health.

For many people, body dissatisfaction is a result of weight stigma—and you may not be consciously aware of its powerful influence. Let's unpack what that means and why it's important.

WEIGHT STIGMA

What is it? Weight stigma is a form of prejudice and stereotyping, which is reported at rates comparable to racial discrimination (Puhl and Suh 2015; O'Hara and Taylor 2018). This statistic doesn't even capture the compounded stigma, when you factor in the intersectionality* of marginalized groups who are also stigmatized, which include but are not limited to: disability, skin color, gender, sexual identity, age, and race. According to the National Eating Disorders Association (NEDA), weight discrimination occurs more frequently than gender or age discrimination. The incidence of weight stigma has escalated 66 percent with the rise in public health campaigns to prevent "obesity" (Daníelsdóttira et al. 2010). It exists across all aspects of society and can look like this:

- Being teased about your shape or size.
- Receiving negative comments about your weight from anyone, including healthcare professionals.
- Being pressured to lose weight to fit in.
- Complimenting someone on their weight loss.
- Being avoided, excluded, or ignored because of your weight.
- Poor treatment by coworkers or bosses because of your size or shape.
- Being charged higher insurance premiums because of weight.
- Mandatory participation in ineffective worksite wellness programs, many of which are weight-centric, in order to reduce insurance premiums.
- Not being able to find clothes in your size at a store.
- Being required to pay extra for an additional seat on an airplane.
- Being denied healthcare because of your size or required to lose weight in order to get a medical procedure such as surgery, joint replacement, organ transplant, or infertility treatment.
- Not getting hired because of the size of your body.

---

* Kimberlé Crenshaw, Professor of Law at UCLA and Columbia Law School, coined the term "intersectionality."

Health consequences of weight stigma

Weight stigma alone is an independent risk for many health problems (Puhl and Suh 2015; Wu and Berry 2017; Messenger et al. 2018), including:

- Increases in high blood pressure, inflammation markers in the blood (C-reactive protein), stress markers (cortisol and F2-isoprostane levels), A1-C (indicator of blood sugar regulation), metabolic syndrome, depression symptoms and disorders, anxiety, lower self-esteem, and higher body image dissatisfaction.
- Increases in the risk of mortality and type 2 diabetes.

Medical care problems

A body of research shows that healthcare is one of the primary sources of weight stigma (Mesinger, Tylka, and Calamari 2018), which leads to major consequences, including:

- Avoidance of healthcare by folks in larger bodies.
- Misdiagnosis. You cannot assess someone just by looking at the size of their body. Yet there have been too many cases of physicians doing that very thing. An egregious example is the death of Ellen Maud Bennett. In her obituary, the final message Ellen wanted to share was about the fat shaming she endured from the medical profession. Over the past few years of feeling unwell she sought out medical intervention, and no one offered any support or suggestions beyond weight loss. When she finally got the correct diagnosis, inoperable cancer, she lived for only a matter of days. Ellen's dying wish was that women of size make her death matter by advocating strongly for their health and not accepting that fat is the only relevant health issue. (This is for you, Ellen!)

Fatphobia

Fatphobia is a prejudice against people in larger bodies. Unfortunately, it has become a cultural norm to stigmatize and bully fat people and treat them unfairly. This affects people in smaller bodies too, because it creates the fear of becoming fat.

• Regardless of your size, when you see a big person on the street do you cast judgment and disdain? That's a form of fatphobia.

• Do you compliment people for losing weight? That's a form of fatphobia too—because it objectifies the body and implies that some body sizes are better than others.

• Do you ever express health concerns online about the appearance or size of someone in a large body? That's called *concern trolling*; it's a form of bullying.

Overall, the greater the weight stigma, the greater the negative impact on health. Shrinking your body size does not put an end to weight stigma; it merely reinforces it! All bodies of varying size deserve dignity and respect.

SAYING GOODBYE TO THE FANTASY

One of the hardest facts many of our clients face is that their weight expectations, based on their survival mechanism for managing weight stigma, are not realistic for their bodies. This includes folks in a variety of body sizes. Our clients do not like to hear this. For some, it shatters a lifelong dream. But we refuse to perpetuate diet culture's agenda and the myth that we can choose our weight. Ethically, we cannot engage in a process that causes psychological and biological harm.

For example, Kathy is a thirty-year-old actress who has been told to lose weight by her agent. She reported healthy eating habits, and she said she worked out most days for one hour. After a soul-searching session, it was concluded that Kathy's body was where it was meant to be. Pursuing weight loss would be detrimental to her metabolism and psyche. She was actually relieved to hear this; she decided she would change agents and keep looking for jobs until someone would cast her as she was—a healthy person.

Many of our clients discover in hindsight that had they lived in a world where they could have accepted their bodies when they were younger, they would have never gone on that first diet, with all of its negative ramifications. They could have been happy then and would continue to be happy now.

You may need to mourn for the fantasy body you've chased and the temporary illusion of peace that came from going down the dieting road. For many people, it begins the difficult work of grieving the loss of a smaller body and all the privileges that may come with it. Consider the price you have paid (energy, time, emotional investment) chasing one diet after another to seek your fantasy body. By saying farewell to the fantasy, you open the door to being at peace not only with your body, but with other facets of your life. This is much easier to do for people who are in culturally accepted body sizes. For larger-sized people, it becomes a journey of how to manage living in a world that oppresses higher-weight people—inner acceptance is not enough. Finding a community of friends and a counselor who can give emotional support for the pain that you may feel from stigma of any kind is the first step in living a fulfilling life.

HEALTH AT EVERY SIZE

Health at Every Size (HAES)* is a concept embraced by many different disciplines. It focuses on health, rather than on how much a person weighs. HAES promotes improved health *behaviors* for everyone, regardless of size (Bacon and Aphramor 2011).

Unfortunately, the weight-focused war on obesity has contributed further to food and body preoccupation, yo-yo weight loss and regain, distraction from other personal health goals, reduced self-esteem, eating disorders, and weight stigmatization and discrimination.

Intuitive Eating is very much HAES-aligned. HAES updated their principles in 2013 to include social justice as follows:

- **Weight inclusivity:** Accept and respect the inherent diversity of body shapes and sizes and reject the idealizing or pathologizing of specific weights.
- **Health enhancement:** Support health policies that improve and equalize access to information and services, and personal practices that improve human well-being, including attention to individual physical, economic, social, spiritual, emotional, and other needs.
- **Respectful care:** Acknowledge our biases, and work to end weight discrimination, weight stigma, and weight bias. Provide information

---

* Health At Every Size and HAES are registered trademarks of the Association for Size Diversity and Health and used with permission.

and services from an understanding that socio-economic status, race, gender, sexual orientation, age, and other identities impact weight stigma, and support environments that address these inequities.

- **Eating for well-being:** Promote flexible, individualized eating based on hunger, satiety, nutritional needs, and pleasure, rather than any externally regulated eating plan focused on weight control.
- **Life-enhancing movement:** Support physical activities that allow people of all sizes, abilities, and interests to engage in enjoyable movement, to the degree that they choose.

Research to date indicates that using a HAES approach is associated with statistically and clinically relevant improvements in health, including improvement in blood pressure, blood lipids, physical activity, and body image. There were also reductions in metabolic risk factors and eating disorder behaviors. Notably, not a single study found adverse changes. This latter finding is important, because some people have expressed a concern that *not* focusing on weight would result in worse health outcomes. Not so.

Chapter 14

PRINCIPLE 9:

Movement—Feel the Difference

Forget militant exercise. Just get active and feel the difference. Shift your focus to how it feels to move your body, rather than the calorie-burning effect of exercise. If you focus on how you feel from working out, such as energized, it can make the difference between rolling out of bed for a brisk morning walk or hitting the snooze alarm.

If you were to classify your attitude toward movement, would it be "just do it" or "just forget it"? Many of our clients fall into the latter category. They are burned out. Working out often went hand in hand with the negative experiences of ineffective food plans and dieting. Our clients were *not* enjoying exercise for two key reasons. Either they had started exercising when they initiated a diet, or they abused their bodies with unrealistic amounts of exercise, which led to injuries. Regardless, both groups felt guilty for not doing enough.

If you began an exercise program while simultaneously starting a diet, it's likely that your energy (calorie) intake was too low. When you don't have enough energy, exercise is not invigorating, let alone fun. It becomes a chore, pure drudgery. When you are underfed, it's increasingly difficult to exercise, especially if carbohydrates are inadequate (which is often the case with our chronic dieters).

Carbohydrates are the preferred fuel of exercise. As you can see in the "Carbohydrate Power Chart," running two miles uses the amount of carbohydrates found in three slices of bread. If you regularly limit carbohydrate foods (such as potatoes, bread, and pasta) and then add exercise, you are burdening the body with a carbohydrate deficit. Remember, for normal biological functions, the body *must* have carbohydrates. If you do not feed your body enough carbohydrates, it will dismantle its muscle protein to create vital energy. This has been demonstrated in studies on endurance athletes. Endurance athletes who did not get enough carbohydrates for their exercise activity burned branched chain amino acids (a component of protein) to help create vital energy to fuel their bodies.

Keep in mind that even very fit and motivated athletes have difficulty working out if they are low on carbohydrates! This effect was illustrated in a classic study of elite college swimmers by exercise physiologist David Costill, of Ball State University in Indiana. He found that swimmers who did not eat enough carbohydrates were *not* able to complete their workouts. If elite athletes had trouble working out because they didn't eat enough, why would you expect to be any different? And while the keto craze is also making its presence in the world of athletics—it goes against the joint recommendations from the American College of Sports Medicine, Academy of Nutrition and Dietetics, and Dietitians of Canada (2016).

If you have never enjoyed exercise, let alone experienced the "runner's high" euphoria from working out, there's a good chance it was because of dieting, or the diet mentality of limiting foods. When a diet fails, exercise often stops

CARBOHYDRATE POWER CHART	
Activity	Equivalent Slices of Bread
Running	
2 miles	3
6 miles	10–11
26 miles	33–37
Swimming	
200 meters	1
1,500 meters	6
Cycling	
1 hour	15–17

Adapted from: D.L. Costill, "Carbohydrates for Exercise: Dietary Demands for Optimal Performance," International Journal of Sports Medicine 9:5 (1988).

because it was only done as an adjunct to dieting. You're left with memories of feeling bad, which makes you less likely to want to exercise in the future.

No wonder the chronic dieter has difficulty with consistent exercise. Who wants to continually subject their body to something that does *not* feel good? Yet clients often blame themselves for not having enough willpower or not possessing the admirable "just do it" mantra of exercise. This is like feeling guilty for not having enough willpower to "will" a car to operate on an empty tank of gas. Yet to reap the many positive results from exercise, there needs to be a consistent effort.

Many of our clients have been burned out both mentally and physically from "crash exercising." Like crash diets and rigid food plans, crash exercising doesn't last long. This typically occurs when someone is determined to get in shape and lose weight quickly. They start with too much activity in a short time period and end up either very sore, or not enjoying exercise, or both.

Others feel intimidated because of the presence of weight stigma in the gym.

There are other reasons that chronic dieters don't feel like starting or continuing to exercise:

- Bad experiences growing up, including being forced to run laps or do calisthenics as a punishment, getting teased for being unco-ordinated, not getting picked for teams.
- Rebelling against parents, spouses, and others who pushed exercise like a "good diet": "You should go run, you should go to the gym," and so forth.

BREAKING THROUGH EXERCISE BARRIERS

Rather than insisting that our clients immediately embark on adding more movement to their lives, we wait until *they* are ready. Postponing activity a few weeks, even a few months, will not make a big difference in a lifelong commitment. Don't worry if you don't feel like strapping on your shoes and running a few laps, especially if you have leaned toward being an over-exerciser. There are several keys to breaking through the barriers that prevent you from exercising.

Focus on How It Feels

We have found that one key to consistent exercise is to focus on how it *feels,* rather than playing the numbers game of counting calories burned. (Any time you are paying attention to the felt sense from within your body, it's a form of interoceptive awareness, which is like cross-training for becoming an Intuitive Eater.) Instead of just biding your time or gritting your teeth when working out, explore how you feel throughout the day (including during exercise and immediately after). How do you feel regarding:

- Stress level: Are you able to handle stress better? Are you less edgy? Is it easier to take situations in stride, roll with the punches?
- Energy level: Do you feel more alert? Is there a little more spunk in your attitude? If you exercise in the morning, does it wake you up instead of making you feel groggy?
- General sense of well-being: Do you have an improved outlook?
- Sense of empowerment: Do you feel more determined? Do you say, "I can do it" and seize the day?
- Sleep: Do you sleep more soundly and wake up more refreshed?

If you are in a period of inactivity, it's especially important to note these feelings. They will serve as your baseline. Compare the difference between when you did and did not exercise. Note how you felt. When you can really feel the difference between moving consistently and being inactive, the positive feelings can be a motivating factor for continuing. Why would you stop doing something that feels good? If instead, you exercise with the dieting mindset, you get used to stopping and starting, just like each new dieting attempt.

Remember, *it's important to shift the focus and intention of exercise away from calorie-burning.* It's about *how you feel*!

Decouple Exercise from Weight Loss

It's well accepted that physical activity is the one consistent element associated with long-term health. Exercise does play a significant role in metabolism and preserving lean muscle mass. But if your prime focus is on weight loss, it won't motivate you to exercise for long. It will only serve as a timecard to be punched by a bored assembly-line employee. And when the payoff doesn't seem quick enough, it becomes discouraging. Researchers also say that it's about time we decouple exercise from weight loss, because it minimizes its myriad significant health benefits (Chaput et al. 2011). Movement is important for its own sake and should be considered as a way to promote health, increase quality of life, and fight off diseases. Using weight loss as the ultimate reason for physical activity could also drive you to exercise abuse.

PHYSICAL ACTIVITY IS THE ULTIMATE STRESS BUFFER

Exercise helps to protect the body from the health-damaging effects of chronic stress. Chronic stress can create a hormonal imbalance, which results in increased production of cortisol in the body, while also rendering insulin less effective (which is known as insulin resistance). Increases in cortisol are also associated with elevated neuropeptide Y release (which, you may recall, increases appetite).

But regular physical activity can counteract this effect by improving the effectiveness of insulin and mood. Additionally, regular movement improves sleep patterns, which is often disrupted during stressful times. Notably, sleep deprivation is associated with insulin resistance and disturbed appetite regulation.

Focus on Movement as a Way of Taking Care of Yourself

Whether young or old, regardless of size, everyone benefits from being active. It makes you feel good and helps prevent health problems later in life. Specific benefits include:

- Increased bone strength.
- Increased stress tolerance.
- Decreased blood pressure.
- Reduced risk for chronic diseases, including heart disease, diabetes, osteoporosis, hypertension, and some types of cancers.
- Increased level of good cholesterol (HDL); decreased total cholesterol.
- Increased heart and lung strength.

• Increased metabolism—helps maintain lean body mass and revs up energy production in the cells.
• Reduced risk for "silent" stroke (Gandey 2011).
• Improved satiety cues and appetite regulation (Chaput et al. 2011).
• Improved mood (Chaput et al. 2011).
• Improved learning and memory (Chaput et al. 2011).
• Prevents or delays cognitive decline associated with aging (Chaput et al. 2011).

Don't Get Caught in Exercise Mind Traps

If you've had a diet mentality for a number of years, there's a good chance that versions of it have permeated into do-not-exercise traps. Let's identify and refute them:

The it's-not-worth-it trap. We know many people who wouldn't walk unless they could get in one hour—anything under that "doesn't count." Therefore, a fifteen-minute walk break during lunch doesn't count. Instead, they do nothing. We commonly see clients discount their workout because they didn't reach their prescribed quota. It "didn't count" because they only exercised three times in a week, rather than five. All the more reason to be focused on how exercise feels, rather than doing it by the numbers.

Besides, over the long term, it all counts. We like to take the power out of numbers, whether those numbers refer to pounds, calories, or even minutes exercising. In this case, however, we use numbers to show how even the smallest amount of movement does matter.

Activity	Time Spent in 1 Year
5 minutes of taking the stairs at work twice daily, five times a week	43 hours
10 minutes of walking your child to school, three times a week	26 hours
15 minutes of mowing the lawn, one time a week	13 hours

Mistaking Being Busy for Physical Activity. Your life may be very hectic, but *being busy is not the same as physical activity.* Most of us spend time "running around" in our cars! Unless you are Fred Flintstone, there is no fitness element to driving. Any of the following could be a component of a sedentary existence:

- Spending hours *sitting* in transit to work (either car, train, bus, taxi).
- Sitting behind a desk all day (pushing papers and telephone buttons is no different than fiddling with the remote control).
- Working at a computer all day.
- Arriving home exhausted, sitting, and reading the mail or paying bills, eating, then going to bed.

The key is to find ways to incorporate movement into your everyday life. Remember, hectic schedules and mental exertion may keep your mind active, but that is not the same as physical activity.

The no-time-to-spare trap. Ask most people if exercise is important, and you'll hear an overwhelming yes. Yet it often gets shoved aside as other details in life vie for your time and attention.

The question we often ask our patients who are in this time-crunch dilemma is: How can you make movement a non-negotiable priority? This is not intended as a rigid guideline, rather a new way of thinking of exercise so that it won't slip through the cracks. In fact, we often substitute the word "movement" for "exercise," as a way to help people see that one of the most important aspects of maintaining good health is to move your body! It's not about going to the gym to exercise; it's about finding a realistic way to provide regular, joyful movement in your life.

If this seems like an impossible task, you may need to evaluate your priorities or compassionately acknowledge that it is a privilege to have enough time for physical activity. Your life may be chronically overscheduled by choice; or if you are living at the poverty line, it may not be possible to add extra physical activity when you are working two jobs and taking public transportation. What are some realistic ways you can take care of yourself? Ironically, many of our overscheduled clients attribute the fact that they don't work out to laziness, when in reality, they are truly too busy!

An option you may want to explore is hiring a personal trainer, if you can afford it. "When I make an appointment with somebody, including my trainer, it automatically becomes a priority on my schedule," said one client. Be sure, however, to check out the credentials. Minimally, a personal trainer should be certified through either the American College of Sports Medicine (ACSM) or the American Council on Exercise (ACE). Do take time to interview them and be sure they are aligned with your fitness goals, which have nothing to do with weight!

The If-I-Don't-Sweat-It-Doesn't-Count Trap. It's easy to believe that the only way to be fit is to engage in activities that make you sweat profusely. But you don't have to invest in sweat equity to reap fitness dividends. It is well accepted that you don't have to perform rigorous workouts to obtain health benefits. You can reap benefits from simple activities such as gardening, raking the leaves, or walking. These no-sweat activities make a physical difference. In a landmark scientific paper, which reviewed more than forty-three studies, the CDC and ACSM concluded that *simply moving* for thirty minutes over the course of most days of the week could reduce the risk of heart disease by half!

All you need to do is accumulate thirty minutes of activity a day, most of the week. The thirty minutes of activity do *not* need to be all at once. (This particular conclusion surprises many people.) For example, the activity could be divided into three ten-minute sessions, or two fifteen-minute sessions, and so forth. In fact, a recent study demonstrated that as little as two minutes of exercise each day significantly alleviated shoulder and neck pain (ACSM 2011). And another encouraging study found that short sporadic activity (defined as incidental, non-purposeful physical activity that is accumulated through activities of daily living) was significantly beneficial (McGuire et al. 2011). Every little bit counts!

GETTING STARTED ON A LIFELONG COMMITMENT

Get Active in Daily Living

Kids are naturally active—squirming, running, and jumping. But as we get older our physical activity declines in spite of fast-paced living.

Unlike children, we need to consciously look for ways to increase our routine activity. Begin by asking how you can become more active in your daily living. For example, consider parking your car down the block from where you work to build in a ten-minute walk. When you factor in the return walk, you've just built twenty minutes of walking into your day. Add a ten-minute walk break during lunch and you've met the minimum level for physical fitness and its health benefits. Remember, ordinary activities do make a difference. (Of course conventional exercise, such as running or aerobics, can also be included.)

Get rid of energy-saving devices and invest in human energy that will help you increase your daily activities.

- Use a hand-push lawn mower, rather than a power-operated one.
- Take the stairs rather than the elevator or escalator.
- Walk your dog (or even consider getting one!).
- Ride your bike to work if you live close enough.

Make Movement Fun

Rather than focusing on fitness targets (like frequency and duration), a growing body of research shows that focusing on pleasure from exercise may be one of the most important factors in sustaining consistent activity. For some people the pleasure factor might mean exercising with a friend, family member, or trainer. It might be the one time of the day you can talk freely with a friend, uninterrupted. Or perhaps your days are so crazed with demands from other people that a little solitude would add to your exercise enjoyment.

One sure way to take the fun out of exercise is to get injured. Do be sure to start slowly in whatever activity you choose. Some further suggestions:

- Be sure to choose activities that you enjoy. Consider playing a team sport such as volleyball, basketball, or tennis.
- Do engage in a variety of activities—you need not dedicate your life to just one sport. By diversifying, you'll also decrease your chance of injuries and increase your enjoyment factor.
- If you exercise at home on stationary fitness equipment, add fun by watching your favorite television show or movie or reading a fun book or magazine (rather than work-related papers).
- Make your walk more enjoyable by listening to music, audio books, or podcasts on your phone.
- Get rid of apps or trackers that get you fixated on a number of calories or steps, etc., because it puts your focus on the numbers, rather than the enjoyment of the movement.

Make Movement a Nonnegotiable Priority

Ask yourself, "When can I consistently make the time to move my body?" Make an appointment with yourself, and honor it as you would any other meeting or appointment.

If you travel a lot:

- Pack your walking shoes. (It's an interesting way to get to know a new city.)
- Pack a jump rope. (It's a lightweight piece of equipment that delivers a cardio-wallop in a short amount of time.)
- Choose hotels that have workout facilities. (They are increasing in number.)
- Take advantage of airport layovers and walk around the airport. (It usually feels good after hours of sitting.)

Be Comfortable

Workout attire does not have to be fashion-show material, but it is important to wear clothes that breathe and allow you to move. This also means dressing for weather. Heavy sweats can make you uncomfortably hot when you wear them to disguise your body. An oversize lightweight T-shirt and leggings or bike shorts with an oversize shirt work well. It's exciting to see athletic apparel creating more activewear for larger bodies.

Don't forget about comfortable shoes as well. Not only will they feel good; they are an investment in injury prevention.

Include Strength Training and Stretching

Strength training helps rebuild muscle wear and tear from dieting. This is also important because our lean muscle mass declines as we get older. After the age of 30, adults lose 3–8% of their muscle mass per decade. (English & Paddon-Jones 2010). Americans lose an average of about 6.6 pounds of lean muscle mass for each decade of life. Therefore, someone who has been dieting for years is losing muscle tissue from both the process of aging *and* dieting. Remember, muscle is metabolically active tissue that helps keep your metabolism revved up. In fact, Bill Evans and Irwin Rosenberg, Tufts University researchers and the authors of *Biomarkers,* estimate that our metabolic rate decreases 2 percent each year from the age of twenty, and they attribute this downward shift of metabolism to decreasing muscle mass.

Ordinary activity, and even vigorous activity such as running, does not leave you immune to muscle-wasting due to age. A ten-year study following master runners (minimum age of forty) showed that while they maintained their fitness from running, they lost an average of 4.4 pounds of muscle from their untrained areas. Their muscles stayed the same size in their legs but decreased in their arms. There was an exception, however, for three runners who did upper-body weights. They were able to *maintain* their muscle weight in their upper body. Therefore, you don't have to lose your muscle mass.

Stretching helps prevent injuries and improve muscle performance, and keeps the tendons flexible, the latter of which is important as you age. Aging often results in substantial loss of tendon flexibility, which limits motion and increases risk for injury.

The American College of Sports Medicine recommends that strength training and flexibility become an integral part of a fitness program for *all* healthy adults (Garber et al. 2011). Specifically, they recommend:

- Strength training at least twice a week.
- One set of eight to twelve repetitions of eight to ten exercises for conditioning of each major muscle group.
- Stretch at least two or three days per week.

BEYOND PHYSICAL FITNESS

Is there anything wrong with wanting to work out more, to feel good? No. Just be careful that you do not fall into the dieting–weight loss trap, where you become a slave to working out and counting calories burned. We have found that increasing exercise can be a way to channel anxiety while becoming an Intuitive Eater. Intuitive Eating can feel foreign, and progress may feel slow in the beginning, especially when the world around you is dieting or extolling the latest food plan. Exercise allows you to feel that you are actively *doing* something to improve your health. You *feel* the benefits.

It's one thing to invest several hours in training if you are getting ready for a marathon or because you are an athlete. It's a problem, however, when exercise consumes you and begins to interfere with your everyday living.

Exercising more isn't necessarily better. How do you know if you are reaching the outer limits of exercise? Signs of *compulsive exercise* include:

- Inability to stop, even when you are sick or injured.
- Feeling guilty if you miss a single day.
- Inability to sleep at night—a sign of overtraining.
- Paying exercise penance for the perception of eating too much, such as running an extra three miles because you ate a piece of pie.
- Being afraid that you will suddenly gain weight if you stop for a single day.

RR—REMEMBER REST

The hardest lesson that I (ET) learned as a competitive marathoner was that rest was as important as training. It's also hard for our clients to recognize this tenet of training. Similarly, if for some reason you are unable to work out on a particular day, it does not mean that you will suddenly become unfit.

Some clients fear that once they stop exercising, they will not continue. That's the all-or-none thinking commonly seen in dieters. There's an easy way to prove to yourself that no exercise today does not mean no exercise forever. Simply resume exercise when you are able. The more you reinitiate an exercise program after a break from it, the more confidence you will have in your ability to continue exercising, even if it's been a few days. After a while it stops being a big issue or worry. Besides, this time it's different. You are not dieting, therefore, it will be much easier to resume training.

Remember, a few days or weeks of no exercise will not make or break your health. After a significant illness, Diane, a client, had to stop exercising. But for the first time, Diane knew that although weeks had passed, it wasn't a big deal. She knew she'd be lacing up her walking shoes again in the near future. Diane missed the stress relief; she missed the freedom from the kids. But she also knew that she had to rebuild her health. Her missed exercise did not become a crisis, and her body was allowed the time it needed to heal.

Sometimes taking care of yourself means choosing *not* to exercise. For example, if you only got four hours of sleep and exercising meant rising at five in the morning, it's best to take that day off. Remember, rest is important. Likewise, if you feel a cold coming on, or you're feeling worn out, take a day off. Listen to your body. Rest will also help keep exercise feeling fresh and fun.

MINDFUL EXERCISE

You can integrate exercise recommendations for health while being attuned to the experience of your body. This type of physical activity is called "mindful exercise," a concept championed by Rachel Calogero and Kelly Pedrotty (2007). Mindful exercise is processed-based and has four components:

- Enhances the mind-body connection and coordination and does not confuse or deregulate it.
- Alleviates mental and physical stress and does not contribute to and amplify stress.
- Provides genuine enjoyment and pleasure and is not used for punitive reasons.
- Is used to rejuvenate the body, not to exhaust or deplete it.

Approaching physical activity with mindfulness helps you to experience your body. When you pay attention to how your body feels, before, during, and after exercise, it helps with attunement. The primary focus is to connect with how your body feels during exercise and to listen to your body's signals indicating fatigue, pain, and when to stop.

When the pursuit of exercise is about feeling good, not about calories burned, or used as a penance for eating, it becomes enjoyable and sustainable.

Chapter 15

PRINCIPLE 10:

Honor Your Health with Gentle Nutrition

Make food choices that honor your health and taste buds while making you feel good. Remember that you don't have to eat perfectly to be healthy. You will not suddenly get a nutrient deficiency or become unhealthy from one snack, one meal, or one day of eating. It's what you eat consistently over time that matters—progress, not perfection, is what counts.

> *We will not be healthier, both psychologically and physically, about our food until we learn to love it more, not less . . . with a relaxed, generous, unashamed emotion. In the process, it may be that we will have to redefine fundamentally the concept of "eating well."*
> —Michelle Stacey, author of *Consumed: Why Americans Love, Hate, and Fear Food*

I keep thinking that someday I'm going to walk in here and you're going to tell me the food party is over." We hear this fear a lot. It's one of the reasons that nutrition is discussed with our clients much later in the Intuitive Eating process, rather than sooner. It's also the reason that *honor your health* is the last principle of Intuitive Eating. You can hardly talk about health and taking care of yourself without discussing nutrition. But our experience has shown us that if a healthy relationship with food is not in place, it's difficult to truly pursue healthy eating. If you've been a chronic dieter or immersed in some form of diet culture, the best nutrition guidelines can still be embraced like a diet.

We don't want to give the impression that just because nutrition is reserved for the last principle of Intuitive Eating, it's not important. We certainly value health. Don't worry, though; we are not going to pull the food carpet from under you.

The role of nutrition in preventing chronic disease has been established by the scientific community. But there are still many other important factors affecting health and longevity, that have an even *more* profound impact—such as:

• *Social Connection*, which includes the quality of your relationships, loneliness, and feeling socially connected to the people in your life. Social connection is associated with a decreased risk in all-cause mortality, as well as a range of diseases. For those of you skeptical of this significance, consider that: psychosocial risk factors are a stronger risk for heart disease than inflammation markers in the blood. Furthermore, social isolation was found to be more lethal than smoking fifteen cigarettes a day according to research published by Julianne Holt-Lunstad of Brigham Young University.

• *Adverse Childhood Experiences (ACEs)*, which are potentially traumatic events that occur in childhood, like growing up with domestic abuse or having a parent with substance abuse. According to the Centers for Disease Control (CDC) at least 5 of the top 10 leading causes of death are associated with ACEs.

• *Social determinants of health* are economic and social conditions that influence the health of people, including these factors: poverty, racism, where you live, having access to healthcare and clean water.

The over-emphasis of nutrition has served to breed a nation of "guilty" eaters—feeling the need to apologize for eating a traditional Thanksgiving meal or a rich dessert. To put this in perspective, the CDC estimates that genes, biology, and health behaviors together account for about 25% of population health.

FOOD WORRY

Our whole culture needs a food attitude adjustment. You don't have to be a chronic dieter to be worried about food. Almost daily there is a new headline or cover story on a nutrition-related topic, from killer biotech foods to research proclaiming that margarine is no better than butter (and may be even worse). At best, the dueling headlines get you confused, and at worst, they contribute to a growing food phobia. With special-interest groups massaging the media, the fear is magnified. Add the food companies that climb onto any nutritional bandwagon that furthers their economic cause, and you get one nation of confused and worried consumers.

The medical nutrition research, as it's reported in the media, easily creates the impression that food will either kill you or heal you. This fuels the fire of magical thinking with food. No wonder some people erroneously believe that drinking a mixture of apple cider vinegar, honey, and cayenne pepper will burn off fat, or that special food combination will raise metabolism. This just isn't so.

Ironically, nutrition stories that blow the whistle on misleading food product ads unintentionally create more fear of food. The message to the consumer is that you can't trust the food companies, or the food label—you've been duped. If you are worried about what's in your food, how can you begin to enjoy it? If you believe that a magical food or pill is around the corner to solve your problems, why would you even look inward for the answers? If you don't trust what's in your food, and have trouble trusting your body's inner signals for eating, how can you begin to eat healthfully without guilt or trepidation?

In tandem with the growing anxiety over food selection, there is a new type of eating disorder that has emerged in recent years called orthorexia, which is characterized by an unhealthy and rigid obsession with eating healthfully. While it's not officially recognized as a medical diagnosis, physician and author Steven Bratman, MD, called attention to this problem in his book *Health Food Junkies—Orthorexia Nervosa: Overcoming the Obsession with Healthful Eating.*

A young case of orthorexia. A few years ago, a ten-year-old who was terrified of eating trans fats came in for nutrition counseling. Part of her treatment was to sit down and eat a Ding Dong during one of her sessions in the office. Can you imagine a dietitian eating a Ding Dong with her client? But this girl needed the opportunity to create a healthier relationship with food by observing a health professional she respected eating a Ding Dong. She began to realize that she wouldn't end up with a clogged artery by eating one Ding Dong!

Contrary to popular belief, nutrition science is not set in stone. Research is a slow, evolutionary process of gathering and validating data, which often overturns widely held theories. Here are a couple of landmark examples:

• The cause of 80 to 90 percent of ulcers is a bacterium called *H. pylori*. But up until that discovery in 1982, food was thought to be a contributing cause, resulting in a diet prescription of bland eating.
• For decades, polyunsaturated fats (PUFA) have been heralded as "heart healthy," but a critical analysis of the data showed that a particular type of PUFA may actually increase heart disease risk (Ramsden et al. 2010).

Similarly, you might believe that eating rich, fatty foods would automatically lead to heart disease. Or perhaps you believe that to be fit, you need to eat a "perfect" diet of "clean" spartan cuisine. Not so. If you keep in mind that the science of nutrition is regularly evolving, you won't get stuck in the belief that you have to choose a perfect array of foods. After all, if information is regularly changing, there can be no "perfect way to eat"!

Before getting into specific nutrition information that may be of interest to some and may be a section to postpone for others, let's take a look at what we can learn from other cultures.

Americans Are Number One in Worrying About Food

"Food worry" has not served the health status of Americans. In fact, it may have an opposite effect. Food psychologist Paul Rozin and his research team, from the University of Pennsylvania, conducted a study of four countries and found that the French are the most food-pleasure-oriented and the least health-oriented (1999). In contrast, Americans had the worst of both worlds: they had the greatest worry over their health and eating, and greater dissatisfaction with what they ate. Americans scored the highest on worrying about the "fattening effects" of food.

Rozin was way ahead of his time and concluded that the negative impact of *worry and stress* over healthy eating may have a more profound effect on health than the actual food consumed. Indeed, it is widely accepted that stress triggers a biological chemical assault in our bodies, which is harmful to our health (McEwen 2008).

France and the Pleasure Principle of Health

The French have a longer life expectancy, take less medication, and have a markedly lower rate of heart disease. (See table 6, "Health Indicators in France Versus the United States.") Yet the French eat a diet that appears to be less than healthy. This health paradox is popularly known as the French paradox. Notably, France has the highest per-capita dairy fat consumption (think cream, butter, and cheese) of any industrial nation (Guyenet 2008).

Less publicized, but just as important, the French have fewer eating disorders and don't engage in dieting as much as Americans. Despite this fact, in 2010, the *New York Times* reported that Jenny Craig planned to open diet centers in France. Unbelievably, the CEO of Jenny Craig, France, believes that Americans have credibility for weight loss! We hope that France's strong aversion to Americanized foods will protect the French people from going down that dieting path.

While it has been speculated that wine consumption and eating smaller portions of food may explain the French paradox, we believe it could be the relationship that the French have with food. The French have a more positive attitude toward eating—it is viewed as one of life's pleasures, not as poison. Food is not revolting; instead, it's something to be revered. Perhaps this is why our clients who have traveled to France, *even before working with the Intuitive Eating process,* describe that they had discovered how much they enjoyed their eating experience and their celebration of food without the worry.

The French pay more attention to the sensory qualities of food, eat for a significantly longer period of time, while eating less—thus creating a more satisfying food experience. Even when the French eat fast food, they take more time to eat, compared to the eating pace of Americans (Rozin et al. 2003). They also cultivate the pleasures of the palate at a very early age. For example, public childcare centers in Paris provide three-course meals for their tots. Can you imagine an American toddler sitting down to braised lamb served with cauliflower au gratin, and enjoying every bite? That's a typical entrée for the French toddlers, who joyfully ate that meal on the day that National Public Radio interviewed the dietitian responsible for the 270 public daycare centers in Paris (Beardsley 2009).

Interestingly, research has shown that the medical practices of French versus American physicians reflect their culture. Consequently, American physicians prescribe more medication, while the French physicians are inclined to suggest rest, vacations, or a stay at a spa (Rozin 1999).

TABLE 6. HEALTH INDICATORS IN FRANCE VERSUS THE UNITED STATES

	United States	France
[a]Life expectancy (rounded to the nearest year)	78 years	81 years
[a]Dollars (U.S. equivalent) spent on medication per capita	$897	$607
[b]Heart disease death rates (per 100,000 people)		
Women	79	21
Men	145	54
[c]Incidence of dieting (% of total population)	26%	16%
[d]Use of light foods and beverages (% of total population)	76%	48%
[d]Consumption of low-fat products (% of total population)	68%	39%
[e]Duration of minutes eating at McDonald's	14 minutes	22 minutes

[a]*OECD Factbook 2010*. [b]OECD Health Data 2009. [c]*Calorie Control Commentary*, 14(1):1–2, 1992. [d]Adapted from Calorie Control Council National Surveys. [e]Rozin 2003.

What We Can Learn from Nutritional Outliers

Despite all that we currently know about nutrition, there are instances in which even the most "unhealthy" food intake does not have a negative effect on people's health.

The Roseto Effect. A remarkable discovery by physician Stewart Wolf found a strikingly low incidence of heart disease and deaths from heart attacks, spanning three generations, in a small Italian immigrant community located in Roseto, Pennsylvania (Stout et al. 1964; Wolf et al. 1994; Egolf et al. 1992). Even more astonishing was the discovery that it wasn't diet that was protecting their heart health. To the contrary, Rosetans embraced westernized foods and cooking, at the expense of their Italian-Mediterranean culinary roots. For example, Rosetans:

- Shunned olive oil, and used lard instead, as the main fat for cooking.
- Dipped their bread in a lard-based gravy, rather than olive oil.
- Ate Italian ham, including its one-inch rim of fat.

The distinguishing protector of their heart health and longevity was found to be social cohesion and social support. This paradoxical discovery became known as the Roseto Effect, and it inspired author Malcolm Gladwell to write his bestselling book *Outliers*. Once again, as with the French, the effect of positive emotional experiences can have a greater impact on health than which foods people actually eat.

Olympic Swimmer: Poster Boy for "Junk Food" Diet

Champion swimmer Michael Phelps made global headlines—not just for his record-shattering, perfect eight-for-eight gold medal performances in the 2008 Olympics. The quality of his food choices also captured the rapt attention of the media. For example, Phelps's typical meals included the following foods:

- **Breakfast:** Fried egg sandwiches, loaded with cheese, fried onions, and mayonnaise.
- **Lunch:** One pound of enriched pasta. Large ham and cheese sandwiches, with mayonnaise, on white bread.
- **Dinner:** An entire pizza and one pound of pasta.

And while his large caloric intake (twelve thousand calories) was no surprise to sports nutritionists, the quality of Phelps's diet was criticized.

A two-page photo spread in *People* magazine, with Phelps in his Olympic Speedo, surrounded by the foods he typically eats, is quite an image. Phelps appears as if he is a poster boy for eating a diet of nutritionally questionable foods. This visual aid has helped many of our clients. When clients see this photo spread and examine it carefully, they are asked, "If foods that some people call junk food could automatically make someone unhealthy—why can Phelps perform so well, eating foods like these?"

The point in this example is to remove the power of the widely perceived belief that eating a particular food will automatically make you unhealthy and unfit—that food is either good or bad. There seems to be a prevalent fear that "I'm one bite away from _____" (a heart attack, getting cancer, and so on). Unless you have a lethal food allergy or a medical condition, such as celiac disease—one bite of food, one meal, or one day of eating will not make or break your health or fitness. Phelps is a good example of the latter.

Paul Rozin, the food psychologist, believes that a key contributing factor to the good-food/bad-food belief is the availability of studies reported by the media. These studies have not been accompanied by education of the basic concepts of probability, risks and benefits, and the difference between cause and association. The average consumer takes these findings as facts, especially when deleterious effects of eating a certain food are reported. In order to take the uncertainty out of every bite, people tend to develop a reductionist belief—that food is either good or bad. Rozin says this type of belief establishes a goal that is both extremely unhealthy and unattainable.

WHAT ABOUT NUTRITION BY THE NUMBERS?

Consider that for nearly two decades, there has been nutrition information on just about every food label, due to the 1990 Nutrition Labeling and Education Act. Yet this has given rise to a cultural obsession with food and body. It's no wonder that eating disorders have doubled, with a growing rise in orthorexia and disordered eating. There's even more nutrition information available today, thanks to the internet and smart phone apps.

"Nutritionism," a concept created by Dr. Gyorgy Scrinis, describes how the overly reductive focus on nutrients in food undermines *how we think about food, how we view the experiences of our own bodies, and how we understand the relationship between food and our bodie*s (2008).

Nutritionism seems to have its roots in an historical misstep. During World War II, the U.S. government formed two committees to jointly help navigate the consequences of food shortages, while trying to ensure the nutritional adequacy of Americans. Anthropologist Margaret Mead led one of those committees, the Committee on Food Habits.

When the war was over, the government discontinued Mead's committee (that's the misstep), while its counterpart remained—the Food and Nutrition Board, which still exists today. Nutrition scientists on that board are entrusted to define and update food and nutrition policy guidelines—but it lacks the social and psychological expertise around eating, which the Committee on Food Habits imparted. We can't help but wonder if this vital missing piece has contributed to the rise of nutritionism, healthism, and the weight stigma that proliferate today.

Unfortunately, we see nutritionism and the perpetuation of weight stigma in many government health policies. The 2015–2020 Dietary Guidelines for Americans is a prime example, which is framed with an emphasis on calories and body weight.

Ultimately, the nutritionism ideology has only served to add a lot of anxiety to grocery shopping and food selection. Our experience has shown that the more a person focuses on a number, the more it interferes with the process of listening to the body.

Eating healthfully should feel good, both physically and psychologically, ultimately resulting in a satisfying experience. But we've lost sight of that feeling, due to the food phobia and fatphobia that's sweeping the country. Michelle Stacey, author of *Consumed: Why Americans Love, Hate, and Fear Food,* concludes that Americans need to change their eating attitude to enlightened hedonism: a balance between information and pleasure, an educated hedging of bets. That's how we approach nutrition and food.

MAKING PEACE WITH NUTRITION:
ACHIEVING AUTHENTIC HEALTH

Critics express concern that encouraging people to eat what they want will lead them to eat with abandon, resulting in poor nutrition. The underlying belief is that self-monitoring is essential for keeping appetite under control. It is thought that without this vigilance, people would make nutritionally poor choices, including eating to excess. Instead, studies show Intuitive Eating is associated with improved nutrient intake, eating a wider variety of food, and reduced eating disorder symptomatology.

Eating Healthfully Feels Good. When you remove the overlay of guilt and morality from eating, it allows you to really feel the physical sensations that you derive from eating. Many of our clients unknowingly create a somatization of guilt from their eating experience. This occurs when the *feelings* of guilt arise, in tandem, with the unpleasant *physical sensations* of eating without attunement. It becomes an intertwined union of uncomfortable feelings from guilt *and* the discomfort from eating, joined into one physical experience. When you know you can truly eat whatever food or meals you want, without guilt, why would you choose to feel physically uncomfortable?

Here is one of my (ET) favorite stories that illustrates how eating healthfully simply feels good. My son was in his rebellious teenage phase and had spent an entire day at an amusement park. When he came home, he rushed into the kitchen and said, "Mom, I ate junky today, will you make me something extra healthy for dinner?" This was not a boy trying to please his mom (or score points). Nor was he uber-health-conscious—he just knew how it *felt* to eat healthy and was seeking that experience for his next meal.

What Is Healthy Eating? We define healthy eating as having a healthy balance of foods *and* having a healthy relationship with food. Of course, there is a nutritional difference between eating an apple versus a piece of apple pie. Having a healthy relationship with food means you are not morally superior or inferior based on your eating choices. It means that both foods have emotional equivalency. Eating selection is not a reflection of your character. Throughout the book, we've focused on the healthy relationship part, because there's been a big whopping gap in American eating that leaves out this important concern.

Intuitive Eating is a dynamic attunement process of your mind, body, and food. The majority of Intuitive Eating principles (1 through 8) deal with attunement to your inner world, which is informed by the inner workings of your mind and body. The inner world includes your thoughts, feelings, beliefs, and physical sensations arising from within your body (such as hunger and satiety cues).

Achieving "authentic health" is a process of dynamic integration of your inner world and the external world of health guidelines, which include exercise and nutrition. You decide if and what of the external world you'd like to integrate, ultimately, to achieve "authentic health." The external world includes health policy (usually a consensus from experts, based on a body of research, which is often misdiagnosed). The external world

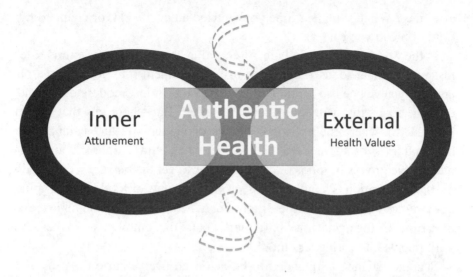

Intuitive Eating: The Dynamic Integration Between Inner Attunement and External Health Values to Achieve Authentic Health *Adapted with permission from Catherine Cooke-Cottone, SUNY Buffalo*

can also include philosophical preferences, such as a desire to eat locally grown foods with a low carbon footprint. If you are truly inner-attuned, you can integrate an external value while paying attention to hunger, fullness, satisfaction, and so forth. If, however, you enter this realm too soon, there is a risk that the new mindset will be embraced as another rigid set of rules.

Food Wisdom Tenets

No doubt you've heard for years of the nutritional merits of variety, moderation, and balance. There's a reason these nutrition mantras have been chanted for decades: they work! It's one of the best ways to hedge your bets for healthy eating. But "eat a variety of foods" sounds like "wear a sensible pair of shoes"—practical but easily ignored advice. A study looking at diet diversity has gotten those sensible shoes tap dancing in the spotlight of health. According to a study reported in the *American Journal of Clinical Nutrition,* adults who ate foods from two or fewer food groups were associated with an excess mortality risk of 50 percent in men and 40 percent in women. But how often do you eat the same meal day after day? When's the last time you've tried a new cereal, or changed the kind of bread you eat?

In the world of dieting and macro-counting, it may seem easier and safer just to eliminate foods rather than to balance them into your meals. Or perhaps you've been so afraid that you couldn't eat just moderate amounts of some foods that you shun them altogether. But where has that gotten you? Here's where the nutritional tenets of moderation and balance can help you. First of all, moderation does not mean elimination. If you eliminate whole groups of foods, it can be harder to get the nutrients your body needs. Moderation is simply eating various amounts of food without going to extremes of either too little or too much. Moderation is also an average over time. Unfortunately, we have seen sneaky diet culture use this term to guilt people into eating less food!

Second, balance is intended to be achieved over a period of time—it does not have to be at each and every meal. Your body does not punch a time clock. Most nutrition recommendations are intended to be an *average* over time, not for a single meal or a single day, and with good reason. You will not suddenly get a nutrient deficiency if you did not eat enough in one day. Similarly, you will not make or break your health from one meal or even one day of eating. It is consistency over time that matters. Our bodies are remarkably adaptable. Here are a few examples:

- If you eat too little iron or calcium, the body starts to absorb *more* of it.
- If you take in too much vitamin C, the body begins to excrete more of it.
- If you eat too little, the body slows its need for calories.

We'd like to suggest another tenet: progress, not perfection. You don't have to eat perfectly to be healthy. This is progress in having a flexible mindset. Regardless of your food choice, however, all foods can offer satisfaction.

In Matters of Nutrition, Consider Taste, Quantity, and Quality

Taste. Eating nutritiously does not have to be about deprivation, although that's what many Americans fear. The problem is that healthy eating for many people has been clouded with regrettable food experiences. How often have you heard, for example, "You'll get used to it," which really means that the food tastes so bad you have to condition yourself to like it! Or, how many times were you told as a child, "Eat your vegetables, then you can have dessert"—which really means that vegetables are so difficult to eat that you deserve a reward for choking them down. Or maybe you've experienced:

- Inferior "new healthy foods"—from food companies scrambling to capitalize on the latest nutrition trend—from fat-free to gluten-free. Rubbery fat-free mozzarella and cream cheese that resembles a caulking agent hardly foster enthusiasm for healthy eating.
- Pretending—where you close your eyes (and taste buds) and pretend that what you are eating is a terrific substitute for what you'd *really* like to be eating. For example, whipping a few ice cubes in a blender with a diet hot chocolate mix and calling it a milkshake—hardly! Or adorning applesauce with graham cracker crumbs and pretending it's apple pie—James Beard is probably rolling in his grave!

The combination of taste atrocities in the name of healthy eating, with the emerging fear of food in the United States, prompted Julia Child to take action in the late 1980s. She spearheaded a revolutionary project through the American Institute of Wine and Food (AIWF) called "Resetting the American Table: Creating a New Alliance of Taste and Health." This venture joined together opinion leaders from both the culinary (taste) world and health community, with the mission to move Americans toward healthier eating, without having to give up the pleasures of the table. Early in my (ET) career, I was fortunate to be included on this task force, which had a big influence on how I work.

Julia's task force had two key conclusions:

1. Negative, restrictive approaches to eating do not work.
2. People need to be steered toward a healthy diet they can live with, *without guilt*. (The italics are our emphasis.)

Ultimately, the key message from the task force was, "In matters of taste, consider nutrition, and in matters of nutrition, consider taste." If a food aficionado can consider nutrition without compromising their gastronomic palate, so can you! We call this approach *gentle nutrition*. Taste is important, but health is still honored, without guilt.

Quantity Issues: Not Too Much—Not Too Little

Portion control is not an issue for Intuitive Eaters. Many public health policy makers consider the inflated size of food portions to be problematic. But if people were truly attuned to hunger, fullness, and satisfaction, it wouldn't matter if they were served a twenty-pound steak or a gallon of ice cream. That's because Intuitive Eaters would stop eating when comfortably satisfied—there would just be a lot more leftovers.

We acknowledge that it's easy to bypass fullness if you are eating while distracted, have a history of food insecurity, or are new to recovering from diet culture. Eating without distraction is especially important for emerging Intuitive Eaters. But, of course, it doesn't need to be done perfectly. Only you can determine where you are in this process.

Eat enough—not too little. Clearly you need to eat. Remember that to stoke your metabolic fire, you need wood, not just kindling. For many of our clients, this means eating more of some foods than they are used to, especially carbohydrates. You may be thinking, "Forget eating more, I'll just exercise." But, as we explained in chapter 14, exercise will not prevent metabolic damage from undereating, even for athletes. In a small study, scientists at the University of British Columbia in Canada studied fourteen competitive female rowers. Half of them were weight-cyclers—another word for dieters. During the study, the weight-cyclers (aka dieters) lost weight during the four weeks leading up to their national championships. Consequently, their metabolic rates plummeted by about 7 percent. They also lost over six pounds of fat-free body mass (primarily muscle). In this particular study, the rowers were fortunate and were able to get back their previous metabolic rate, *when they began eating more.* If athletes can lose precious muscle from undereating, why would you be any different? Remember, the more muscle you have, the higher your metabolic rate. It is one reason that men need more energy intake than women; they naturally have more muscle.

How do you make peace with feeding your body? This is a scary prospect for most of our clients. To help you overcome this fear, keep reminding yourself that by feeding your body you are feeding your metabolism, which will allow you to eat more food, with all the nutrients your food provides. This is a win-win!

Quality Issues

Some people are eager to hear what the nutrition community is recommending in the realm of food to promote optimal health. So, we'll offer suggestions. Please be sure to take out of the following sections what suits you and be sure to let go of any guilt feelings that might emerge if you find that this information triggers any discomfort. In fact, if you find yourself being triggered while reading this section, it might be best to skip this chapter until you truly feel ready. It's really okay! Remember, we are not pulling the rug out from under you and suddenly telling you what we think you *should* eat. We are simply providing information for those who would like to learn more about nutrition.

Eat enough fruits and vegetables. People who eat higher amounts of fruits and vegetables have lower risks of many chronic diseases, especially cancer. In almost every study looking at plant food and people (more than two hundred studies to date), plant food is associated with lowering the risk of cancer. These foods are loaded with antioxidants and fiber, which offer many other health benefits. There is a growing body of research that shows fruits and vegetables have special food factors, called phytochemicals, that have added health benefits. See the chart on page 244.

There are hundreds and maybe even thousands of phytochemicals. Research is just scratching the surface on their health benefits. This is one reason why we can't rely on getting all of our nutrition in a bottle. You can't manufacture compounds that have yet to be identified and put them into a supplement!

One problem we've seen with our chronic dieters is that they've been "veggied out." For example, nearly every diet regimen prescribes celery and carrot sticks as the safe and approved snack of choice. If that's your case, ask yourself how you can incorporate vegetables (and fruit) in a manner that's *pleasing* and does not smack of a weight loss diet, such as adding grated carrots to a favorite pasta sauce. Think of possible ways in which you can eat fruits and vegetables as a built-in component to a meal, such as:

- Vegetable lasagna
- Ratatouille
- Potato pancakes spiced with various chopped vegetables

Phytochemical	Plant Food	Potential Benefit
Limonene	Citrus fruits	Helps increase enzymes that get rid of cancer-causing agents.
Sulforaphanes	Cruciferous vegetables: broccoli, cauliflower, Brussels sprouts, cabbage	Helps amplify the body's own defense against chemicals that can lead to cancer.
Allyl sulfides	Leeks, garlic, onion, chives	Increases the production of enzymes that make it easier for the body to excrete cancer-causing compounds.
Ellagic acid	Grapes	Scavenges carcinogens and may prevent them from altering the body's DNA.

- Stir-fried vegetables on rice
- Stuffed baked squash
- Stuffed peppers
- Stuffed baked potatoes
- Fajitas (they're usually loaded with vitamin-rich peppers)
- Pancakes topped with a fresh fruit medley
- Fruit compote
- Fruit smoothie

One client, Sally, was averse to fruit, though she didn't know why; she just had trouble eating it. But one day she found she was having no difficulties whatsoever. What had changed? Two things. First, she was rid of her diet mentality and second, she began eating fruit in a "non-diet" manner. All of her past diets had prescribed eating a spartan single fruit for a snack or with a meal, such as a plum, an apple, and so forth. When she tried fruit salads of all sorts and fruit smoothies, her interest in fruit was renewed.

Frankly, we've never seen anyone get into trouble eating fresh fruits and vegetables (unless that's all they eat, or they have an eating disorder). In fact, research results also show this to be true. John Potter, a physician and researcher out of the University of Minnesota, has been studying a group of people who were told to eat up to eight servings a day of fruits and vegetables. His data suggests that people eating more fruits and vegetables actually like it and *feel better doing it.*

Eat enough grains, preferably half of which are whole. Grains (especially whole grains) are a rich source of carbohydrates, fiber, and B vitamins.

Eat enough fish. There is a bounty of research that shows a multitude of benefits from eating seafood—from improved mood to lower risk of chronic diseases. This health benefit prompted the 2010 U.S. Dietary Guidelines to include a recommendation for eating fish, and while not as prominent in the 2015–2020 Guidelines, fish consumption is still encouraged.

Drink enough fluids—primarily water. Water actually doubles as both a beverage and a nutrient. Water is essential for living—we can only survive a few days without it. We included it because it often gets overlooked. The need for getting plenty of fluids is no secret, but many of our clients wind up short in this department. The traditional 8-ounce cups of fluid a day is the same as drinking a half gallon (that's the size of your typical milk carton). Other fluids, such as milk, coffee, and tea, can help meet your water quotient.

The issue of processed foods. Generally, the less a food is processed, the more nutrients are retained, and less sodium and sugar are added. If possible, choose the following types of foods to eat more often:

• Nutrient-dense foods: These foods naturally provide more nutrients per bite. These include: whole grains, beans, fish, avocado, nuts, and calcium-rich foods, such as milk, cheese, yogurt, and calcium-fortified soy milk.

• Protein-rich foods: Eat a variety of these foods. They include beans, seafood, chicken, turkey, nuts, eggs, and lean meats. In addition to its role in building and maintaining muscles and hormones, protein helps provide a feeling of fullness.

• Quality fats: Fat is also a nutrient required by the body. Notably, when the essentiality of fats was first discovered, they were called "vitamin F" (Evans et al. 1928). Too bad this nomenclature didn't stick—if it had, it would help remind people that we do need some fat in our diet. We need fat in our diet for a number of reasons, including making neurotransmitter receptors, to promote satiety, and to help absorb fat-soluble nutrients, such as vitamins A, E, and D. The brain is made up of mostly fat and functions best with omega-3 fats, which are found in seafood, fish oil, algae, and seaweed. Other quality fats include olive oil, avocado, nuts, seeds, flaxseed oil, and canola oil. And for satisfaction purposes, fat is the molecule that gives flavor to foods and promotes satiety.

• Whole foods: These are the unprocessed foods, which include, for example: brown rice, oatmeal, millet, beans, quinoa, and fresh fruits and vegetables.

A Word About Food and Diet Trends

Vegetarianism. Before we get into trends that could be problematic, many people have moved toward vegetarianism. As long as you are conscious of supplying enough protein each day, you will be able to get in all the nutrients you need, if you choose this path. If you are a lacto-ovo vegetarian, and dairy and eggs are complete protein sources, while beans and nuts will offer protein, which, when combined with grains and vegetables, will offer a sufficient amount of protein in the day.

We have witnessed the popular pendulum swing from eating fat-free to carb-free, and when viewed as a trend, it's easier to unpack the inherent problems they bring.

The fat-free trap. Back in the 1980s and '90s, low-fat eating was very popular. The low-fat message went to extreme levels for many chronic dieters and created the fat-free trap. Dietary fat was viewed as the national enemy, which spawned a profitable cottage industry of fat-free foods—from fat-free cheese to fat-free potato chips and ice cream.

One of the most common problems created was the idea that "if it's fat-free, it doesn't count, I can eat as much as I want." The problem with this thinking is that it is a form of disconnected eating, which can lead to overeating. Instead of responding to satiety levels, it often becomes an eating affair—"I'm going to eat it all." When inner satiety cues are bypassed, it perpetuates further dissonance from your body. In addition, *fat-free does not mean calorie-free*. Ironically, during that era, many of our clients discovered that if they were to have the real version of a food, they'd end up eating much less, because it's more satisfying, and they would remain in touch with satiety cues.

Many of the fat-free products are low in whole grains and, thus, low in fiber. For example, Rice Krispies cereal used to proclaim on its label that it's always been fat-free. But it's also always been low in fiber. If your prime mission in eating is selecting processed fat-free foods, you could easily end up with a nutritionally weak diet. There's nothing wrong with eating fat-free foods as an adjunct to a healthy diet. But you cannot assume that just because you've been eating 100 percent fat-free foods, your diet is healthy.

The carb-free trap. The fat-free pendulum swung from exonerating fat to demonizing carbohydrates in just about all forms. So here are a couple of key points to consider:

- The brain uses carbohydrates exclusively as a fuel. Your brain needs carbs!
- Several large studies have found that low-carbohydrate diets are associated with early deaths from all causes and more health problems! For example, a meta-analysis study by Mazidi and colleagues (2019) found that folks eating the lowest amount of carbohydrates had the highest risk of heart disease, cancer, and stroke.

So where's the chocolate group? As we have said, we're not going to pull a fast one. There are no forbidden foods, because deprivation doesn't work. All of the above guidelines are intended as a balance over time—which means even if you eat a candy bar, it will eventually average out. When you have let go of the diet mentality and have made peace with food, you will discover that you sometimes have a desire for food that has few nutritionally redemptive powers. We call this food *play food.* We prefer this term to one of the most commonly used terms to describe what's considered unhealthy foods—junk food. The term "junk food" implies that there is no intrinsic value in this food—in fact, that it probably should be thrown in the garbage can. But we feel that this thinking is unwarranted. There are times when a piece of red velvet cake or a stick of licorice is just the food that will satisfy your taste buds. And eating these types of foods doesn't mean you are an unhealthy eater. Here's a favorite story I (ER) like to tell that illustrates this point.

One day, when my son was a teenager, he asked me, "Mom, what happens to people who don't eat as healthfully as you do?" His question sparked a sense of pride in me that, as a nutritionist, I had taught him the virtues of healthy eating. My response to him included some lofty comments about how people who didn't pay much attention to nutrition probably had a higher incidence of heart disease, diabetes, cancer, and so forth. But before I could get the words fully out of my mouth, he pointed to me with his best adolescent "got you" finger and said, "But sometimes I see *you* eating French fries and other junk foods!" I had to stop and laugh for a moment and then said, "You're right, honey. Much of what I eat considers my health, and sometimes I eat things just for pleasure." I explained that for true satisfaction in my eating, those foods that he called junk can be part of balanced eating. From that point on, the term "junk food" has been replaced with "play food" for its role in the world of eating satisfaction.

But how can eating play foods be healthy? This is where you pull together all the Intuitive Eating skills, which means, in a nutshell, listening to your body. This is key. For example, if you were to eat chocolate all day long, there's a very good chance that by the end of the day, you would experience the following physical feelings: nausea, heaviness, dullness, and so forth. The question to you is, do you want to continue feeling this way? The truth is, if you listen to your body, you will not feel good eating this way. Even kids exposed to gobs of Halloween candy do not want to eat it endlessly. And when you know that you can truly have the food again (chocolate, or whatever else), it doesn't take too much to satisfy you. The bottom line is that we want to make all foods emotionally equivalent, even if they're not nutritionally equivalent.

One client, Joe, was extremely fond of chocolate. He had truly made peace with food and was also at the stage of honoring his health. He was grocery shopping and discovered a new *triple* chocolate ice cream dessert, which was very rich. He chose not to buy it, not because it was loaded with fat, but because he did not want to experience what he calls headache food. He did not feel deprived; he knew he could have chocolate whenever he wished, and instead bought a bag of M&Ms and was satisfied.

Making Informed Food Choices

Clients often ask us if there is any value in knowing the nutrient content of food. The answer to this question can be tricky. If you have any remnant of diet mentality lingering in your mind, looking at a food label might trigger some of your old diet thoughts. If, on the other hand, your food choices are based on deriving satisfaction from your meal, then having a general sense of the nutrient content of foods—such as fiber, fat, and sodium—can help guide your eating decisions.

For example, if you know that including high-fiber foods in your meals will be beneficial to the functioning of your gastrointestinal tract, and you notice that one type of whole wheat bread is higher in fiber than another, then by all means choose the higher-fiber product. Using nutrition information in this manner helps to honor both your palate and your health.

Or suppose you discover for the first time that a particular canned soup is very high in sodium, and you're concerned that it might have an adverse affect on your blood pressure. You may feel that you could take or leave the soup, because you don't enjoy it that much and wouldn't feel deprived by choosing a lower-sodium soup. You might also decide that, if you were going to eat something high in sodium, you'd rather have pizza! Or perhaps you discover that a beverage you drink contains a high amount of sugar, and you would equally enjoy mineral water—then, by all means, opt for the mineral water.

There may come a time in your journey back to your Intuitive Eater when eating with regard to nutritional quality becomes a priority for you. The key to knowing if you're ready for that decision is based on the following:

- In making your food choices, are you considering the sensual qualities of the food, while at the same time honoring how you will physically feel when you eat this food?
- Do you have a medical condition that will be helped by paying attention to nutrition? Intuitive Eating can integrate medical nutrition therapy, but you might find it helpful to work with a registered dietitian nutritionist who is trained in both to help you.
- Does thinking about nutrition feel neutral to you, rather than stirring up any old diet thoughts?
- Are you able to choose a food that may not have a high nutritional value, but will simply give you pleasure, without any old guilt feelings?

If you can answer yes to these questions, then making choices based on health and nutrition will not betray your ability to be an Intuitive Eater.

How to Keep the Pleasure in Healthy Eating

If we are to change our eating attitudes to enlightened hedonism, we need to balance information with the pleasure of eating. The information part comes from two sources: listening to your body and the nutrition guidelines we shared in this chapter. Listening to your body means not only staying in touch with satiety levels, but also assessing the following questions:

- Do I really like the taste of these foods, or am I being a diet/ health martyr?
- How does eating this food or type of meal make my body feel? Do I like this feeling?
- How do I feel when eating consistently in this manner? Do I like this feeling—would I choose to feel this way again?
- Am I experiencing differences in my energy level?

If eating healthfully is a pleasurable experience, *and* it makes you feel better, you are more likely to continue honoring your health with your food choices. The key, however, is *not* to turn the idea of healthy eating into an all-or-none prospect based on deprivation. Deprivation does not work in the long run.

It's hard to enjoy eating a meal when the people around you are engaged in dieting talk or body bashing. To keep the pleasure in eating, consider your Intuitive Eating Bill of Rights:

1. You have the right to savor your meal, without cajoling or judgment, and without discussion of calories eaten or the amount of exercise needed to burn off said calories.
2. You have the right to enjoy second servings without apology.
3. You have the right to honor your fullness, even if that means saying "No, thank you," without explanation, to dessert or a second helping of food.
4. You have the right to stick to your original answer of no, even if you are asked multiple times. Just calmly and politely repeat, "No, thank you, really."
5. It is not your responsibility to make someone happy by overeating, even if it took hours to prepare a specialty dish.
6. You have the right to eat pumpkin pie for breakfast (or cereal for dinner!), regardless of judgmental comments or rolled eyes.

Remember, no one, except for you, knows how you feel, both emotionally and physically. Only you can be the expert of your body. This requires inner attunement, rather than the external well-meaning suggestions from family.

Don't Let Yourself Be Put on a Food Pedestal

At first our clients think we must be perfect in our eating habits—after all, we are dietitians. We do not want to be placed on a pedestal. Some of the best information we've passed on to our patients is not about how nutritiously we eat, but rather that we ate a whole piece of tiramisu and enjoyed each bite. Or how we got stuck with our food down, so to speak, and gobbled the nearest candy bar. And in spite of these times, we balance out our nutrition. We still honor our health, and our taste buds, and our humanness.

Many of our clients have been elevated to a place of specialness among their friends, colleagues, and family members, because they *appear* to eat so well. "She is the health-conscious one." In the beginning, it's fun to garner the extra attention, because they have attached a value to this identity. After a while, however, most of our clients no longer want this notoriety. It adds more pressure. When you are on this food pedestal it can intensify feelings of deprivation. It often means sneaking around to eat, which doesn't feel good and can create fears of "getting caught." My goodness, to get caught "cheating" on your diet! Horrors!

I'll (ET) never forget attending a dinner hosted by a professional group at an incredible French restaurant. I was a stranger, seated among twenty people at the same table (I was a guest of one of the members). As the meal was winding down, the server presented us with a bounty of beautiful desserts. When the last dessert was described, someone asked, "Let's see what the nutritionist thinks—which one of these desserts is the *healthiest* to choose?" This was a food pedestal moment. As I opened my mouth to speak, all heads turned toward me, and I replied, "What's more important is whatever dessert is the most *satisfying*!" There was a very loud and collective sigh of relief!

Our clients usually feel relieved when they voluntarily dethrone themselves as the food-fitness czars. Others might feel a loss of their special identity, and that's okay too. It's important to grieve the loss and explore other identities that align with your values. What this means is they are no longer closet eaters—they no longer put on a false food face. If they feel like ordering dessert with a meal, they will. It's their opportunity to show how appearing to be a perfect eater does not equate to the value of optimal health and fitness. Remember, balance is the key!

Chapter 16

Raising an Intuitive Eater:
What Works with Kids and Teens

We are often asked if it is possible to help children return to the Intuitive Eaters they were at birth. Not only is it possible, but it is often easier than with adults—since children are generally less dubious and far more open and eager.

Let's begin with prevention. I (ER) was fortunate enough to visit a friend's daughter, who had given birth just two weeks prior. Alexis was just getting comfortable with the overwhelming task of figuring out how to take care of her newborn daughter—which cry meant that she was sleepy, which one said a diaper needed changing, and which one cried hunger? If you have ever spent time with babies, you know that their most recognizable cry is that of hunger. If a hungry child is ignored, they'll scream and scream until offered the breast or bottle. The hunger signal is acutely recognizable for the majority of babies, and there is a natural instinct to make the need for nourishment known. I was sitting and talking with Alexis, when little Lily made noises that let her mother know that she was hungry. Lily nursed until she was full, turning away her precious head and falling asleep. Alexis was in awe of this beautiful connection with her child and how intuitive the feeding experience was.

Parental attunement to children's hunger signals nurtures a sense of self-confidence that their needs are appropriate and will be consistently met. When children are hungry and quickly fed, they learn that hunger is a natural, normal, and "correct" sensation. Their hunger will then elicit a sense of safety, eliminating any fear of deprivation. If, instead, hunger is criticized or ignored, the child will begin to fear that there won't be enough food. In response, this child risks muting hunger signals and developing an inability to trust the messages the body sends.

Imagine an infant on a feeding schedule, a common recommendation from generations past (and sometimes, even today). Many caregivers were counseled that feeding every two to four hours would be best for the child, while allowing them to plan the whole day in advance. Unfortunately, this has the potential to create a number of problems. If the infant got hungry and cried a half hour before the scheduled time, the parent was prompted to wait to feed them. If, on the other hand, the infant was not yet hungry, they might be coaxed to eat anyway. Since hunger and fullness signals were not consistently being reinforced, both the hungry and not-yet-hungry baby were on their way to mistrusting and disconnecting from their body's powerful messages. For the hungry infant, fear of future deprivation takes root. For the infant encouraged to eat in the absence of hunger, confusion and resistance to eating can emerge.

For a child fed on schedule rather than according to hunger signals, moving into the toddler years can initiate a disordered relationship with food. Children who experienced feelings of deprivation during infancy may develop a tendency to eat beyond fullness when food is available, storing up for the next potential famine. Conversely, toddlers who were regularly persuaded to eat more than they needed as an infant may continue to eat more than their bodies ask for or get into "food fights," refusing to eat much at all.

The fundamental steps in ensuring that a child retains their innate ability around hunger and fullness are consistency and trust, in infancy and beyond. It is this internal wisdom that forms the basis of Intuitive Eating.

BABY-LED WEANING/SOLIDS

When my (ER) son was an infant, I was instructed to begin spoon-feeding him at two months old. Yes—two months! So I bought brown rice, ground it in a nut grinder, cooked it, then put it through the blender. I was so excited to put that baby spoon filled with this mush into his tiny mouth! As you can probably guess, this ended in disaster. He pushed the spoon right out of his mouth with his tongue thrust, sending the spoon and the rice flying. He certainly gave me the clear message that he wasn't ready for solid foods! Yet I and all of my contemporaries continued to feed our babies the way we were told was "right" by our doctors.

Fortunately, progress is being made in the realm of feeding solid foods through "baby-led weaning" (BLW), or sometimes called "baby-led solids."

We call it Intuitive Eating for Babies! While BLW is trendy, it has been around for eons—there were no jars of pureed foods in primitive cultures or before modern food processing. Some advanced societies have continued this natural process—however, the modern world seems to believe that spoon-feeding purees is what is meant to be. Most pediatricians believe this as well, with strong beliefs about when the "right" time is to start this transition.

Gill Rapley and Tracey Murkett describe BLW in their book *Baby-Led Weaning: The Essential Guide to Introducing Solid Foods and Helping Your Baby to Grow up a Happy and Confident Eater.*

The authors explain that BLW is the intermediate stage between exclusive milk consumption and the introduction of solid foods and other liquids. The goal here is for the infant to direct their eating journey from instinct, rather than being led by parent or doctor authority. In this way, BLW embraces the understanding that "baby knows best." This nourishes and protects their inner Intuitive Eater, as they learn to trust internal cues instead of external regulations and rules.

There is nothing that could be more aligned to Intuitive Eating as a child is ready for solids than BLW.

Here is a short guide to BLW:

1. Set the intention of giving your child the opportunity for a lifetime of satisfying eating and a sense of autonomy, self-trust, and freedom in their relationship with food.
2. The baby's digestive system is ready for BLW by six months old. Before that, all the baby needs is breast milk or formula, both easily digestible and dense sources of energy for their small stomach capacity.
3. The main focus will be on honoring the baby's cues that they're ready to start eating solid foods. They'll show this when they start to grab food and put it in their mouth.
4. The baby will share meals with the family, rather than being "fed," in order to enhance social skills and develop an increased sense of confidence and independence. (Family can mean one caregiver and one baby.)
5. "We focus on finger foods." When feeding themselves, food enters into the front of their mouths. This makes it easier for the child to chew and manipulate food, as well as better detect taste, and spit

out what they don't like. By contrast, spoon-feeding delivers food to the back of the mouth, which makes it more difficult to spit out and can trigger a gag response. This increases the likelihood of food refusal.

6. Learning and practicing chewing is important for the development of speech, proper digestion, and safe eating. Manual dexterity and hand-eye coordination will also improve with baby-led weaning. By feeling the food in their hands, babies learn what size foods are easier to chew and move around in their mouths.

7. Babies who eat with their hands have far more fun while feeding themselves than when spoon-fed. They get to touch and feel the food, exploring different textures and being more willing to eat a wider variety of food.

8. By widening the family's range of foods, the baby will learn to include and experiment with a diversity of nutritious eating. After all, babies love to copy their parents and siblings. As a result, the whole family may end up with an increased focus on balanced eating.

Ellyn Satter outlines the "Division of Responsibility" for eating between parent and child in her groundbreaking book *Child of Mine: Feeding with Love and Common Sense*. Beautifully complementing the BLW framework, Satter explains that it's the parents' job to provide and prepare the food, while the child's job is to eat as much or as little as they need.

Your job as the parent includes the following:

- Having the baby sit with the family while eating.
- Allowing them to pick up food, whether they can actually eat it yet or not.
- Providing foods that are cut in small pieces that the baby can handle.
- Allowing the baby to feed themself—no spoon-feeding by caregiver.
- Allowing the baby to eat as much or as little as they like and to move on to other foods when ready.

For more specific directions about BLW, here are three excellent resources:

- Rapley and Murkett will guide you through the process.
- *Born to Eat,* by two dietitians—Leslie Schilling and Wendy Jo Peterson.
- @feedinglittles on Instagram (especially videos of baby-led weaning in their stories).

Lastly, please keep in mind that there is no one way that works for every baby. You can still raise an Intuitive Eater if you don't do baby-led weaning.

FAMILY EXPERIENCES

Here, you will find stories from real-life clients on some victories and challenges that come with adopting Intuitive Eating as a family. We incorporate tips and guidelines for protecting your child's inborn intuitive signals and for addressing some common roadblocks.

As you've been reading so far, you may be thinking, "How can I trust that my child will be an Intuitive Eater? How can I allow my child to make these decisions on their own—all they'll want to eat is candy!" To address these concerns, let's first explore the stories of some children who have been able to grow up with Intuitive Eating signals intact. We have the great honor to hear about many children raised by parents who have healed their own food and body relationships through Intuitive Eating, committing to raise their children with the same philosophy.

Andrea and Allie

Andrea was referred to me (ER) for counseling by her pediatrician when her baby, Allie, was seven months old. Andrea told her doctor that she had no idea how to feed her child, having suffered with anorexia, bulimia, and binge eating throughout her teens and twenties. Allie was more than ready to eat solid food, but Andrea was terrified of creating an eating disorder in her own child. She arrived in the office with a big hug of hope and gratitude, saying, "Please teach me how to feed my daughter." In those first few months of counseling, Andrea was not only supported in learning how to feed Allie, but she was also introduced to Intuitive Eating to help heal her own disordered eating.

Through Allie's toddler years, she had the advantages of being offered a wide range of nutritious foods that her mother would prepare and sitting at the table with her parents while eating. She wasn't introduced to play food in her home as a baby, but no restriction was put on her exploration of foods in other people's homes. Carrots, ice cream, spinach, and candy were all treated equally. Andrea made no comments and gave no judgmental glances at Allie's choices. As a result of this freedom, Allie has a true desire for a wide range of food. When it was her turn to bring a snack to nursery school, she wanted to bring bok choy! When she was about five, she woke up one morning and asked Andrea for tofu and hearts of palm for breakfast. When asked at school to draw a picture of her favorite food, Allie drew Brussels sprouts. But don't get the wrong impression—Allie also loves candy and cookies. She simply has no need to fill up on these foods, because they're never restricted and never judged.

Allie is now fifteen and retains her love of a variety of foods. From seven months to her teenage years, Allie has been the model Intuitive Eater. Her mother no longer suffers from her eating disorder—both mother and daughter sustain positive relationships with food and body.

Tanya and Naomi

Tanya is a mother of two and had struggled with anorexia and exercise bulimia for most of her life, until she found Intuitive Eating. With healing, came the commitment to raise her children with an Intuitive Eating, body-positive approach. She related a story about an experience that six-and-a-half-year-old Naomi had in school. A little boy came up to Naomi and made some judge-y comments about her size. After several remarks, Naomi responded, "I'm myself, and I'm exactly the way I'm supposed to be!" Tanya was so proud, not only that Naomi spoke up for herself, but that she had taught her that everyone's body is the way it's "supposed to be."

ROLE MODELING

Parents most often serve as the primary role models for their children in the realm of eating. There is great power in setting an example of eating when hungry, stopping when full, and enjoying a wide array of satisfying foods. This is a case of "do as I do," rather than "do as I say," as some well-intentioned parents intending to help their children with Intuitive Eating don't actually practice it themselves. Speaking about food, whether it's excessive pressure to try something new or judgments about the amount a child eats, heightens the risk for a child's resistance toward or rebellion against the "authority" figure. Less talk and more role modeling mean it is more likely the child will try new foods, find vegetables interesting, and have more balance and satisfaction in the entire eating experience.

Jill and Billy

Jill is a client who sought nutrition counseling after a lifetime of eating and body image disturbances. Growing up with a mother who was always dieting propelled Jill into restrictive eating, which ultimately led to a diagnosis of anorexia nervosa and a mind that could think of nothing else but food and body. At the time she sought counseling, Jill was thinking about having children. She was worried that if she didn't heal her own problems with food, she would transmit them to her future children, as her mother had done. She was finally ready to make some changes.

Jill worked very hard to reject the diet mentality thinking and start feeding herself according to her body's hunger and fullness signals. She eventually became pregnant, crediting her improved eating for her ability to conceive. She also credits Intuitive Eating for the profound effect it has had on the raising of her two sons. She recently told a story that exemplified this. Her oldest son, Billy, was sitting at dinner with the family at age four. He turned to his father and said, "Daddy, you need to eat your vegetables—they're good for you!" Jill has cooked and served her children a wide array of nutritious foods since they were able to eat solids. She also keeps play food in the house and does not restrict the foods they eat at other children's homes. Jill never commented on how much or how little food the children eat or classified foods as "good" or "bad." Above all, she has never told Billy that vegetables are healthy or that he should eat them. She has no idea how he got the thought to tell his father to eat his vegetables and that they're healthy!

Jill is raising her boys with the trust that they will get a wide variety of food and nutrients, if they are allowed to make their own decisions about what they eat and how much. There are no food fights in this home. Both boys are growing appropriately and getting the full spectrum of foods that they need to thrive.

SUPPORTING YOUR CHILD'S INNATE
RELATIONSHIP TO FOOD AND EATING

Below, you'll find some of the basic concepts of a child's innate relationship with food, along with some practical tips:

Children are self-regulating. For the most part, children are self-regulating in terms of how much food they need. Some children have a slower growth rate and some faster and, given the opportunity, both will eat what they need in order to meet their body's needs.

- Children grow in spurts. Sometimes they eat as much as an adult and sometimes as little as an ant. If left alone and not nudged, they'll get everything that they need over time.
- If children are physically active, they will be hungrier than if they are sedentary.
- Children's food preferences vary regularly. Don't worry if your child only wants peanut butter and jelly for many weeks and then won't look at it for months afterward. If no judgment is made (such as, "You've always loved this—why aren't you eating it now?"), the child is quite likely to go back to this food sometime in the future.
- Conversely, if you serve the same food every day, the child might become disinterested in it. Remember habituation—too much of a good thing can become boring and rejected. Alternate foods every few days to maintain children's interest in different foods.
- Look at the whole week, instead of a particular meal or day of eating, and you will see that your child will get everything that they need.

Children seek autonomy. An important developmental task of childhood is the quest for autonomy. This can show up as early as eighteen months old and continues throughout childhood, peaking in adolescence. Honoring children's developing autonomy is key for nurturing their inner Intuitive Eater.

- Allow your children to serve themselves as soon as they are developmentally able to do so. If you serve them, you are presuming

how much they need to satisfy their hunger. They will take what they need, without feeling pressured to "clean the plate."
• Saying no to eating is often a way for a toddler to show their independence, especially if they're not hungry. Don't worry, they'll eat when they're hungry!
• If you have raised your children as Intuitive Eaters, you can feel safe allowing them to order for themselves in a restaurant.
• Involve children in food shopping and meal preparation—they'll be more interested in eating the foods they pick and prepare.

Introducing new foods is an art. Parents often expect their children to try a new food when offered, even if it's only a bite. Feeding conflicts can arise if foods are introduced without understanding how children can react to this new experience.

• Around age two, children often become fearful of new things, including new foods. Trust that if the child isn't pushed, they'll eventually be willing to try new things when they're ready—especially if they see the family eating them too.
• Allow small children to experiment with food, especially if introducing a new food or a food prepared in a different way at the family meal. A child might put it in their mouth, take it out, play with it, and then try it once again. Or they might not be ready to eat it at all at that time. Let children be a little messy—this sensory experimentation phase is part of normal development.
• It can sometimes take over twenty exposures for a child to accept a new food. Don't give up just because you introduce something new once or twice and the child doesn't choose it. Keep serving it from time to time, without any pressure. At some point, the child might try it.
• When presenting a new food, be sure to have some familiar foods at the table as well. Presenting several new foods at once can be overwhelming for the child, and they might refuse everything.
• There are going to be some foods that your child simply doesn't like, just as adults have particular food preferences and dislikes.

Talk about foods in non-moralistic terms, rather than "good" or "bad." Telling children that some foods are "bad" can instill feelings of guilt.

Instead, tell children that "play food" isn't necessarily nutritious for the body, but exists just to taste good. Don't talk about "junk food," as that could elicit shame for eating something perceived as having no value. These kinds of discussions, paired with unrestricted access to a wide range of foods, reduce the risk of your child gravitating toward and fixating on the play food at another child's home.

Your role as the parent is powerful. Parenting is an awesome task. In the realm of feeding your children, following some basic guidelines will help pave the way to healthy food relationships.

- Stay neutral when serving food, rather than pushy. If you're invested in what or how much your child eats, your child will react to you instead of to their inner signals.
- Eat a variety of foods yourself and enjoy and appreciate food together as a family.
- Above all, do not bribe, reward, or attempt to comfort with food. Food is for hunger, satisfaction, and nourishment. Help your children learn how to endure feelings. Let them know that their feelings are real and valued and that there are ways to comfort oneself without using food.

THE POWER OF RESTRICTION

The examples above illustrate the best outcome of raising children with respect for their body's intuitive signals. Other clients, especially those who are still struggling with their own disordered eating, encounter more challenges in giving this message.

Mary, Denise, and Molly

Mary has thirteen-year-old twin daughters, Molly and Denise. Molly has always been extremely active, while Denise is more sedentary. From the time they were toddlers, Mary worried about Denise's inactivity.

Problems began to arise when the children were about four years old. When the girls learned about play food, Mary marveled at what limited interest Molly had in these foods. Denise, on the other hand, loved play food! Since Molly didn't care much for play food and was so active, she was left alone, while both parents began setting limits on how much play food Denise was allowed to have.

After learning about Intuitive Eating, Mary began liberalizing her message about play food to her daughters. Her husband, Danny, was unfortunately not on board. One day, Denise found two bags of M&Ms and offered one of them to Molly. Molly wasn't interested, so Denise took the second bag and brought it to her room. This appeared to have a happy message. Denise was willing to share with her sister, not needing to eat both bags at the same time.

A little later that day, Mary found Denise hiding in her room, secretly eating her stash of candy. When Denise shared that she feared her parents would be angry if she ate too much candy, Mary said, "Denise, you can have as much candy as you want. I won't get mad. I know that you eat plenty of nutritious foods and that some days you want candy, and some days you don't."

Mary expressed concern to her husband about Denise sneaking candy out of fear. She explained that attempting to micromanage Denise's eating was sending the clear and harmful message that her body cannot be trusted. After returning to her inborn Intuitive Eater and encouraging her husband to do the same, Mary learned how to speak about food with her children. Today, both Molly and Denise are young teens who know that their bodies are worthy of their trust—with play food and all foods.

This poignant story shows what can happen when an anxious parent believes that they must control the amount of play food a child can have.

Numerous studies explore how dietary restriction can have serious consequences for children. These include disconnection from hunger signals, preoccupation with food, and lowered self-esteem. Attempting to rigidly control children's eating teaches them to mistrust their bodies, moving them further away from the Intuitive Eaters they were at birth. Ellyn Satter believes that "overcontrol" and "undersupport" are at the basis of many childhood eating problems.

THE IMPACT OF DEPRIVATION

Nancy

As we've seen, the power of deprivation can lead to dysfunctional food behaviors. A client of mine (ER), who is an early childhood educator, told me a frightening story about a little girl in her preschool class. Little Nancy's mother believed that sugar was dangerous and forbade her from eating any food that contained it. One day, my client noticed that Nancy had not gone onto the playground to play with the other children. Instead, she stayed back in the classroom to pick up crumbs on the floor left behind from other children's sugar-containing snacks. She also picked up and gobbled pieces of dirty raw rice and dried beans, which the children used for play. This child was so desperate to taste what she couldn't have that she went to this extreme to fix her feelings of deprivation. After seeing this behavior continue, my client approached Nancy's mother to request she stop restricting Nancy from eating what the other children were eating. Even after being told what Nancy had done, her mother remained vehement that her daughter was never allowed to have sugar.

HEALING DEPRIVATION

Pamela and Eric

Fortunately, many parents are more receptive. Pamela, the mother of a healthy five-year-old, was referred to work with me (ER) to address a lifelong history of restrictive eating. In the early part of her treatment, she mentioned that her son, Eric, was hyper-focused on dessert. After each bite of dinner, he would beg for dessert, without appreciating the tastes of the other foods served to him. Pamela's husband was very adamant that Eric finish his dinner before having dessert, and the dinner table became a battleground. Pamela and her husband came in for counseling together and were astonished to hear the recommendation of putting all of the foods on the table at once—yes, including dessert, along with the chicken and the broccoli and the bread. Although Pamela and her husband were skeptical, they were open-minded about this new approach.

It didn't take very long before Eric stopped seeking the desserts over all other foods. Did he still eat the cookies? Of course! But instead of reaching for them first each time, he began to eat and enjoy most of the foods served to him with the confidence that cookies would be available to him any time.

Fear of deprivation is a powerful force in the seeking and overeating of restricted foods. The surest way to disinterest a child in the food a parent wants them to eat is to tell them that they can't have their dessert until they finish their dinner. Dinner then becomes the enemy—the barrier to getting what they really want. Limited access, conditional availability, and rigid serving sizes can also create a food fight or an overvaluation of dessert. Releasing control about the minutiae of what goes into a child's mouth and allowing them to make those decisions themselves brings an amazingly rapid "cease-fire," calming the feeding experience for both parent and child.

STEPS FOR PROTECTING AND REINFORCING YOUR CHILD'S INTUITIVE EATING

If your child is thirsty, offer water rather than juice. Juice was only introduced into the food supply during the early 1900s. Before that time, people mainly ate fruit and drank water. Too much juice can fill up a child's stomach and disconnect them from true hunger signals. Filling up with juice within an hour before a meal will lead the child to feel too full at the next meal.

Postpone introducing play food to very young children. There is no need to introduce play food to very young children before they've had a chance to experience a variety of more nutritious foods. They'll have plenty of opportunities to experience these foods later. If, however, someone offers a play food to a toddler, allow the child to eat this food without comment (either negative or encouraging). If your child has already been oriented to a wide assortment of foods when they begin to eat solids, play food will not become overvalued. It will take its place in the child's healthy and unselfconscious relationship with food.

Share the benefits of nutrition early on. Teach your children that food can have the power to give them energy to play, can help them sleep well at night, and help them think clearly at school.

Put a variety of foods on the table. Prepare balanced meals for your children and try to eat together as a family whenever possible. When the children have become aware of play food, occasionally put some on the table alongside all of the more nutrient-dense foods. Make no comments about which foods or how much food a child should eat. Remember that some days they may only want the play food, but most often they'll eat an array of everything that is served. Remember, your child's food choices may change from meal to meal, day to day. In the big picture, they'll get all the nutrients that they need.

Pack lunches that have a variety of choices, including a little play food. If your child never gets a cookie in their lunch, you can be sure that they'll trade something with another child to get what they want.

Make nutritious snacks available for your children. Have nutritious snacks readily available for when your child gets hungry between meals. These snacks might include cut-up fresh fruit and vegetables, nuts, cheese, hummus, and whole grain crackers. If these foods are ready to eat and visible in the refrigerator or on the counter, there's a good chance that they'll go for them when they're hungry.

Do not be a short-order cook! Make one meal for the whole family, including a number of side dishes. This ensures that each child has something to eat, even if they don't like the main course. Tell them that you will be preparing well-balanced meals to help them grow and be strong. Let them know that you won't be making several dinners for the family, but assure them that you will be serving some foods that you know they each like. Reassure them that you will not be monitoring which of the foods or how much of the foods they are eating. That will be their job.

Trust your child's innate abilities. Children know how much to eat to satisfy their hunger and meet their body's needs. In the big picture, Intuitive Eating supports your child in getting their biological needs met and maintaining a positive relationship with food.

HEALING YOUR CHILD'S BATTERED
RELATIONSHIP WITH EATING

Parents often seek nutrition counseling to help their young children learn to eat a wider variety of foods or avoid overeating. Oftentimes, it's unnecessary to actually work with the child. Instead, we teach the parents about Intuitive Eating and provide practical guidelines. Sometimes, however, it is appropriate to directly help a child to change eating habits and feelings about food.

Here are some strategies we commonly teach parents who come to our offices:

Tips for Parents for Making Changes at Home

1. Tell your child that you have read a book or talked to a professional who has given you some very different ideas about how to approach eating in the home. Acknowledge that parents can learn new things and change, and that you are eager to make some of these changes. This will intrigue your child and get the soil ready for planting the new ideas.

2. Tell your child that from now on, their job is to choose how much and what to eat at mealtime, and that you will provide a variety of foods at meals—including previously forbidden foods.

3. Ask them if there are any foods that they would like to have in the house that are not usually present. You'll see a great deal of excitement and disbelief in the child's face at this point.

4. Most important: stick to your promise. Your child will test you to see if this is too good to be true. Your child might wait for you to slip and say that they don't need more food, that "they should eat some vegetables," or that they have to finish dinner before having any dessert. It may take time before your child believes that you really aren't going to interfere with their eating.

This advice can be scary for many parents. Fears stem from worrying that others will think that they're not good parents because they're not enforcing strict eating rules and worrying that the child will never stop eating, will only eat desserts, or won't eat enough food.

To ease the transition, it may be helpful to seek counseling with a nutrition therapist or a psychotherapist who is well versed in Intuitive Eating. It is also important that all parents are aligned on the family's eating philosophy to allow the child to feel safe and avoid confusion.

Meeting with an Intuitive Eating professional also supports each parent to examine their own beliefs about food, eating, and body. Supporting a child to eat intuitively is extremely challenging if disordered eating lingers in the family elsewhere. If there is any form of disordered eating in the family, it can be difficult to heal a dysfunctional eating experience in a child. Remember, parents are important role models to help a child return to their Intuitive Eating roots.

WHEN YOU'RE TOLD YOUR CHILD
IS "OVERWEIGHT"

Incessant cultural fear-mongering messaging around the so-called "obesity epidemic" warns that children living in larger bodies are at higher risk for many health issues, without evidence to show causation. For example, in the United States, a child is 242 times more likely to have an eating disorder than type 2 diabetes!* Rather than promoting health, public health campaigns to end "obesity" reinforce weight stigma—and increase the risk of eating disorders, the impact of which is not benign.

As you have learned, imposing rules and restrictions on food often contributes to the development of disordered eating and body image disturbances. Leann L. Birch, a professor of human development at Pennsylvania State University (retired), and her research group have extensively evaluated these issues. Their studies show that parents using restrictive feeding practices backfires, leading children to eat when they aren't hungry, often resulting in extensive overeating:

- In a study of five-year-old girls of varying size, those whose mothers used restrictive feeding patterns were shown to have the greatest level of overeating behavior by age nine.
- In another study of five-year-old girls, those who perceived parental pressure and control around food began to restrict certain foods and eat emotionally.

It can be very difficult and even terrifying for parents to let go of monitoring their children's eating when they've been told that their child is overweight.

In children of all sizes, limiting the amount or the type of foods they eat can only lead to feelings of deprivation and rebellion, just as diets do for adults. They are more likely to sneak food, eat as much as they can at a friend's house, or, eventually, develop a serious eating disorder. Feelings

---

* For every 100,000 kids in the United States, there are 12 incidences of type 2 diabetes, compared to 2,009 cases of eating disorders. Linda Bacon, *Body Respect: What Conventional Health Books Get Wrong, Leave out, and Just Plain Fail to Understand About Weight* (Dallas: BenBella Books, (2014), p. 30.

of shame can emerge in a child who breaks the rules in an overcontrolling eating environment, and the child-parent relationship may be harmed.

To stop monitoring a child's eating and trust their body's wisdom might feel like taking an impossible leap of faith. Perhaps Michele's story will help reassure you that it can be done.

Michele

Many years ago, the parents of an eight-year-old girl called (ER), seeking help for her overeating. They were concerned about their child's weight and physical discomfort and worried about potential adverse health issues to come. The parents reported that they were both dieters but knew this was the wrong approach for their daughter. They didn't think that they were ready to change their own habits but said they would do anything they could for their daughter. After a few sessions with the parents, it became clear that this child would benefit from counseling of her own.

The first time that Michele came into the office, she said that she wanted to have her parents present during her session. Their presence was wonderful, allowing Michele to feel safe to speak about her feelings with the confidence that her parents would support her. She was excited to hear that her parents were willing to make changes to help her start feeling better. Michele revealed that she often ate too many desserts, especially chocolate, at parties, would get "a very bad tummy ache," and would have to leave. When asked why she thought that she ate enough dessert to make her feel sick at other people's houses, she said that her parents wouldn't allow any desserts at home, unless they were low in calories. She didn't like the diet desserts, so she felt the need to eat as much as she could when delicious desserts were available.

During our sessions, there was never a word spoken about weight. The emphasis was always on how Michele felt, both physically and mentally. In this way, Michele could feel more in tune with her body and bolster her self-esteem. Any focus on a child's weight, either by her parents or by any professional, whether doctor or dietitian, runs the risk of giving some very damaging messages to the child. Also, worry about future health issues does not have the power to motivate behavior change and gives a fear-mongering message. Feeling physically better in the moment, however, can provide a strong impact.

We spoke with the family about how allowing Michele access to desserts she loved on a regular basis could help her learn to enjoy them without the stomachache. Michele wrote a list of her favorite desserts, with a promise from her parents to go grocery shopping after the session.

Michele also learned that her body sends messages to let her know when she is hungry and when she is full. She said that she knew when she was hungry, and she usually knew when she was full. Then she asked a provocative question: "How can I stop eating when I know that I'm full?" I asked her, "If your tummy is full, does your body need more food?" She replied, "Well, no." I then asked, "So, if your body doesn't need any more food, then what do you really need?" This eight-year-old child got it, right there, and answered, "I need to know that I'll be able to get the sweets I want at my own house."

Michele then added, "Sometimes I need to eat when I'm feeling bored or sad or lonely or scared." Many adults can't make that connection! After it was explained that some people think they need food to help soothe their feelings, Michelle was asked if she could think of anything else she could do to help herself when she feels bad. Michele proposed that she could color in a coloring book, play with her dog, or talk with her mom. This was the beginning of helping Michele heal her feelings of deprivation about food and start to separate her physical cues from her emotional cues for eating.

Over time, Michele started trusting that she would have sweets at home when and if she wanted. Her feelings of deprivation vanished, and she found that she only needed moderate amounts to satisfy her. She stopped overeating at parties, talked about balancing nutritious foods with play foods, and grew into a young woman with a healthy relationship with food, body, and self.

Ten Steps for Working with Your Child Who Eats Well Beyond Fullness

Note: If you feel uncomfortable doing this on your own, don't hesitate to seek the counsel of a nutrition therapist who is trained in Intuitive Eating. (See the link to the list of Intuitive Eating Counselors in the Certified Intuitive Eating Counselor Directory on p. 360.)

1. Have a discussion with your child about what hunger feels like in their body. (See chapter 7, principle 2, on page 84 to review how to "honor your hunger.")
2. If your child is too young to get food on their own, teach them to make sure they tell an adult when they're hungry.

3. Have a discussion about what fullness feels like in their body. (See chapter 11, principle 6, on page 167 to review how to "feel your fullness.") Ask them if they know what fullness feels like. Tell them that their stomach is like a balloon filled with air. The balloon can be filled a little bit, leaving lots of space to fill it with more air, just as their stomach can be filled a little bit, leaving room for more food. The balloon can be filled with a little more air to make it bigger, just as their stomach can be filled with a little more food to make them fuller. Or either of them can be filled with so much air/food that it feels uncomfortable.

4. Explain that satisfying their hunger with enough food will give them plenty of energy to run and play, but too much food could make them feel uncomfortable or even sick. You can illustrate that just as the car needs gas/fuel so that it can drive, their body also needs fuel to be active. If the car gets filled with too much gas, there's no more room in the gas tank for the extra.

5. Ask them if they think that their body needs more food after they feel comfortably full. If they say no, present a question about what they really need. If they don't know, tell them that sometimes people eat too much food because they're bored or to feel better when they're sad or scared. Assure them that you'll be there with them while they express their feelings. You can also help your child come up with some alternatives to eating to soothe uncomfortable emotions, if they aren't quite ready to talk about their feelings.

6. Above all, don't criticize your child about weight, and don't put them on a scale—better yet, remove scales from the house altogether! Talk about the immediate benefit of feeling more comfortable in their body, if they eat according to their hunger and fullness signals. Please, do not talk to them about future health problems in relation to food.

7. Ask them if there are foods that they'd like to have that have previously been forbidden. Tell them you will buy and keep these foods in the house.

8. Assure your child that you are not going to tell them what to eat, what not to eat, or how much to eat. Share that you will provide them with a variety of foods at a meal—some that are more nutrient-dense and some play foods. It will be up to them to decide what they want in a meal and how much they need to take care of their hunger.

9. Let them know that you trust their own internal voice about hunger, fullness, and food preferences to guide their eating decisions. The more that your child knows you trust their inner wisdom, the more they will eat in an attuned way, rather than in reaction to you.

10. Ask them if there is any kind of help that they would like from you. Reassure them that you aren't abandoning them; you simply will no longer attempt to control their eating. They may say that they would like you to remind them to pay attention to their hunger signals, or to remind them to eat slowly, so that they can notice their comfortable fullness. Or they may ask you to stay out of it. Honor their wishes.

WHEN YOUR CHILD IS UNDERWEIGHT OR RESISTING FOOD

Addressing the early stages of food resistance in your child can greatly reduce the risk of a full-blown eating disorder in the future. (See chapter 17 for more information on treating eating disorders.)

We frequently receive calls from parents who report that their children are not eating enough or that they can't get them to eat anything but "white carbs." They tell us that the dinner table has become a battleground between parent and child. Not to worry; these food fights are both preventable and treatable when properly addressed.

Steps for Reestablishing Peace Between You and Your Food-Resistant Child

Your child's need to exert their autonomy by rebelling against eating enough or eating nutritious foods can often take precedence over their biological or nutritional needs. Here are a few strategies to consider in order to reestablish peace with your food-resistant child:

1. If you stop pressuring your child to eat more or to eat "better," it is likely that their rebellion will diminish and eventually vanish. Hunger is a very powerful motivator for seeking food, if the more potent psychological need to rebel isn't present. Trust that your child's relationship with food will heal, and that they will once again eat to meet their needs. Know that it might take a while for your child to trust that you mean it when you say you will leave the food decisions in

their hands. Seek help, if necessary, to support you during this stressful time.

2. Let your child know that you love them and believed you were doing the right thing by trying to direct their eating. Tell them that you have found that your suggestions have only led to tension between the two of you and share the changes that are about to take place.

3. Explain that one of the exciting things that you have learned is that their body has inner knowledge to guide them to eat in a balanced and enjoyable way. Their job will be to listen to the signals their body sends about how much they need to eat and to check in with how they feel physically after making their food choices.

4. Be prepared for the child's excitement about this lifting of pressure, followed by distrust about whether you will really stick to your word. The more time that goes by without your comments, the more your child will trust that the food fight is over. You will see a remarkable transformation take place before your eyes: your child's food intake will increase, and the ratio of play food to more nutritious food will begin to balance.

Surrendering and accepting that what they've been doing isn't working are the first steps to healing their relationship with their children and, by extension, their children's relationship with food. Some parents may worry that others will think that they're neglectful parents if they no longer direct their children's eating, especially if they see that their children are underweight or not eating in a balanced way. But the benefits of this healing process must outweigh the fear of others' judgments.

Caveats

Unfortunately, we're hearing about more and more very young children being diagnosed with anorexia nervosa. If you feel that your child's eating refusal is deeper than a rebellion against being pushed to eat, then please seek help from a psychotherapist who specializes in children's behavior and/or eating disorders. Also, if you suspect that there may be sensory integration problems (for example, a child having extreme reactions to different textures of food), then you may need to seek the help of an occupational therapist specializing in sensory processing dysfunction. And one last caveat, there are some children who may have experienced trauma or medical problems early in life, which may disconnect them from their innate eating instinct.

ADOLESCENTS

We frequently receive calls from parents who are worried about their adolescents' eating. We hear concerns ranging from parents hoping to help their teens avoid the unhappiness that they had experienced as adolescents, and parents who have been told by the doctor to monitor their teens' eating to lose weight to avoid medical problems. We also work with many adolescents who have put themselves on diets.

Adolescents are filled with contradictions. One day they can be delightful and almost childlike in their openness and trust. On other days, they can be sullen and barely talk. Understanding the developmental stage of adolescence is tantamount to helping teenagers heal their relationship with food.

In order to find their own identity, teens need a sense that they are emotionally independent from the adults in their lives. They attempt to achieve independence in many arenas. Eating in a way that they know will anger and frustrate their parents may be one way of asserting their autonomy.

Having fed my (ER) son an array of nutritious foods throughout his childhood, I admired how well he ate compared to some of his friends. When he became a teenager, however, I was astonished to see how often he would stick a candy bar or some other play food under my nose, just to taunt me! I later learned, of course, that this was one of the ways he was trying to exert independence from his nutritionist mother!

If a teen goes on a diet, regardless of whether it comes from the doctor or the parent or is self-imposed—it will inevitably have the same unfortunate results that are found in adults who diet, including being at higher risk for developing an eating disorder. This also strongly perpetuates diet culture and weight stigma.

- A 2003 study found that dieting was associated with binge eating among both preadolescent and adolescent young people.
- A 2007 study found that teen girls who dieted had an increase in binge eating and a decrease in breakfast eating. Teen boys were also found to have an increase in binge eating, as well as a decrease in physical activity.

Since dieting is not the answer, how can we help our teens maintain their innate Intuitive Eating or help them get back on the right tract to rediscover their intuitive signals?

TEN STEPS FOR PROMOTING INTUITIVE EATING DURING ADOLESCENCE

Just as in the "terrible twos," adolescents are fighting for their autonomy. They are likely to rebel against anything that is forced upon them.

1. Provide easily available, balanced food for your teens. Keep a variety of nutritious foods in the house, as well as the play foods that your teen enjoys. Involve teens in food shopping and in the preparation of meals. Many teens love to cook and are happy to be included in this experience.
2. Ask your teens how you can help them. They may appreciate your help in making breakfast or lunch and by providing snacks that can be taken on-the-go.
3. Don't fall into the trap of telling your teen that they can only watch television or be on their phones or computers after school while they're having their afternoon snack. If you connect relaxation with snacking, they might learn to overeat as a procrastination technique. Encourage them to eat a snack if they're hungry, and then suggest they do a nonfood-related activity to relax before starting their homework.
4. Talk to your teens about the people they're following on social media. Help guide them away from people who endorse dieting or weight-stigmatizing messages.
5. Maintain family mealtime as often as possible, even if only a few times a week.
6. Do not make mealtime the time to reprimand or interrogate. It is best for mealtime to be calm and peaceful, allowing for optimal satisfaction and recognition of fullness signals. The best way to get a teen to overeat or to refuse to eat is to begin a fight at dinner!
7. Make no comments about what or how much your teen is eating. Also be aware of your own body language or body scanning of your teen. Adolescents are highly sensitive to criticism and judgment.

Even the slightest perception that their body or food choices are unacceptable can lead to shame, attempts at dieting, rebellion, or even eating disorders.

8. If you notice that your teen is binge eating or barely eating, recognize that this may be a sign of emotional distress or unmet needs. Spend quality time with them, be patient, and let it be known that their feelings are appropriate and may be expressed as much and for as long as needed.

9. If your teen is over- or undereating, and it becomes clear that they need further support, seek a counselor, psychotherapist, and/or nutrition therapist who is trained in Intuitive Eating and eating disorders. Many teens have reported the onset of an eating disorder coinciding with seeing a professional who has prescribed a diet or a meal plan. You can also offer *The Intuitive Eating Workbook for Teens* to help guide them through this process.

10. Be highly aware of your own relationship with food and your body. Never make disparaging comments about your body, spend time talking negatively about what you've eaten or haven't eaten, or weigh yourself. It will be extremely beneficial for your teen if you remove a scale from the house.

To illustrate the process of helping a teen move from resistance to Intuitive Eating, take a look at Bobby's story.

Bobby

Bobby was fifteen when he first walked through the door for nutrition counseling. His doctor referred him with the prescription to lower his cholesterol and lose weight. When he was asked what his goals were, he said that he was only there because the doctor had sent him, but he guessed that he would like to be healthier. Similar to many teens, Bobby exhibited a high level of sophistication and appeared to be capable of understanding the tenets of Intuitive Eating. As sophisticated as he was, however, when he heard that no foods were going to be forbidden, the grin that came across his face was priceless.

When I (ER) explained the psychological concepts of deprivation and drive for autonomy, he relaxed and was eager to share his story.

Bobby described parents who were overly focused on "healthy" food and exercise, alongside their countless attempts to get him to lose weight, and he told poignant tales of emotional eating that felt uncontrollable to him.

Bobby's initial treatment was centered on helping him find satisfaction in eating. This meant paying attention to eating when he was moderately hungry, so that he wasn't experiencing primal hunger when he started a meal. We spoke about finding foods that truly satisfied him and eating them slowly, so he could appreciate all of the tastes, textures, and aromas. He set his own goals, honoring his need for independence. Bobby reported that he was eating "unhealthy foods," which he was buying at school but not really enjoying. One of the first goals that he set was to find more satisfying foods to replace these foods.

It was remarkable to see his sudden interest in eating in a more balanced way, after he had been told that all foods were fair game and that nothing would be forbidden. He had regularly bought only play food at school, where his parents couldn't scrutinize his eating. There is that adolescent rebellion at work! Bobby soon felt his urgency to eat the foods his parents previously forbade lessen, because there were now no foods off-limits. He also decided that he wanted to focus on stopping eating, after he noticed that he was full. He had recognized that the food wasn't as satisfying after he was full, and he was committed to working on ending his meal at this point.

Sifting out eating triggered by defiance and rebellion freed Bobby to look at the times he was eating for deeper emotional reasons, such as when he felt overwhelmed by schoolwork. He saw that the anxiety that came with striving for excellence in school was the hardest emotion to handle. Now that he had a license to eat whatever and whenever he wanted, he found that he could deal with his emotions without using food, and realized that he no longer needed a justification to eat previously forbidden foods based on emotional distress. Bobby identified ways in which he could find joy, realizing that these things soothed him more than food ever had. He also got more support for his schoolwork, which reduced his anxiety in that area.

As Bobby returned to his inner Intuitive Eater, his blood cholesterol went down to a normal level. He learned to respond to his body's wisdom to guide his eating choices, as well as how to separate physical hunger cues from emotional ones.

Bobby proudly said that his cardiologist was so impressed by his progress that he asked him if he would talk to his other patients and teach them what he had done. He then shared his experience, including:

- "This wasn't a competition. There was no pressure to lose weight or get on a scale. There was no concrete number that I was trying to achieve, so there were no expectations. No one focused on weight loss or said that I wasn't doing enough."
- "I never felt any deprivation, and I never felt guilty about what I ate." In fact, when talking about what he had eaten that day, he mentioned that he had ice cream.
- "Before this work, my mother told me that I would have to watch what I eat for the rest of my life."
- "Teens don't respond to fears about health."
- "When people overeat, they're doing it for a reason. They don't want to be told that they're a bad person. It doesn't help. It hurts and creates shame. Then they eat to push down that feeling."
- "When people say a food is bad and you shouldn't eat it, you don't get the good taste of the food—you get the feeling of rebellion when you eat that food. And that feeling of rebellion feels good!"

MOVEMENT

In chapter 14 we talk about exercise, or as we prefer to call it, movement. We can see the propensity toward movement throughout the lifespan. Most newborns can be seen flailing their arms and legs. As infancy progresses, they learn to turn over in their cribs, sit up, and eventually crawl. Soon, they're walking and running. No one who has been around a small child can deny this natural desire to move. There are many explanations as to why so many children ultimately become inactive, but we won't reiterate them here. Living in an active family helps children and teens maintain their innate desire to move. Just as serving and eating a wide variety of foods yourself models Intuitive Eating, playing outside with the family or dancing together inside the house does the same job for movement.

If there were less focus on trying to control children's eating and more focus on families being active together, we might see far fewer sedentary children and teens. Just as eating is intuitive, our intuitive desire to move needs to be treasured and nurtured!

The Intuitive Eating Approach to Physical Activity
for Your Children and Teens

By following these five guidelines, you will ensure that your children establish a lifelong appreciation for movement.

1. To promote and maintain movement in the teenage years, build on your infants' and toddlers' intuitive sense about movement. When possible, engage in family activities, such as taking walks, hiking, playing sports, rollerblading, biking, skiing, or swimming.
2. Encourage your children to be involved in group sports, dance, martial arts, or other forms of movement as early as possible. Help your child find an activity that gives them a sense of identity, joy, and self-esteem, without promoting competitiveness.
3. Just as with eating, role modeling movement is imperative. Find an activity that gives you pleasure, so your children will see you enjoying movement. On the other hand, be sure that you're not engaged in compulsive exercise. Watching a parent who over-exercises can be a surefire way to turn a child off from exercising altogether or adopt that dangerous habit themselves.
4. Be aware of the effect of extended media use on children and teens. Whether they're watching too much television, playing excessive video games, checking their social media feeds, or even working too many hours on the computer, these activities will affect their chances for engaging in regular movement. The American Academy of Pediatrics (AAP) recommends that "parents prioritize creative, unplugged playtime for infants and toddlers. Some media can have educational value for children starting at around eighteen months of age, but it's critically important this be high-quality programming. For school-aged children and adolescents, the idea is to balance media use with other healthy behaviors."
5. Finally, physical activity should not be promoted as a means for weight loss. If a child recognizes a parent's anxiety about weight, any talk about movement being for purposes of health will be interpreted as movement for weight loss (and is sure to be harmful, resented, or rejected).

PULLING IT ALL TOGETHER

Whether you have a newborn with Intuitive Eating intact or an older child who has strayed from their body's inner wisdom, the happiness and peace of both family and child resides in a commitment to Intuitive Eating. Give your child the confidence to trust in their innate ability to eat and move. Base your own relationship with food on Intuitive Eating. Parents are the primary role models for their children. Provide a wide array of nutritious foods to your children early in life. Avoid the labels of "good food" and "bad food" to help children make neutral food choices and prevent the sense of shame around eating. Eat together as a family, whenever possible, and engage in an active life together to put your children on the path for a happy, healthy, and well-balanced life. All you have to do is trust!

Chapter 17

The Ultimate Path Toward Healing from Eating Disorders

> *Eating Disorders are not just a fad or a phase. They are serious, potentially life-threatening conditions that affect a person's emotional and physical health.*
>
> —National Eating Disorders Association

As you have explored this book, you may have noticed a number of references to eating disorders, especially comments about how dieting has been found to be one of the most provocative and powerful catalysts in the development of an eating disorder.

We have yet to meet a patient who declares, "I wanted to have bulimia, anorexia, or a binge eating disorder." It usually starts off with "I just wanted to lose a few pounds," which evolves into dieting, disordered eating, and, finally, to a full-syndrome eating disorder. Dieting is known to be one of the most important predictors of developing an eating disorder. In fact, 35 percent of so-called "normal" dieters progress to pathological dieting. Of those, 20 to 25 percent will progress to partial or full-blown eating disorders. A systematic review of 94 studies found that the prevalence of eating disorders more than doubled, from 3.5% for the 2000–2006 period to 7.8% for the 2013–2018 period (Galmiche et al. 2019). The bottom line, according to the researchers, is that eating disorders are highly prevalent worldwide.

While the causes of eating disorders are multi-factorial, dieting and body dissatisfaction are known risk factors. We believe that the normalization of diet culture, masquerading as wellness, health, or lifestyle, is creating the conditions for eating disorders to manifest and thrive.

THE INCORPORATION OF INTUITIVE EATING IN THE TREATMENT OF EATING DISORDERS

Most patients in the throes of an eating disorder have lost touch with their innate signals of hunger, fullness, and taste preference. For some patients who are medically compromised, residential treatment may be the only appropriate setting to begin the healing process. For others, intensive outpatient treatment programs (IOPs) may be the solution that is prescribed. For some who are more stable, the appropriate course is to work with an outpatient team of a physician, psychotherapist, nutrition therapist, and sometimes a psychiatrist. There is one caveat, however, when someone who is healing from their eating disorder and is working with a registered dietitian or nutrition therapist in private practice—*they must be given the clear message that attempting to follow the Intuitive Eating principles of hunger and fullness in a literal sense will lead to negative results!* This is true especially for those who are suffering from anorexia nervosa. The physical starvation associated with anorexia is often so grave that an attempt to rely on certain intuitive signals can only lead to confusion and maintenance of the underfed state. Some patients love to say to us: "I'm only eating when I'm hungry, because that's what the book says (and I'm hardly ever hungry!)" or "I'm full after a few bites, so I don't need to eat more." We reassure them that they will someday be able to trust their hunger and fullness, but at the moment, their starved bodies are not able to give them accurate signals. One of the troublesome symptoms of starvation is slowed stomach emptying, or gastroparesis. As a result, ingesting even the smallest amount of food can create a false sense of fullness and push away signs of hunger. At this point in their healing process, we consistently emphasize the unreliability of waiting for the hunger signal as a cue to eat.

In the early treatment of anorexia in the private practice setting, we attempt to refeed patients in a slow, deliberate fashion, so as not to physically overstress the body. We also don't want to overstress a patient's emotional state and create excessive fear. We teach them about the body's physiology and drive toward homeo-balance, the role of brain chemistry, the fundamentals of nutrition, the mechanism of metabolism, and the potential dangers of undernourishment. We guide them toward making choices that will nourish them and promote a return to health.

Along with our role as teachers, we strive to help patients feel empowered by becoming part of the "nutrition team." They are encouraged to give their input about food likes and dislikes, uncover what is a feared food rather than a disliked food, and plan the eating risks that they're willing to take. They can talk freely about their food fears and body image struggles and can reveal their eating "secrets," knowing that they will never be judged. They feel free to reveal the outcome of undereating versus eating enough, as not eating enough is often the constant theme.

In other words, the members of the "team" bounce the ball back and forth as they move forward to the common goal. Conversely, if we were to give them a prescribed meal plan, written authoritatively by us, without their input, it would reinforce their anguish of having all of the control taken away from them. This feeling can lead to rebellion, anger, and a lack of cooperation. It also creates the risk that this meal plan will become cemented in their minds as the only "correct" way to eat. Throughout their healing process, we support them, advise them, and steer them toward finding a flexible way to eat. As time goes on, their eating choices are increasingly driven by their own internal signals, with little external guidance.

(It's important to note that for a varying period of time after refeeding is established, many of those healing from anorexia develop "hypermetabolism," meaning that their metabolism speeds up once they begin to nourish themselves. As a result, their energy needs can rise extraordinarily, and with our encouragement, they learn to increase their food intake to meet these escalated needs. The metabolism will often settle down to a more normal rate after about six months—although it takes longer for some.)

Our patients are taught to take each setback as a learning experience rather than a failure. They are consistently reminded that the healthier they become, the more they will be able to trust their signals of hunger and fullness and finally reclaim their ability to eat without anxiety.

For anyone with an eating disorder, Intuitive Eating can be presented as a model of eating that will give them full trust in their body's eating wisdom. The vision of a future, free of obsessive thinking and compulsive behaviors, is very powerful. This hope can facilitate the patience it will take to get through the period of time that is needed for healing. The body and brain must heal physically, and the mind must heal emotionally. We must emphasize the importance of working with a treatment team, which will require a commitment to working with a psychotherapist and a physician who have been trained in the treatment of eating disorders and, optimally, Intuitive Eating. The physician will monitor the physiological state of a patient and, for some, a psychiatrist may be involved to evaluate medication need. In our work, we, as nutritionists, are a part of a well-oiled and communicative treatment team.

Now let's explore the lives of Carrie, Skylar, Lila, Dana, Laurel, and a couple other of our patients to see their journeys toward developing an eating disorder and ultimately their healing through Intuitive Eating. This philosophy has led them each to a happier and fuller life experience.

TREATING ANOREXIA NERVOSA WITH INTUITIVE EATING

Carrie's Story—Healing Persistent Anorexia Nervosa

One Friday afternoon, the telephone rang, and the answering machine began to record a powerful plea from Carrie, who apologized for calling so late. She became filled with emotion as she said that she knew that the only way that she would ever be able to fully heal from her anorexia nervosa was to learn how to become an Intuitive Eater. She had heard about *Intuitive Eating* on a website and, after reading it, was taken by its focus on autonomy and was convinced that this was her last chance.

Carrie was almost twenty-two years old at the time and reported that she had been hospitalized eleven times in the past four years. Each time, she was kept in the hospital until she reached a normalized goal weight, yet upon release she would immediately lose all the weight she had gained, only to be re-hospitalized once again. At the point that she made this call, she had returned to a very low weight (not her lowest) and was dropping weight by the day. She was determined to never allow herself to go back in the hospital again and that it was time to finally get well. She also knew that she could not keep doing the same things and expecting different results. Carrie explained that each time that she had committed to regaining weight, she was haunted by the fear that she would physically heal, without feeling the freedom to eat and trust that her body wouldn't betray her. A lightbulb turned on in her head when she read *Intuitive Eating*. For the first time, she had hope that there was a solution!

During her first session (with ER), Carrie described her understanding that her eating disorder served her as a method of control, distraction, tension release, and running away from life. She believed that a big factor in the development of her eating disorder was a fear of growing up, getting married, and leaving her parents' home. In her words, "Contrary to the common belief about eating disorders, I had a very secure childhood and did not come from a dysfunctional family. I grew up in a loving family and had a very happy childhood." (What this doesn't say, however, was that her family and community were steeped in diet culture!)

Carrie was confident, easygoing, and liked herself and felt that she had never had any big eating and body image issues. She reported being a picky eater but ate enough of the foods she liked to grow and be healthy. She tried dieting on several occasions, "just because it was what people around me were doing, and it was kind of an activity." The majority of the women talked about needing to lose weight and about which foods needed to be restricted.

In the midst of high school, she was prescribed medication for a medical condition that had to be taken with food. To avoid side effects, she forced herself to eat a large amount of food and drink a lot of juice, late at night. At this point, she also began to do some emotional eating to calm her fears. Soon, she saw her body dramatically change, and decided that she needed to go on a diet.

It's not difficult to predict the outcome of this story. The longer Carrie dieted, the more she liked having the feeling she got from controlling her food and her body. Her fears about growing up were pushed down by the false sense of control that food restriction gave her. At first (unfortunately as often happens in our culture), her weight loss was admired and complimented by friends and family. It soon became evident, however, that she was in a serious health crisis. She also went from being a popular girl who loved school to one who was irritable, moody, and grumpy. She became someone who only cared about what she did or didn't eat and the number on the scale each morning. Eventually, she was diagnosed with anorexia nervosa and hospitalized for the first time.

In some of Carrie's early hospitalizations, she had no desire to get better. She also said, "Hospitals are not the answer for me. It's all a quick fix. I did not get to work on my mind or my eating long enough for it to have any lasting outcome." One problem was that, just as the thought of going on a diet led her family and friends to Last Supper eating, the thought of having to increase her food intake in the hospital led Carrie to "Last Supper restricting" before each readmittance.

As a result of effective psychotherapy, Carrie eventually felt ready to get better, and went into one of her hospitalizations with that goal. But it didn't work out as she had hoped. All she knew how to do was to gain weight when she was in and how to subsequently lose it when she was out. After each discharge, she would restrict food, over-exercise, compulsively weigh herself, and lose weight—all the things she was not allowed to do in the hospital. She knew that if she didn't learn how to trust her body, she would always be afraid of eating and feeling out of control.

So, where does one begin to help a young person with a chronic history of anorexia nervosa who wants to learn to become an Intuitive Eater? The first step was to capitalize on what motivated her, and this was the freedom that she hoped she could achieve by trusting her body. Here are some of the guidelines that formed the foundation for how the principles of *Intuitive Eating* were used in Carrie's treatment:

1. *Honor your hunger*: Carrie could always trust that if she felt hunger, her body was giving her a message that she needed to eat. This did not, however, mean that if she didn't feel hunger, she was getting an accurate message that she didn't need to eat. If this guideline was not emphasized, reemphasized over time, and believed—then the "contract" would be broken.
2. *Feel your fullness*: Carrie needed to accept that until she was renourished—body and mind—her fullness signals were not reliable! Envisioning this future trust in her fullness signals strengthened her motivation to heal.
3. *Make peace with food*: A commitment to taking risks and eating the foods that she had been restricting for years was something she could practice, even at her low weight. (When she began, Carrie was eating only a limited variety of safe foods each day.)
4. *Discover the satisfaction factor*: Eating foods that she wanted to eat and that were satisfying her palate would empower her and remove the rebellion that came from having been told what to eat. Rather than a rigid meal plan, there would be guidance in helping her figure out what she liked and encouragement to take risks incorporating these foods into her eating life. She would also be supported in

gradually increasing the amounts of satisfying foods she'd eat, in response to her healing body's needs.

5. *Cope with your emotions with kindness*: In Carrie's case, this would shift to learning to cope with her emotions without restricting food or getting on the scale. She would learn that pushing down her feelings by counting calories, cutting out foods, or getting on the scale could only give her a false sense of control and offer no solution to her problems. She would learn to talk with her psychotherapist, nurse practitioner, religious leader, family members, and, of course, her nutrition therapist, instead.

6. *Respect your body*: Carrie needed to accept that starving her body was the antithesis of respecting her body. In order to honor her body, she needed enough food to re-nourish her mind and body. Respecting her body would also mean radically accepting her DNA-programmed size and shape without trying to change it. She also needed to throw away her "anorexia" clothes and make peace with the fact that they would never again fit her. She needed to buy comfortable clothes that would fit a nourished body.

7. *Reject the diet mentality*: Carrie had seen the ill effects of dieting on her family members, and she especially saw how diet culture was one of the driving forces toward her eating disorder. All of the people she knew who were dieting were continually weight cycling. As a result, she knew that diets didn't work and that she never wanted to diet in order to manage her body—but she had never known an alternative!

8. *Challenge the food police*: Oh, and there were many Food Police in Carrie's head. The Food Police spoke from the voice of her anorexia. She would have to challenge her distorted thoughts and replace them with thoughts that came from the logical emerging Intuitive Eater within. She would have to let go of valuing perfectionism. She would learn to get right back on track toward her goal, every time she would revert to a restrictive behavior—this was a process, not a perfect, straight line to recovery!

9. *Movement—feel the difference*: Carrie would have to learn that any exercise beyond her normal walking would be counterproductive to her healing process. She would learn to look forward to the time when she could trust her body to tell her how much movement was just right for her and to feel the positive effects that movement would offer her.

10. *Honor your health—gentle nutrition*: The healthier Carrie's body would become, the more she had cravings for healthier foods. Ironically, Carrie had no problem eating play food. At first, it was mainly play food that she craved. Eventually she would want to add more protein and fruits and vegetables.

During her treatment, Carrie was repeatedly reminded that she could not trust her fullness until her body and mind were re-nourished, but she was also told that any hunger signal could always be honored. In her process toward this goal she used every experience as a learning opportunity rather than as a failure. In this way, she stopped beating herself up for not "doing it" perfectly. When she would get extremely hungry very late at night, she would take that as a message that she had not eaten enough during the day. When she would get on the scale after being advised to abandon that practice, Carrie learned that she would suffer for days with an increase in obsessive thoughts about her weight. Carrie also learned that her meals did not sustain her if she didn't eat enough protein, or, at other times, enough fat or enough carbohydrates at a meal. Most important, when she had intermittent instances of losing weight, the message became very clear—eat more! Carrie directed her own recovery. She was counseled about what would constitute a sustaining and balanced meal, but she was never told what to eat or exactly how much to eat.

Carrie didn't have the need to feel rebellious, because she was always led to evaluate her own decisions and decide whether they worked for her. In other words, with the goal of freedom ahead of her, she was motivated to stay on her journey to becoming an Intuitive Eater. Having reached her goal, Carrie never again had a regression into anorexia, ultimately married and became pregnant, and now has a little girl in elementary school. She wants to shout her relief and excitement to the world. She is convinced that the gift of being an Intuitive Eater and the freedom it brings surpass any benefit she ever gained from anorexia!

Skylar's Story—Coming to Treatment for Anorexia Later in Life

Skylar was referred for treatment of atypical anorexia by her psychotherapist at the age of fifty-seven. In atypical anorexia, although people do not appear underweight, they have the same eating disorder characteristics, fears, and body-image distortions as those with anorexia nervosa.

To look at Skylar at that time, one would see a well-dressed woman who did not appear emaciated. Even though she looked somewhat listless and had no sparkle in her eyes, she did not present the "typical" image of someone with anorexia nervosa. Yet the thoughts and behaviors of this woman mimicked those that had imprisoned her from the age of fifteen.

They had followed her through a hospitalization for anorexia at an extremely low weight, through gradual, although inadequate refeeding over the years. Although her body was no longer wasted, her pattern of restriction, with its lack of sufficient energy intake, and her obsessive thinking about and fear of food and eating certainly qualified her as having an eating disorder.

As a child and young teen, Skylar's mother and grandmother made judgmental comments about her weight and put pressure on her to diet. After restricting food and losing weight, she received praise and, ultimately, a diagnosis of anorexia nervosa. In her late thirties and early forties, she was subsisting mainly on frozen yogurt. At last, at age fifty-seven, she was referred for nutrition therapy. She was still in an extreme state of food restriction, had gained weight without increasing her caloric intake or variety of food, as a result of slowing her metabolism, and was living with an enormous fear of food and further weight gain.

With some of the same guidelines that helped Carrie, Skylar recovered from the symptoms of her anorexia before she hit sixty. In her late seventies, she continues to eat a wide variety of foods and restricts nothing. She has said that she actually prefers eating a normal meal, finding it far more satisfying than her two pints of frozen yogurt. She moves her body consistently, but not excessively, and takes in enough food to sustain her during exercise. Sufficient food and exercise have helped her build muscle. Honoring her body's need for proper nourishment has also sped up her metabolism. Skylar loves the freedom she has as an Intuitive Eater and truly believes that her years of being afraid to eat are gone forever!

Skylar did not have the typical case of anorexia nervosa when she began her Intuitive Eating journey. She did, however, have an extreme fear of eating and a loathing of her body. Without treatment, this could have lasted a lifetime. Regardless of age, however, Intuitive Eating can help one feel the freedom and trust in their body to be able to live a fulfilling and healthy life.

TREATING BULIMIA NERVOSA AND BINGE EATING DISORDER WITH INTUITIVE EATING

The treatment for binge eating disorder and bulimia begins in a slightly different way. If patients with these disorders are not in a starved state, they will more rapidly be able to tune in to their intuitive signals of hunger and fullness than those healing from anorexia. With bingeing disorders, they have become accustomed to eating quantities of food that are larger than their body's needs. As a result, their interpretation of fullness is initially highly skewed. As they rarely feel hungry, asking them to listen to hunger signals can feel alien and frustrating. They often have ignored hunger and fullness and are eating for many other reasons. These reasons can include boredom, loneliness, anger, and often guilt about what they're eating. We help them let go of their guilt by teaching them to be self-compassionate and understand that they developed these coping mechanisms as the only way to get through their difficult emotions. As their journey through Intuitive Eating progresses, staying present when eating and focusing on satisfaction will help these signals to return.

Also, as we do with those healing from anorexia, we put on our nutritionist caps. We give them scientific information in order to challenge their cognitive distortions and myths about food and their body, and we help them build nurturing coping mechanisms. We also keep the focus on satisfaction, body respect, joyful movement, and all the other Intuitive Eating principles.

For Lila, Dana, and Laurel, we'll see how their experiences with restricting led them down the path to their eating disorders. We'll then see how making Intuitive Eating their own has freed them completely from their fear of eating and feeling out of control. Ultimately, this philosophy has led them to happier and fuller life experiences.

Lila's Story—How Bulimia Nervosa Can Develop

Bulimia nervosa, or the attempt to purge calories after they have been consumed, often becomes the desperate solution to "failed dieting." Predictably, there is an inevitable rebound of overeating that occurs after someone has restricted—either a particular food, or quantity of food. This rebound that accompanies a semi-starved body can be physiologically/neurochemically triggered as a result of the secretion of brain chemicals, such as neuropeptide Y and others. Or it can be psychologically triggered due to the rebound from deprivation that results from restrictive thoughts or behaviors. In addition, their emotional state can drive them to binge eating for comfort or numbing. More often, we see all of these precursors. Once overeating takes hold, subsequent to dieting, people often feel out of control and terrified that all of the weight that was lost will return. Or, even worse in their minds, they fear that they'll end up at a higher weight than before they began dieting. In this desperation, they will look for ways to rid themselves of the calories consumed from overeating or from a binge. Purging attempts include excessive, compulsive exercise, vomiting, the use of laxatives, diuretics, diet pills, or even medically prescribed drugs that have a side effect of weight loss, or starving for a period of time after overeating. (As a note, laxatives and diuretics mainly remove water from the body, not calories. The resultant dehydration gives someone with bulimia a false sense that they have lost weight. This dehydration is inevitably followed by rebound water retention. This then leads to a recurring cycle of dehydration, followed by bloating, followed by further use of these drugs to rid the body of bloat—and on, and on, and on. There are extremely serious medical consequences accompanying the overuse of these drugs, as there are with diet pills, purging, and even compulsive exercise.)

For Lila, dieting began when she was a senior in high school, as she and her girlfriends were preparing for the prom. Prior to this time, Lila always felt that she was a "bigger" girl, but she wasn't overly concerned. Lila describes this time as one in which she was enjoying the "bonding" experience of going on a diet together with her girlfriends, so that they would "look good" for the prom. The daily meal plan for the girls included an apple for breakfast, salad with vinegar for lunch, and chicken and vegetables for dinner. They decided that they would do this for one week before the prom to "see what would happen." Lila, having underfed her body, remembered seeing an immediate change—and she was elated.

Graduation came after the prom, with a subsequent trip to the Caribbean for three and a half weeks. For the first time in her life, she felt completely free and independent. It was a time for partying and eating and losing her virginity. She drank many piña coladas and ate copious amounts of foods that she had previously been restricting, such as French bread and desserts. When she got home, her body size had grown and she barely fit into her clothes.

Rebounding from her diet experience, she continued her overeating during the summer before college. At the same time, she was navigating a multitude of emotions—anxiety about her newly found independence and sexuality and her impending move away from home, which resulted in emotional overeating to try to cope with these feelings.

Immediately after arriving at college, Lila became involved in a romantic relationship that lasted through her college years. She found herself transitioning from a very active, athletic high school student who wasn't worried about life to an inactive college freshman. She continued overeating, began actual bingeing, and had episodes of secret eating. She found herself thinking, "I can't believe I've eaten so much!" and panicking, which led to her purging her food, in an attempt to undo her out-of-control behavior. Lila never thought of bulimia as a weight control mechanism—instead, she saw it purely as a means of erasing the results of her bingeing. (Note that quite a significant amount of calories are still absorbed, even if one vomits after a binge—it's the brain and body's attempt at survival.)

Frequently, the experience of feeling out of control and consuming an enormous amount of extra food can become horrifying to a person. As a result, the impulse to eradicate any remnant of the behavior can become as compulsive as the behavior itself. As purging becomes a regular part of life, the sense of responsibility for one's actions disappears. As we have seen, coping with feelings without using food and with kindness can be a very difficult challenge for many people. Bulimia, once discovered, sometimes begins as a seemingly exciting alternative to overeating and eventually evolves into another means of pushing away feelings. Some report feeling as if they're "getting away with murder." Of course, as bulimia progresses, with its physical and mental side effects and its influence on one's normal pattern of eating, this "solution" ultimately becomes one's nemesis. Very quickly, shame emerges. Hiding the food wrappers, isolating in order to find time for the bingeing, or stealing away to the bathroom when eating in public become daily rituals, as well as a source of stress.

By Thanksgiving, Lila's bingeing and purging had continued to spiral out of control. Although still in her romantic relationship, she felt increasingly insecure about her body. She began an intense workout program, once or twice a week, with alternating periods of starving and binge-and-purge incidents. By the end of freshman year, Lila's normal exercise turned into compulsive over-exercising. Before going back to school, she sought the help of a nutritionist who helped her to curb her bulimia. During sophomore year, she joined a sorority and began a crusade to save her sorority sisters from the dangers of developing an eating disorder.

For the rest of her time in college, Lila was able to manage her eating and her exercise and was free of bulimia. Unfortunately, after graduation, she moved into an apartment with two roommates, one of whom was a binge eater and the other a restrictor. It was a highly emotional year, as her relationship ended, and she was facing the stress of postgraduate life. Living with roommates who had eating disorders, combined with the problems in her life, she felt depressed and went back to some of her old behaviors of restricting, then bingeing and purging.

In the healing of a serious eating disorder, we often see periods of time when the symptoms of the eating disorder return. These times are associated with periods of increased stress. This stress can be greater than the person's ability to cope with it. When this happens, one needs to see the return of symptoms as a red flag that should not be ignored. It represents a need to seek help in order to get back on the path of healing. And Lila did just that.

Although Lila had had a respite from her eating disorder during her last three years of college, she had not truly made peace with food. She had become a careful eater and a diligent exerciser. As her stress levels increased dramatically, she again sought the behavior of controlling her food as a way of giving her a false sense of control of her life. She also began overeating again, as a physical and psychological rebound of renewed dieting and as a way of comforting herself and numbing her pain. And, once again, the bulimia had returned. At this point, she sought a psychologist at an eating disorder clinic who helped her to stop purging once again. Directly afterward, she began doing the work required to help her find her way back into Intuitive Eating. This included a commitment to never diet or restrict again. As a result, Lila discovered that eating primarily for hunger, and respecting her body's signal of fullness, gave her an inner sense of empowerment. Choosing to eat what was appealing to her allowed her to receive satisfaction from her meals. She began to spend time with her feelings rather than pushing them down. She found that by developing her "emotional muscle," she was far better able to cope with life than she had ever been while engaging in bulimic behaviors.

Lila became a happily married woman, with three children, eating intuitively, including healthy movement in her life, and swearing off weighing herself. She became fully secure in her recovery and in her sense of inner trust.

Dana's Path to Binge Eating Disorder

There are many influences that can become the catalyst for entering the world of an eating disorder. Dana's story begins with feeling self-conscious about her body and comparing herself to her schoolmates at about age twelve. (This can often be a vulnerable time for a little girl who's beginning puberty. Her body is changing, and she can become fearful and unhappy about the changes.) By the time she was fifteen and in the beginning of ninth grade, Dana decided that she had to "do something to make a difference in her body."

In a perfect storm, this thinking coincided with several emotional traumas. Her parents got divorced, her mother subsequently remarried and then suffered a heart attack (from which she fortunately recovered). To complicate matters further, when Dana was at her dad's house, he regularly made comments about portion sizes and often told her that she had "had enough," even though she usually still felt hungry. Dana's mom had a resolute interest in nutrition and regularly bought what she thought were healthier foods. As a result of her mom's focus on "healthy" food and her dad's investment in the amount of food she ate, Dana developed an excessive consciousness about food. All of these conditions set the stage for eating and body image problems for Dana.

Dana had regularly enjoyed ice-blended chocolate drinks from the local coffee bar. Her first attempt at "making a difference" began by cutting out these drinks and was followed by cutting out one small item after another. As a result of these restrictions, she soon found that her clothes were beginning to fit looser. Concerned about her behavior, Dana's mother took her to see a nutritionist, who, unfortunately, turned out to be unqualified. The nutritionist inappropriately and incorrectly told her that her body couldn't handle carbohydrates. When she told her to cut down on her carb intake, Dana was eager to agree to the restriction. Dana complied even further, by believing that she should also restrict fruits, and even some vegetables, such as carrots! (In many states, there are no legal requirements to call oneself a "nutritionist." Be sure that your nutritionist is, at minimum, a registered dietitian nutritionist [RDN] and preferably trained in Intuitive Eating and Health at Every Size. Dietitians must have at least a bachelor's degree and postgraduate training, pass a national exam, and maintain continuing education.)

Predictably, Dana continued restricting what and how much she ate and began to feel fearful of many foods. Fueled by her sense of accomplishment, her search for identity, and a false sense of control, she continued to restrict. Dana became very weak, and by the time she reached nutrition therapy, her thinking was blurred by malnutrition.

(As a note, a journey into the Intuitive Eating process must begin not just with a motivation to heal, but also with a mind that is clear enough to understand what is taught and retain the information. Dana, at this point, was far beyond this ability.)

Dana was subsequently referred to a higher level of care—first, day treatment, and ultimately to an inpatient treatment at a hospital that had an adolescent eating disorder program.

After six months, she was discharged and greatly improved. With more sufficient nutrition, Dana began to grow again, and grew a couple of inches. Her menstrual cycle also returned.

Unfortunately, this was not the end of Dana's story. Although Dana's weight was restored, she still held the fear of eating certain foods and of eating early in the day. Undereating during the day led to excessive overeating at night. It's not hard to understand why she felt a total lack of control of her body and her life. Dana was now dealing with all of her previous emotional issues. In addition, being back in school, she experienced all of the normal issues of being a sixteen-year-old in high school. With this emotional angst, Dana continued to distract herself from these feelings by focusing on her battle with food and body.

Dana's compensatory eating at night scared her so much that she began once again to restrict her food intake. Fortunately, she was unable to maintain this serious restrictive behavior for more than three weeks. She then returned to her pattern of daytime undereating, followed by the inevitable nighttime overeating.

At this point, extremely frustrated and frightened, Dana was open to returning to nutrition therapy. Unhappy with her excessive hunger during the day and the discomfort that resulted from overeating at night, she finally had the motivation to make peace with food and eating. When her body was consistently nourished, she very quickly began practicing the principles of Intuitive Eating and was overjoyed by the results. She learned that by not eating enough for her body's needs during the day, she had quickly fallen into primal hunger and was inevitably set up to overeat at night. As soon as she committed to eating sufficient amounts during the day, the nighttime overeating diminished. Added to this, once she embraced the belief that no food was her enemy and allowed herself free access to foods she had been avoiding, she found that those foods took a normal balanced place in her eating life. While working on Intuitive Eating principles, she also continued in her psychotherapy with her psychologist. In this setting, she was able to deepen her ability to cope with her feelings instead of pushing them away with restriction and overeating.

By the time she was a high school sophomore, Dana had become a stable Intuitive Eater. Dana's path began with a dangerous and frightening slope to climb. Because she was far too malnourished, her initial introduction to appropriate nutrition therapy expectedly suffered a quick demise. She required medical stabilization and nutrition rehabilitation in an inpatient hospital setting in order to be ready for this journey. For the many patients we've seen—of all genders—the willingness to change entrenched habits and let go of old coping mechanisms could only begin with trust.

The Importance of Safety and Trust

The nutrition therapist must provide an atmosphere of safety and hope. Trust can only be developed when there is a belief that everything that is shared will be heard, absorbed, and not be judged. There needs to be confidence that the nutrition therapist understands that any behaviors that are revealed, no matter how dangerous or even life-threatening, were developed as a way to cope with a private world that was very scary or lonely or sad. Letting go of these coping mechanisms requires patience, a leap of faith, and a learning of new ways to think about food, body, and life. All of this is possible—the stories that we've related are just a few of the many people who have healed their eating disorders with this work.

An eating disorder can potentially have a short course and be resolved without permanent physical and/or psychological damage if it is treated with both psychotherapy and nutrition therapy in the early days of its inception. Unfortunately, there can be lifelong suffering and anguish and even death for those who go without proper treatment. This can also be the case for those who drop out of treatment before they are fully able to embrace the Intuitive Eating philosophy. But, on the bright side, let's look at a few cases where the eating disorder was caught early enough, given appropriate treatment, and healing took a rapid course.

Laurel—A Case of Rapid Healing

In the previous case histories, we've seen many influences that triggered the development of an eating disorder. Comments by family members frequently have a powerful effect on a young person's body image. School pressures, transitions into new phases of development, and other life experiences often create anxieties that are calmed or even numbed by the underuse or overuse of food. Dealing with these emotional issues can also be avoided by putting the focus on obsessional thinking about food and body. In Laurel's case, a combination of illness and personal trauma set off her eating disorder.

Laurel was a healthy girl without eating issues until she was almost seventeen years old. Just before her seventeenth birthday, she became very ill with tonsillitis, which decreased her normal appetite. The subsequent shrinking of her body led to positive comments by her friends. Liking this attention, Laurel found herself dieting for the first time in her life. She would tell herself that she didn't need "that cookie" or "that bag of chips." One month later, she got sick again, this time with the flu, leading again to a loss of appetite. Back to school, she received even more attention.

Soon after this, Laurel discovered that her boyfriend was cheating on her with her best friend—news that understandably devastated her. Feeling betrayed, she completely stopped eating and began to isolate from her friends. After that, even though her hunger returned, feeling so unhappy, she chose not to eat at all and began using laxatives. Laurel was trying to feel some semblance of control in her now out-of-control life.

Deeply concerned about her well-being, her parents sent her to a psychotherapist, with whom she had a wonderful relationship. She was also sent to a nutritionist, with whom she did not connect. She was given a high-caloric meal plan by the nutritionist, was told to weigh and measure her food, and to keep a food log. Unfortunately, this excessive amount of food caused "refeeding edema" (water retention that occurs when eating begins again after a period of starvation). In order to get some relief from her physical discomfort, Laurel began purging her food. Ultimately, she stopped seeing the nutritionist, stopped her bulimic behaviors, and stopped any kind of healthy eating. Instead, she began to eat nothing but candy!

At this point, Laurel was referred to nutrition therapy to learn Intuitive Eating by her psychotherapist. As in other cases previously mentioned, the safety that Laurel felt in this new experience led to a strong feeling of trust. With this trust, she became willing to absorb information that would help her change her thinking about eating and begin the journey to rebuilding a healthy relationship with food. Laurel was treated as part of the team in her recovery. She was told that, ultimately, her body was hers to protect and that a decision to get healthy again had to come from within. Clearly, it hadn't worked for her to follow an authoritarian recommendation. In her new treatment, she felt respected as an individual who was intelligent and capable of making wise decisions. She also appreciated hearing that all of the behaviors she had attempted in her eating disorder were created as coping mechanisms to deal with emotional and physical feelings.

Laurel was taught about starvation's effect on her energy levels, immune system, sleep patterns, cognitive functioning, and metabolism. She was taught the many advantages of eating in a balanced way that would be respectful to her body but still include the play foods that she had come to love. If she chose to eat this way, she would prevent large blood sugar fluctuations, and she would be providing her body with the nutritional building blocks for making hormones, strong bones, immunoglobulins, muscle tissue, neurotransmitters, and more. She soon began to examine the trade-off between what she would be getting by maintaining her disordered eating and what she would be giving up.

Part of Laurel's disordered behavior included isolating, out of a fear of eating in public. Soon, she was able to see that this emotionally damaging isolation, along with her potentially physically dangerous current patterns, was far more frightening than actually learning to eat again. This time around, however, she began by taking tiny baby steps, rather than giant leaps. Adding a bit of protein to her day, such as a string cheese in the morning or some cottage cheese or yogurt at lunch, was acceptable to her. It was not too much food to encourage excessive bloating, but it was a step in the right direction. Little by little, she added new foods, working toward a balance of protein, carbohydrates, and fats. She began to include fruits and vegetables, waffles and brown rice and pizza, nuts and beans, beef jerky and avocados. She also came to trust that she could include play food in the day. Little by little, she progressed, with very little physical discomfort.

She practiced and rehearsed what it would be like to go to dinner with friends. Although feeling scared, she took the risk and got through the initial experience, feeling triumphant. Her friendships were renewed, and she accomplished the task of college applications, the joy of the senior prom, and graduation. Eventually, Laurel left for her first year at college, where she was preparing and providing food for herself, as well as eating out with friends. She was able to again experience normal hunger signals and began, once again, to regularly get her period.

At college, as was to be expected, Laurel experienced a few emotionally uncomfortable situations. These experiences led her to an initial loss of appetite and a fleeting thought that controlling her eating might give her a sense of emotional control. But she very quickly remembered the conversations she had in the early days of her psychotherapy and nutrition therapy and was able to get right back on track. She stayed in touch through weekly calls and felt that this support was an important part of her transition into independence and full healing.

DEFINING MOMENTS

Regardless of what triggered the eating disorder, the most important course of action is to connect with a psychotherapist and a nutrition therapist. These professionals should be trained to understand the psychology of eating disorders and be able to offer a safe arena for the exploration of the thoughts and feelings that form the basis of one's relationship with food. Sometimes, during the treatment, there can be one defining moment that can affect the healing process profoundly. The following two vignettes illustrate defining moments:

Kelly is an example of someone who was fed up with her eating disorder and ready to do what it would take to fully heal. After her initial treatment, the time had come to work on refining Kelly's sense of satisfaction in eating. When asked if there was any one thing that particularly helped her during this period, Kelly's face lit up, and she said, "Yes, it was your [ER] story about eating a chocolate truffle during the movie *Chocolat*"— her defining moment! She loved hearing about the sensual experience of slowly tasting and savoring a delicious piece of chocolate, while watching a film about a chocolate shop in Paris. She had also seen the film, wishing that she could enjoy the chocolate—a food she had forbidden for herself. With a commitment to making peace with food, as well as trust in her nutrition therapist as a role model, Kelly began an exploration of all the foods she had restricted for years—especially chocolate!

Kelly continues to maintain her recovery and eats with a freedom that she hadn't felt since before her eating disorder began. Kelly's remarkable progress was attributed to challenging her destructive thoughts, honoring her hunger, and making peace with food.

Della, a six-foot-tall twenty-three-year-old, who had always been taller than her peers, had been in a battle with food all her life. She always felt "bigger" than others and self-conscious about her body, in comparison with her sister and, also, her mother, who was hyper-focused on appearance. Della began dieting at age fourteen, beginning a roller-coaster ride of drastic weight fluctuations, diet pills, food restriction, compulsive overeating, laxative abuse, and purging, which lasted until she began nutrition therapy at the age of twenty-two.

In her first session, Della was asked about her favorite foods. She mentioned many nutritious foods, such as beans and soups and vegetables and meat, and then, guiltily, acknowledged that she liked candy, but could only eat it in excess. As the Intuitive Eating process was explained to Della, she heard that she would always be able to eat any food that she desired, even candy. At first, she had a sense of disbelief, which was soon followed by a sense of calm. Della has since said that this moment of hope was one that has changed her life forever—her defining moment! She knew that all of her attempts at dieting had not worked and decided to give up the battle and focus on "just feeling good and enjoying all foods."

She left the office with a resolve to quit dieting once and for all. Immediately, she experienced a quieting of her mind and a feeling of peace, which she had never remembered feeling in relationship to eating.

Although past experiences with the excitement of each new diet gave her a temporary feeling of well-being, this couldn't compare with what she ultimately felt as an Intuitive Eater. After a year and a half of this work, Della still loved candy, but she no longer needed to eat the whole box—in fact, she never even thought about doing that again. Eating became a pleasurable experience. As she followed her hunger and fullness and taste preferences, she received satisfaction from her meals, enjoyed the play food that she desired, and never felt stuffed. All remained quiet on the front of Della's war with food and body, and her concerns disappeared—what a surprise!

As we have seen in hundreds of people, becoming an Intuitive Eater can have a powerful effect on many aspects of one's life. Many people have spent the majority of their waking moments thinking about what they've eaten and about their perceived physical inadequacies. Some have used these obsessions as a way to distract themselves from difficult thoughts and feelings. Others have literally numbed themselves from traumatic experiences. Many have felt shame about aspects of their eating disorders or about a body that doesn't meet society's unrealistic standards. For some people, the only emotion that triggers overeating is one that is associated with a feeling of guilt about eating itself. To their disbelief, once they are able to release this guilt, by making peace with food, their overeating vanishes.

Regardless of the root cause or trigger of binge eating, undereating, or other behaviors associated with eating disorders, an unhealthy or uncomfortable relationship with food can impede moving forward in life. Through their journey on the path of Intuitive Eating, we have seen people change jobs, leave abusive relationships, mend bad feelings with friends or family, and simply regain or achieve, for the first time in their lives, peace and joy and contentment. Just ask Della, or any of the others mentioned in this chapter—each would tell you, without a moment's hesitation, that the tradeoff is worth far more than anything they could have ever imagined!

READINESS FOR INTUITIVE EATING

Healing an eating disorder can take from a few months to many years. This depends on how long you've had the eating disorder, when you're ready to seek help, and other mitigating factors. It's important to be patient and compassionate with yourself. It's unlikely that anyone with an eating disorder can fully dive straight into Intuitive Eating. If you start too soon, without professional help, you may end up feeling scared, frustrated, and overwhelmed.

Here are some of the indicators of when you are ready to move into work on Intuitive Eating. Remember, this should be done in conjunction with your healthcare team:

- *Biological restoration and balance.* If you have anorexia, this means weight restoration to your genetic blueprint, which is different for different bodies. It's not realistic to expect yourself to be able to regularly hear hunger signals, let alone honor hunger and fullness before you're fully nourished. If you have bulimia or a binge eating disorder, this means moving from a pattern of chaotic eating to regular meals. Regardless of the eating disorder, it will usually take some sort of nutrition counseling with a nutrition therapist trained in Intuitive Eating and HAES to get you back into balance.
- *Recognition that the eating disorder is not about weight stigma or food, but rather a symptom of something deeper.* Once you begin to accept this, eating will move into the realm of self-care, rather than a staunch attempt at defending the eating disorder's existence.
- *Ability to recognize and willingness to deal with feelings.* As you are able to identify and appropriately cope with your feelings, the need to turn to eating disorder behaviors will decrease.
- *Ability to identify your wants and needs.* The more you are able to identify your wants and needs, the less you will need your eating disorder behaviors to fill that void.
- *Ability to take risks.* As your body begins to heal, both physically and psychologically, you will be ready to take and tolerate risks with your eating. For someone with anorexia, it may simply be eating a food without knowing its exact calorie content. For someone with bulimia, it might be savoring chocolate for the first time.
- *Willingness to give up diet culture forever.* Even the slightest thought of restriction can set into motion feelings of deprivation that can be the stepping-stone to an eating disorder.

INTUITIVE EATING CHART
How Intuitive Eating Principles Apply To Eating Disorders

Core Principle	Anorexia Nervosa	Bulima Nervosa/ Binge Eating Disorder
1. Reject the Diet Mentality.	Restricting is a core issue and can be deadly.	Restricting does not work and triggers primal hunger, which can lead to binge eating.
2. Honor your Hunger.	Weight restoration is essential. The mind cannot function and think properly. You are likely caught in an obsessional cycle of thinking and worrying about food, and have difficulty making a decision. Your body and brain need calories to function. Your nutrition therapist will work with you to create a way of eating that feels safe to you.	Eat regularly—this means three meals and two or three snacks daily. Eating regularly will help you get in touch with gentle hunger rather than the extremes that often occur with chaotic eating. Ultimately, you will trust your own hunger signals, even if they deviate slightly from this routine.
3. Make Peace with Food.	Take risks; add new foods when ready. Do this gradually with baby steps.	Take risks, try "feared" foods when ready and not vulnerable. (Vulnerability includes being overhungry, over-stressed, or experiencing some other feeling state.)
4. Challenge the Food Police.	Challenge the thoughts and beliefs about food. Take the morality, judgment, and rigidity out of eating.	Challenge the thoughts and beliefs about food. Take the morality and judgment out of eating.

INTUITIVE EATING CHART		
How Intuitive Eating Principles Apply to Eating Disorders		
Core Principle	Anorexia Nervosa	Bulima Nervosa/ Binge Eating Disorder
5. Discover the Satisfaction Factor.	Frequently, there are fears of or resistance to experiencing the plea-sure from eating (as well as other pleasures of life).	If satisfying foods and eating experiences are included regularly, there will be less impetus to binge.
6. Feel Your Fullness	You can't rely on your fullness signals during the beginning phases of recovery, as your body likely feels prematurely full, as a result of slowed digestion and stomach emptying. There is also a feeling of being bloated from "refeeding edema."	A transition away from experiencing the extreme fullness that is experi-enced with binge eating. Once regular eating is established, gentle fullness will begin to resonate. Note: If you are withdrawing from purging, especially from laxatives, the feeling of fullness may temporarily be distorted by feel-ing bloated from water retention.
7. Cope with Emotions with Kindness.	Often emotionally shut down. Food restriction, food rituals, and obses-sional thinking are the coping tools of life. With re-nourishment, you will be more prepared to deal with feelings that emerge.	Binge eating, purging, and excessive exercise are used as coping mecha-nisms. Can begin to take a time-out from these behaviors to start experi-encing and dealing with feelings.
8. Respect Your Body.	Heal the body image distortion.	Respect the here-and-now body.
9. Movement—Feel the Difference.	Will likely need to stop exercising or substitute gentle movement like yoga.	Over-exercising can be a purging behavior. Moder-ate exercise can help man-age stress and anxiety.

Cont.

INTUITIVE EATING CHART		
How Intuitive Eating Principles Apply to Eating Disorders		
Core Principle	Anorexia Nervosa	Bulima Nervosa/ Binge Eating Disorder
10. Honor Your Health.	Learning to remove the rigidity of nutrition— where there is a strict adherence to "nutritional principles," regardless of their source. Recognize that the body needs: Essential fat, Carbohydrates, Protein, Variety of foods	Learning to remove the rigidity of nutrition. There is a strict belief as to what constitutes healthy eating, and if this belief is violated, purging consequences can ensue (if bulimic). Recognize that the body needs: Essential fat, Carbohydrates, Protein Variety of foods

Eating Disorders Resources

ORGANIZATIONS

National Association of Anorexia Nervosa and Associated Disorders
P.O. Box 7
Highland Park, IL 60035
Crisis hotline: 847-831-3438
Website: www.ANAD.org
  An association of lay and professional people dedicated to alleviating the problems of eating disorders through advocacy, education, and prevention. One particular benefit of this group is that it offers more than three hundred *free* regional support groups throughout the country.

National Eating Disorders Association
603 Stewart Street, Suite 803
Seattle, WA 98101
Hotline: 800-931-2237
Website: www.nationaleatingdisorders.org
  The National Eating Disorders Association (NEDA) is the largest nonprofit organization dedicated to supporting individuals and families

affected by eating disorders. NEDA serves as a catalyst for prevention, cures, and access to quality care. They offer a free eating disorder screening tool on their website.

PROFESSIONAL ORGANIZATIONS

Academy for Eating Disorders (AED)
6728 Old McLean Village Drive
McLean, VA 22101
Phone: 703-556-9222
Website: www.aedweb.org

The Academy for Eating Disorders is a multidisciplinary association of academic and clinical professionals with expertise in the field of eating disorders. Their official peer-reviewed publication is the *International Journal of Eating Disorders*. AED's objectives include advancing research, advocacy, and prevention of eating disorders, and promoting effective treatment and care of patients with eating disorders and associated disorders. AED has some limited public information on their website.

International Association of Eating Disorders Professionals (IAEDP)
P.O. Box 1295
Pekin, IL 61555
Phone: 309-346-3341
Membership: 800-800-8126
Website: www.iaedp.com

IAEDP offers education, training, and certification for professionals treating eating disorders. The organization also promotes public awareness of eating disorders and assists in prevention efforts.

National Eating Disorders Association (NEDA)
Helpline: 800-931-2237
Crisis Text Line: or crisis situations, text "NEDA" TO 741741 to be connected with a trained volunteer.
Website: www.nationaleatingdisorders.org

OTHER WEBSITES

Eating Disorder Hope

www.eatingdisorderhope.com

> Offers articles about eating disorders, recovery stories, and a Facebook Live series.

Anorexia Survival Guide

www.anorexiasurvivalguide.com

> Offers a very helpful (and *free*) monthly e-newsletter *Eating Disorder Survival Guide for Parents*. Archives of past newsletters are available on the website. Especially valuable for parents with a child with an eating disorder.

Eating Disorder Referral and Information Center

www.edreferral.com

> An easy-to-navigate site with many helpful topics on eating disorders. This site is free to the public, but professionals pay a fee to get listed on the referral list.

Eating Disorder Resource Catalogue

www.EDcatalogue.com

> A catalogue of self-help books, professional resources, treatment facilities, and national organizations.

Gurze Books

www.gurzebooks.com

> Run by a small publishing company that specializes in eating disorders publications, including newsletters, books, and workbooks. Free catalogue upon request.

Epilogue

This may be the end of the book, but if you choose to become an Intuitive Eater, it becomes a new beginning.

Take the journey to becoming an Intuitive Eater, and you will go through a process that is bound to challenge some of your most entrenched thoughts, and perhaps stir up some deeply hidden feelings and fears. You know that living in a world of dieting chaos, with its self-blame and failure, doesn't work. It doesn't work metabolically or emotionally, and it certainly doesn't work spiritually. Clients talk over and over about feeling beaten down, defeated—as if their souls are actually hurting. By the time they come to this process, many have given up hope of ever being a normal eater.

Intuitive Eating is an empowering process that not only promotes health, but is your gateway to freedom. When you are freed from the tyranny of food and body anxiety, you have the space and renewed energy to pursue your dreams and discover your purpose in life. But becoming an Intuitive Eater requires a highly conscious decision and commitment. It means letting go of the old way of surviving and opening up to a new way of viewing life. It might take soul searching and introspective work to decide whether diet culture has been keeping you from your deepest appreciation of life. Making this perspective change can be difficult to accomplish initially but can ultimately become a way of living that defies reversal.

To begin this paradigm shift, you'll need to consider that there are many tradeoffs in the eating world. Having the "willpower" to stay on a diet can give you a temporary sense of power and control, while being an Intuitive Eater can give you a lifelong sense of self-empowerment. The acts of dieting and rebound bingeing can offer excitement. So does eating forbidden foods. But when excitement no longer comes from food or dieting, other aspects of life are free to be experienced. When you are using food or the obsession that dieting creates to numb yourself or to distract yourself from your feelings the majority of the time, you might feel calmer and less stressed, but your life can seem like a blurred, out-of-focus home movie. You know you're alive and racing through life, but you rarely experience its highs, lows, and nuances of sensation. Once you peel off the layers of dieting and disconnection from your feelings, you'll discover a richness in life that might have been buried for decades.

When you become an Intuitive Eater who responds to those innate bio-logical and food preference signals, you become acutely in touch with your body, thoughts, and feelings. Ultimately, this awareness and responsive-ness can extend to the rest of your life.

You also learn to operate from a framework of curiosity rather than judgment. When dieting, every digression from the food plan becomes an opportunity to become critical of yourself. And criticism can become deadly and infectious. It's not unusual for this critical viewpoint to spill over into other behaviors or even to family members and friends. As an Intuitive Eater you see the food experience as an opportunity to learn more about your thoughts and feelings. You may find that this curiosity stimu-lates other explorations in your life. You may even decide to make serious changes in other parts of your life that have been making you stressed or unhappy. Some clients have decided to change jobs or remove themselves from abusive relationships, as a result of going deeper into the meaning of life. Others decide to get into counseling with a therapist.

One of our clients aptly suggested that Intuitive Eating is about *waiting* and learning to be patient. She finds herself *waiting* to eat until she is hungry. Then she describes *waiting* during a time-out in the midst of her meal to see if she is full. When she is experiencing a difficult feeling that she used to cover up with overeating, she now sits with the feeling and *waits* it out until she feels better. And in the bigger picture, she is *waiting* for her eating to normalize so that she feels the freedom and peace in her life that she has so badly craved. She says that this process has taught her to be more patient than she has ever been in her life. She has decided that patience is golden, that what she has learned about herself as she "patiently *waits*" is more valuable than all the hope that dieting had offered her (and, of course, ultimately taken away) and all the money she has spent on her failed diets. Learning to *wait* has freed her from the burden of dieting and from a life in which she felt locked in and trapped, with no escape.

We deeply hope that you will be able to free yourself from diet culture by reclaiming the Intuitive Eating ability with which you were born.

We also want to acknowledge that while Intuitive Eating can be a profound transformational process on an individual level, there is a lot of work that needs to be done on a cultural and policy level in order to dismantle the systems of oppression for all bodies.

Common Questions and Answers About Intuitive Eating

We have compiled some of the most frequently asked questions by our clients as they go through the process of Intuitive Eating. We hope that these answers will also be answers to some of your questions.

Question #1: How long will this process take?
Answer: Unfortunately, this question has no pat answer. It depends on how long you've been dieting and how entrenched the voices of the Food Police are. It also depends on how willing you are to place your focus on the messages your body gives you about hunger, fullness, and satisfaction and concentrate on honoring your body with respect and self-care. We have seen some people connect quite rapidly with the concept and take only a month or two to be eating in a new way. For others, it's taken two or three or even five years to be ready and motivated to work on the principles and make serious change.

Question #2: If I let myself eat whatever I want, won't I eat uncontrollably?
Answer: When you have made complete peace with food and trust that what you like will always be available to you, you'll naturally be able to stop eating. If you're only giving yourself pseudo-permission, it won't work, because you don't really believe you'll always have access to this food. So, check out how genuine your permission giving is. Remember, guilt is what tends to make people eat uncontrollably. Intuitive Eating means having no guilt in your eating. When you first begin the healing process, you may find that you're eating more of the foods that you have

previously restricted. This restriction has led to deprivation, and you may end up eating more of these foods for a while. Once the deprivation has healed, these foods will take a balanced place in your eating life.

Question #3: Won't my friends be judgmental and question my eating?
Answer: You may find that many people won't understand what you're doing. Most of our society is conditioned by diet culture. In fact, some people are perpetually talking about being on diets or saying that they should be on diets. So, yes, some people will be judgmental. You may find that it's hard to explain what you are doing, but if you mention that you're just trying to get back to your inner wisdom about eating that was lost due to diet culture, there's more of a chance that they'll drop their judgment. Remember, this is an intuitive process. Some of the time, you'll just be feeling your way through it as you become secure in the knowledge that it feels right to you.

Question #4: Should I try to explain what I'm doing?
Answer: You can try, but it might be frustrating. Key phrases to give out would be:

- Dieting leads to deprivation, deprivation leads to craving, and craving can lead to out-of-control behavior.
- I give myself permission to eat whatever I want when I'm hungry and find that I'm more easily able to stop when I'm full.
- When I feel satisfied with what I eat, I eat just what my body needs.
- I'm learning to cope with my emotions with kindness, instead of relying on food.

Question #5: Will I ever lose weight doing this?
Answer: The most important statement that we can make is that if you focus on losing weight, it will interfere with Intuitive Eating. Remember, Intuitive Eating is an internal process, while weight loss is an external process that pulls you away from tuning in to your inner wisdom about eating. We are not shaming you for your desire to lose weight (it's understandable, given the omnipresent diet culture)—we simply hope that you will embrace a fulfilling life in your here-and-now body, rather than putting it off while you chase weight loss.

Question #6: What if I stop focusing on weight loss? What's this all worth?
Answer: You will derive a great deal of peace and contentment from this process and let go of weight stigma. You will get off the "treadmill" of deprivation and guilt. You will eat in a way that's pleasurable and satisfying. You will stop feeling guilty about your eating and stop shaming yourself for your body. All in all, achieving an Intuitive Eating style will free your time for more enriching thoughts and feelings (rather than food worry and guilt). For many people, that means ultimately feeling happier.

Question #7: What if I never feel hungry?
Answer: Some people report that they don't feel hunger in their stomachs, but ultimately get raging headaches or some other sign of not having eaten. For some people, they've dieted and/or binged for so long that they've completely lost touch with hunger. If this is the case for you, you can give yourself a period of time where you purposely eat every three to four hours to try to reestablish your hunger signals. Your body needs food in these intervals, and you may find that after a while your body trusts that it's going to get fed and will respond by expressing hunger.

Question #8: How will I know when I'm full?
Answer: When you have full food security by *making peace with food* and have learned to *honor your hunger,* you'll find that your fullness signals are much more apparent to you. If you eat all the time and don't feel hunger, it's hard to experience fullness. You'll have no base with which to start to discern the difference. It's helpful to take a time-out in the midst of your meal to test your fullness.

Question #9: Can I ever eat something if it just looks good, but I'm not hungry?
Answer: The Intuitive Eating process is not another diet with a set of absolute rules. Although *honoring your hunger* is one of the first principles, there will be many times when you'll choose to eat something just for its taste or sensual pleasure, without being hungry. We call this taste hunger. If you give yourself permission for occasional responses to taste hunger, you'll feel more satisfied with your entire eating experience.

Question #10: What about sweets? Should I eat them when I'm hungry?
Answer: In general, if you wait until you're hungry to eat sweets, you'll find that you may end up eating a larger quantity than you might need to

satisfy your sweet tooth, because you'll be trying to satisfy your biological hunger. Most cultures offer sweets after the meal to please the palate and to punctuate the end of the meal. Having something sweet, then, is usually in response to taste hunger.

Question #11: What if I want to eat when I can't handle my feelings?
Answer: Generally, the quickest route to resolving emotional conflict is to allow yourself to experience your feelings to their utmost. But sometimes this can be overwhelming. Some people need to be with a friend or a therapist to feel safe enough to let their feelings come out. Others are able to tolerate their feelings for some period of time, but then need an escape for a while until they feel able to deal with them again. If that is where you find yourself, then search for kind ways to comfort and distract yourself from the feelings so that you don't end up numbing with food as your only way of coping.

Question #12: What about good nutrition? If I eat whatever I like, I won't be healthy, right?
Answer: We have found, in case after case, that giving yourself permission to eat whatever you like ultimately results in a balance of food choice. You'll find, after you have finally made peace with food, that the majority of your food choices will be nutrient dense, and a smaller portion will be play food. The more nutritious foods take care of your body, while the play food takes care of your soul! After all, if you never have to be deprived of a favorite food again, you won't have insatiable cravings for it. You'll want to feel good, and feeling good comes from eating according to your hunger and fullness signals, without overfilling yourself.

Question #13: Do I have to exercise to make this work?
Answer: We have put our chapter on movement toward the end of the book, because we find that an emphasis on exercise in the beginning of this process can make some people feel as if they're on another diet. Moving your body is something that you'll probably want to do, because it makes you feel good. If you disconnect your eating from movement, you'll find that you don't get into the old trap of feeling that exercise is for the purpose of weight loss. Movement is a benefit for all people, young and old. It's part of a healthy existence. Look for opportunities to move that are fun and enjoyable. If, on the other hand, you are someone who is adamant about not

exercising, this process will still be of benefit to you, because it frees you from the world of diet culture and its unending demands. But wait and see, you may find yourself moving despite yourself!

Question #14: Should I tell others that they should try this process?
Answer: Most people don't like being told what to do. It usually makes them feel rebellious. You're probably better off just enjoying being an Intuitive Eater living this new lifestyle. If people ask you why you seem so calm and not obsessed about food or why you look so radiant, you can tell them what you're doing. They might then ask about doing it themselves.

Question #15: What do I do if a host or hostess tries to push more food on me when I don't want any more?
Answer: This person is not respecting your boundaries and does not have a right to pressure you. Say, "No, thank you" firmly. Say that you're full and don't want to feel uncomfortable. Remember, your intuitive signals are what count, and you have the right to honor them.

Step-by-Step Guidelines

If you're someone who cooks, you'll know that before you learned how to cook, just pulling out a recipe card might have caused you to feel anxious about whether the finished concoction would ever resemble any cooked dish you'd ever before seen. In order to gain a comfort level in your kitchen, you probably needed to understand some of the basic concepts of cooking. If the recipe said "simmer," you wouldn't have known the difference between boiling, simmering, or sautéing. The following guidelines are similar to your recipe card. If you look at them before you read the rest of the book, you might get confused and misunderstand the purpose of each. Once you've become comfortable with the Intuitive Eating philosophy, however, these guidelines can become a quick and easy reference when you need to reconnect with the process.

STEP 1 — PRINCIPLE 1:
REJECT THE DIET MENTALITY

Throw out the diet books and magazine articles that offer you false hope of losing weight quickly, easily, and permanently. Get angry at a diet culture that promotes weight loss and the lies that have led you to feel as if you were a failure every time a new diet stopped working and you gained back all of the weight. If you allow even one small hope to linger that a new and better diet or food plan might be lurking around the corner, it will prevent you from being free to rediscover Intuitive Eating.

1. Make a firm commitment to give up dieting for the rest of your life. As long as you hold on to even the slightest thought, promise, or hope that

dieting is in your future, you will sabotage your ability to become an Intuitive Eater.

2. Throw out all of your diet and tracking apps, calorie counters, and old diet books and articles. Unfollow those who promote dieting, and follow those who promote Intuitive Eating and Health at Every Size.

3. When friends talk about the newest fad diet, or you see a TV commercial or magazine article on dieting—avoid getting drawn into the excitement that might arise. Instead, take a deep breath and gently assure yourself that you are committed to a new way of thinking and feeling about food and eating, and that dieting is not a part of this new process.

4. Protect your food boundaries by refusing to allow others to tell you what to eat, when to eat, or how much to eat. Protect your body boundaries by refusing to allow others to make comments about your weight and body.

5. If you notice that you're feeling rebellious or beginning to eat unconsciously, check in with yourself to see if you're still holding on to diet thinking and diet rules that are triggering this reaction or if you're being bombarded by any outside boundary invaders.

Step 2 — Principle 2:
Honor Your Hunger

Keep your body biologically fed with adequate energy and carbohydrates. Otherwise you can trigger a primal drive to overeat. Once you reach the moment of excessive hunger, all intentions of moderate, conscious eating are fleeting and irrelevant. Learning to honor this first biological signal sets the stage for rebuilding trust with yourself and food.

1. Begin to listen to any noise or bodily sensation and mood that indicates that you are experiencing hunger, such as a growling or grumbling stomach, a slight headache, a lack of mental focus, grouchiness, lack of energy, and so on.

2. As soon as you recognize your biological hunger, make the time to eat.

3. If you neglect this most basic signal and get over-hungry, it will be very hard to identify what you really want to eat or when you've had enough. Experiment with the "Hunger Discovery Scale" on page 99.

4. If you don't seem to experience hunger signals over long periods of time, you might want to try eating every three to four hours. Eventually, your body will get used to being fed regularly and will begin to provide you with dependable hunger signals.

5. Keep in mind that if you are sick or stressed, hunger signals may be blunted. It's important to feed your body on those days, too, even if you don't feel the hunger.

6. Be prepared—be sure to make time for shopping for food, cooking or picking up pre-made food, and for gathering snacks or even meals to put in a lunch bag or to carry in the car. In this way, you show respect for your body's signals and can provide for your needs.

STEP 3 — PRINCIPLE 3:
MAKE PEACE WITH FOOD

Call a truce, stop the food fight! Give yourself unconditional permission to eat. If you tell yourself that you can't or shouldn't have a particular food, it can lead to intense feelings of deprivation that build into uncontrollable cravings and, often, bingeing. When you finally "give in" to your forbidden food, eating will be experienced with such intensity, it will usually result in Last Supper overeating, and overwhelming guilt.

1. Give yourself unconditional permission to eat whatever you really like. Make avocado emotionally equivalent to lettuce and peach pie equivalent to a peach.

2. Beware of giving yourself "pseudo-permission" by telling yourself that you can eat what you like but continuing to hold guilty thoughts about your food choices. It won't work!

3. Do not eliminate any food that sounds appealing to you, unless you have a medical condition, such as celiac disease.

4. Observe how your body feels when eating this food and how satisfying it is to your tongue. Make a mental note of these experiences for your memory bank.

5. Keep an ample supply of all the foods that you think you might like to eat. (Restock the supply when it gets low.)

STEP 4 — PRINCIPLE 4:
CHALLENGE THE FOOD POLICE

Scream a loud no to thoughts in your head that declare you're "good" for eating minimal calories or "bad" because you ate a piece of chocolate cake. The food police monitor the unreasonable rules that diet culture has created. The police station is housed deep in your psyche, and its loudspeaker shouts negative barbs, hopeless phrases, and guilt-provoking indictments. Chasing the Food Police away is a critical step in returning to Intuitive Eating.

1. Identify your distorted food, dieting, and eating thoughts and beliefs. Throw them out and replace them with the truth.

2. Listen for the destructive voices that can speak harmful thoughts:

- **The Food Police** voice is harsh and critical and is driven by diet culture. It can be stimulated by listening to the media, parents, and peers. It keeps you at war with your relationship with food and your body.
- **The Nutrition Informant** voice is judgmental and colludes with the Food Police. It gives you nutrition facts to help justify your dieting.
- **The Diet Rebel** voice is angry and is born in response to boundary invaders who cross over the line into the private space that holds your Intuitive Eating signals and feelings about your body. It protects your autonomy while also causing some destructive eating behavior.

3. Develop the helpful voices that can get you through hard times and make your eating relationship more comfortable:

- **The Food Anthropologist** voice makes neutral observations. It notes your thoughts and actions with respect to your food world to help you make choices about what you want to eat, when you want to eat, and how much you need to eat. It can also record these thoughts in your memory bank, so they will be easily accessible when needed in the future to help you make eating decisions.
- **The Nurturer** voice is compassionate and gentle and provides soothing and reassuring statements that support you through this process.
- **The Rebel Ally** voice evolves from the Diet Rebel voice and helps you protect your boundaries against anyone who invades your eating space.

• **The Nutrition Ally** voice replaces the Nutrition Informant voice when the Food Police are exiled. It is interested in nutrition with no hidden dieting agenda.

• **The Intuitive Eater** voice speaks your gut reactions. You were born with this voice, and it gives you messages and answers about your eating that only you can know. It also helps you make decisions that only you have the right to make.

4. Watch out for negative self-talk based on the following irrational beliefs and distorted thinking:

• Dichotomous thinking—thinking in an all-or-nothing, black-and-white fashion.
• Absolutist thinking—magical thinking that believes that one behavior will absolutely affect and control a second behavior.
• Catastrophic thinking—thinking in exaggerated ways.
• Pessimistic thinking or "the cup is half-empty"—where a given situation is seen in its worst-case scenario.
• Linear thinking—inflexible thinking in a straight line, allowing for no variables.

5. Replace negative self-talk with positive self-talk based on rational thinking. Some examples of rational thinking include:

• Living in the gray—moderate thoughts, not black and white.
• Permissive thoughts and statements.
• Accurate, nonexaggerated thoughts.
• "The cup is half-full" thoughts—creating the best-case scenario.
• Process thinking—focus on continual change and learning, prioritizing the means rather than the end.

STEP 5 — PRINCIPLE 5:
DISCOVER THE SATISFACTION FACTOR

The Japanese have the wisdom to promote pleasure as one of their goals of healthy living. In our compulsion to comply with diet culture, we often overlook one of the most basic gifts of existence—the pleasure and satis-

faction that can be found in the eating experience. When you eat what you really want, in an environment that is inviting, the pleasure you derive will be a powerful force in helping you feel satisfied and content.

1. Give yourself permission to seek pleasure in your eating. The more pleasurable your food is, the more satisfaction you'll derive from your eating experience. (The more satisfied you feel, the more you'll eat just what you need—especially if you know that this food will never be forbidden.)

2. Figure out what you *really* want to eat by paying attention to the following sensations associated with eating:

- Taste—sweet, savory, salty, sour, bitter
- Texture—hard, crunchy, smooth, creamy
- Aroma—sweet, acrid, mild
- Appearance—color, shape, eye appeal
- Temperature—hot, cold, icy, temperate
- Volume or filling capacity—airy, light, dense

3. Think about how your body might feel when you finish eating:

- Will you be physically satisfied by your choice?
- Will a dense food make you feel uncomfortably full later or an airy food leave you feeling empty?
- Will an overly rich meal give you stomach distress?
- Will a primarily sweet meal send your blood sugar on a roller-coaster ride?

4. Make your eating environment enjoyable:

- Eat when gently hungry rather than over-hungry.
- Make time to appreciate your food.
- Create an aesthetic environment—try pretty placements, candles, colorful dishes, classical music.
- Sit down to eat.
- Take several deep breaths before you eat.
- Savor your food.

- Pay attention to eating as slowly as you can.
- Taste each bite of food that you put in your mouth.
- Provide variety in your meal.
- Avoid tension while eating.

5. Don't settle. Eliminate the unenjoyable—*if you don't love it, don't eat it, and if you love it, savor it!*
6. Check in with your taste buds in the midst of your meal to see if the food still tastes as good as it did when you began.
7. Remember, it doesn't always have to be perfect—sometimes meals are not in your control. There are many more opportunities ahead for satisfying meals.

STEP 6 — PRINCIPLE 6:
FEEL YOUR FULLNESS

In order to honor your fullness, you need to trust that you will give yourself the foods you desire. Listen for the body signals that tell you that you are no longer hungry and observe the signs that show that you're comfortably full. Pause in the middle of a meal or food and ask yourself how the food tastes, and what your current fullness level is.

1. Pay attention to your fullness signals. But remember, the only way that you can do this is to give yourself unconditional permission to eat, if you have food security. You must firmly believe that you will be able to eat again when you get hungry in order to be able to stop when you're full.
2. Be sure to honor your hunger. If you're over-hungry, your urgency to eat will create great difficulty in recognizing your fullness signals. Equally, if you begin eating before true hunger arises, your fullness signals will be muted—you're likely to be guided by your tongue instead of your stomach.
3. Discard the notion that you must finish everything on your plate because you fear wasting food.
4. Increase your consciousness in order to help you identify satiety.

- Try eating without distraction so that you can be fully present during your meal.

• Pause in the middle of a meal or snack and take a time-out to check your fullness level. This is not a commitment to stop eating but a commitment to check in with your body and taste buds.

    —Take a taste check. Ask: How does the food taste? Does it meet my expectations? Is it satisfying my taste buds? Or am I continuing to eat just because it's there?

    —Take a satiety check. Pay attention to the signals that your stomach gives you to indicate that you're becoming comfortably full. Ask: What's my hunger or fullness level? Am I still hungry? Is hunger going away? Do I feel insatiable? Am I beginning to feel satisfied?

    —Practice self-connection using the "Fullness Discovery Scale Journal" for self-connection on page 177.

• Identify the last few bites threshold. This is the endpoint. You know that the bites you take are the last. Don't worry if you can't do this at first—it will ultimately become intuitive. If you feel disappointed that you have to stop at this point, remember, you can eat this food or another food again, when your hunger returns. Eating is actually more satisfying when you're comfortably hungry, rather than already full. You're giving yourself a gift by stopping now.

• Make a concrete statement to yourself that you've reached the threshold bite by putting your fork and knife on your plate or by moving your plate forward a little bit.

• Give your leftovers to the server to wrap up if you're at a restaurant or put them in the refrigerator if you're at home.

• Say, "No, thank you" firmly to your host or hostess if more food is being thrust upon you. You have a right to say no.

5. Make sure that you have plenty of food available for your meals. If you give yourself too little to eat, you'll never feel satisfied or full. You don't need "too much" food, but "too little" food will sabotage this process.

6. Select foods that have some substance. If you only choose "air foods" such as rice cakes and raw vegetables, you'll get a false sense of satiety, only to get hungry again much too quickly.

STEP 7 — PRINCIPLE 7:
COPE WITH YOUR EMOTIONS WITH KINDNESS

First, recognize that food restriction, both physically and mentally, can, in and of itself, trigger loss of control, which can feel like emotional eating. Find kind ways to comfort, nurture, distract, and resolve your issues. Anxiety, loneliness, boredom, and anger are emotions we all experience throughout life. Each has its own trigger, and each has its own appeasement. Food won't fix any of these feelings. It may comfort for the short term, distract from the pain, or even numb you into a food hangover. But food won't solve the problem. You'll ultimately have to deal with the source of the emotion.

1. Ask yourself: Am I biologically hungry? If your answer is yes, honor your hunger and eat!

2. When you find yourself searching for food but know that you're not biologically hungry, take a time-out to ask yourself: What am I feeling?

> • Are you scared, anxious, angry, bored, hurt, lonely, depressed? Or are you happy, excited, need a reward, or want to celebrate?
> • To help identify your feelings, spend some quiet time writing in your journal or talking into your phone. Or if it's easier to get in touch with your feelings with another person, call a good friend or understanding relative. You might even need to call your psychotherapist or nutrition therapist. Use email or text, if that's an easier way to communicate.

3. Then ask yourself: What do I need?

> • Do you actually need sleep, a hug, some intellectual stimulation, or something else? Food doesn't satisfy any of those needs.

4. In order to get your needs met, ask: Would you please? Sometimes, for needs to be fulfilled, you'll have to speak up and ask for help.

5. Meet your needs without using food in the following ways:

• Nurture yourself by taking bubble baths, listening to soothing music, getting a massage, taking a yoga class, buying yourself some flowers, and so on.

• Deal with your feelings. Acknowledge what is troubling you. Allow your feelings to emerge. This will reduce your need to push them down with food.

• If necessary, provide yourself with a temporary distraction. It's okay to get away from the feelings from time to time, but you don't have to use food for this purpose. Try watching a movie, reading an absorbing book, listening to music or an audio book, gardening, and so on.

6. If you have an episode of using food to cope, see it as a sign that something is going on in your life that needs attention. Whatever you do, don't beat yourself up for this behavior. Most people do it at times—just take it as a learning experience and move on.

STEP 8 — PRINCIPLE 8:
RESPECT YOUR BODY

Accept your genetic blueprint. Just as a person with a shoe size of eight would not expect to realistically squeeze into a size six, it is equally futile (and uncomfortable) to have the same expectation with body size. But mostly, respect your body so you can feel better about who you are. It's hard to reject diet culture if you are unrealistic and critical about your body shape. All bodies deserve dignity.

1. Appreciate the functions and miracle of your body.
2. Take bubble baths, and use lotions and creams that feel soothing as you rub them in.
3. Get massages and hugs and caresses that give your body the opportunity to be touched.
4. Get comfortable. Buy comfortable undergarments. Buy clothing that is flattering and fits you without being tight.
5. Don't hide your body in clothes that are too large.
6. Quit the body-check game. Stop comparing yourself to everyone else in the room. It blinds you from appreciating yourself and is a setup

for more body dissatisfaction. It might even create a temptation to return to dieting.

7. Don't compromise for the "big event." Don't succumb to the pressure of "dieting down" to squeeze into that special outfit—it will only backfire.

8. Stop body bashing. Every time you focus on your perceived "imperfect" body parts, it creates more self-consciousness and body worry. It's also a form of objectification. When you hear yourself making disparaging comments about your body, replace these comments with kind body statements.

9. Stop weighing yourself. It can only make you feel discontented with your body.

10. Respect body diversity, especially yours.

11. Be realistic about your genetic makeup. Accept your body type and size. You can't fool Mother Nature!

12. Be understanding of yourself. Respect the fact that you may be someone who has used food to cope when you knew no other way to handle your feelings, or because you've been a victim of diet culture. Be gentle with yourself and accept your here-and-now body.

Step 9 — Principle 9:
Movement — Feel the Difference

Forget militant exercise. Just get active and feel the difference. Shift your focus to how it feels to move your body, rather than the calorie-burning effect of exercise. If you focus on how you feel from working out, such as energized, it can make the difference between rolling out of bed for a brisk morning walk or hitting the snooze alarm.

1. Break through exercise barriers:

   • Discover all the reasons behind any exercise resistance that you might have. It may be due to having been teased as a child, having rebelled against authority, feeling intimidated as a result of weight stigma, and so on.

   • Focus on how it feels. Movement is primarily for feeling good. It so happens that the better you feel, the less you'll need to use food as a way to cope. It can also give you increased energy, a general sence of well-being, a sense of empowerment, and sounder sleep.

• Decouple exercise from weight loss. Erase the tape of how exercise felt when you were dieting. You probably weren't getting enough calories or carbohydrates to give you the energy to exercise and feel good at the same time.

• Focus on movement as a way of taking care of yourself, feeling good now, and preventing health problems later in life.

• Don't get caught in exercise mind games such as:

  ○ *The It's-Not-Worth-It Trap*: feeling it's not worth it if it doesn't last a specified amount of time.

  ○ *Busyness*: being busy is not the same as physical activity.

  ○ *The No-Time-to-Spare Trap*: learn to prioritize.

  ○ *The If-I-Don't-Sweat-It-Doesn't-Count Trap*: physical fitness doesn't have to mean rigorous workouts.

2. Get active in daily living. Make movement convenient and fun:

• Park your car a few blocks from your destination, so you can add some walking to your day.

• Walk up or down stairs instead of using the elevator.

• Ride your bike or walk to work if you live close enough.

• When you travel, take walking shoes or a jump rope. Consider choosing hotels that have workout facilities.

3. Make movement fun.

• Consider playing a team sport such as volleyball (beach volleyball during the summer), softball, basketball, soccer, or tennis.

• Join a gym, if having others around you will motivate you and if it doesn't trigger you to start comparing yourself to others.

• Buy a treadmill or other home exercise equipment and put a TV in front of it so you can watch movies or interesting programs. Listening to music or an audio book might also make the movement more fun.

• Find a partner with whom you can take walks. Talking and walking can make the walk more enjoyable.

4. Make movement a non-negotiable priority.

5. Be comfortable while moving.

6. Include strength training so you can rebuild muscle that was lost from dieting.

7. Include stretching as part of your routine.

8. Remember rest. Make sure you give yourself days of rest within your exercise week. It will prevent burnout and give your muscles a chance to refresh and repair.

Step 10 — Principle 10:
Honor Your Health with Gentle Nutrition

Make food choices that honor your health and taste buds while making you feel good. Remember that you don't have to eat perfectly to be healthy. You will not suddenly get a nutrient deficiency or become unhealthy from one snack, one meal, or one day of eating. It's what you eat consistently over time that matters. Progress, not perfection, is what counts.

1. Consider the tenets of food wisdom: variety, moderation, and balance. As with movement, consider nutrition as your passport to feeling good.

2. Be sure you are eating enough to feed your metabolism. Be sure to stoke your metabolic fire by getting sufficient fuel throughout the day by eating whenever you're hungry.

3. Eat plenty of whole grains, fruits and vegetables, and beans for their fiber content, so your digestive tract works well. They're also a powerhouse of vitamins, minerals, and phytochemicals.

4. Eat sufficient protein for cellular repair and production of hormones, enzymes, hair, nails, and so on.

5. Eat plenty of carbohydrates and sufficient calories, so your protein can be used as a protein source and not be burned as an energy source.

6. Drink plenty of water to aid digestion, prevent constipation, have sufficient blood volume, and cleanse your kidneys.

7. Eat an adequate amount of fat, such as avocado, olive oil, nuts, and so on. We need fat in our diets for these reasons:

- To promote satiety.
- To help build cell walls, including brain cells and neurotrans-
mitter receptors.
- For absorption of fat-soluble vitamins.
- For production of hormones.

8. Allow for some *play foods* in order to balance your good health with pleasure and satisfaction. Let most of your food choices be made for nourishing your body, and allow some of them to be for simple pleasure.

9. Get off the food pedestal. You don't have to be perfect. Honor your health, your taste buds, and your humanness.

These guidelines summarize the chapters of this book. The order in which they're presented is not an absolute, just as nothing in this book is absolute, except for giving up the pursuit of dieting. Use them as your recipe card, as we suggested at the beginning of this appendix. But just as you might improvise in cooking your dish from the written recipe, be creative with these guidelines. Use what feels right for you, add to them if you like, and discard what doesn't fit. The bottom line is to trust your gut—use your intuitive talents to feel comfortable with eating and to release yourself from the prison of dieting.

If you'd like to dive deeper into the practices of becoming an Intuitive Eater, you might find our *Intuitive Eating Workbook* a valuable tool.

References

Intuitive Eating Studies

Avalos, L., Tylka, T., and Wood-Barcalow, N. (2005). The body appreciation scale: Development and psychometric evaluation. *Journal of Body Image* 2:285–297.

Anderson, L., et al. (2016). Contributions of mindful eating, intuitive eating, and restraint to BMI, disordered eating, and meal consumption in college students. *Eating and Weight Disorders* 21(1):83–90.

Andrew, R., Tiggemann, M., and Clark, L. (2016). Predictors and health-related outcomes of positive body image in adolescent girls: A prospective study. *Developmental Psychology* 52(3):463–474.

Andrew, R., Tiggemann, M., and Clark, L. (2015). Predictors of intuitive eating in adolescents. *Journal of Adolescent Health* 56(2):209–214.

Augustus-Horvath, C., and Tylka, T. (2011). The acceptance model of intuitive eating: A comparison of women in emerging adulthood, early adulthood, and middle adulthood. *Journal of Counseling Psychology* 58:110–125.

Barak-Nahum, A., Haim, L.B., and Ginzburg, K. (2016). When life gives you lemons: The effectiveness of culinary group intervention among cancer patients. *Society of Science and Medicine* 166:1–8.

Barraclought, E.L., et al. (2019). Learning to eat intuitively: A qualitative exploration of the experience of mid-age women. *Health Psychology Open* 1:6(1): doi: 10.1177/2055102918824064.

Bas, M., et al. (2017). Turkish version of the intuitive eating scale-2: Validity and reliability among university students. *Appetite* 114:391–397.

Bégin C., et al. (2018). Eating-related and psychological outcomes of health at every size intervention in health and social services centers across the province of

Québec. *American Journal of Health Promotion*, January 1:890117118786326. doi: 10.1177/0890117118786326

Boucher, S., et al. (2016). Teaching intuitive eating and acceptance and commitment therapy skills via a web-based intervention: A pilot single-arm intervention study. *Journal of Medical Internet Research Protocols* 5(4):e180 [http://www.researchprotocols.org/2016/4/e180].

Bruce, L., and Ricciardelli, L. (2016). A systematic review of the psychosocial correlates of intuitive eating among adult women. *Appetite* 96:454–472.

Bush, H., et al. (2014). Eat for life: A work site feasibility study of a novel mindfulness-based intuitive eating intervention. *American Journal of Health Promotion* 28(6):380–388.

Camilleri, G., et al. (2016). Intuitive eating is inversely associated with body weight status in the general population–based NutriNet-Santé study. *Obesity*. doi: 10.1002/oby.21440.

Camilleri, G., et al. (2017). Intuitive eating dimensions were differently associated with food intake in the general population–based NutriNet-Santé study. *Journal of Nutrition*, January 147(1):61–69. doi: 10.3945/jn.116.234088.

Carbonneau, E., et al. (2016). Validation of a French-Canadian adaptation of the Intuitive Eating Scale-2 for the adult population. *Appetite* 105(1): 37–45.

Carbonneau, E., et al. (2017). A Health at Every Size Intervention Improves Intuitive Eating and Diet Quality in Canadian Women. *Clinical Nutrition* 36(3):747–754.

Carbonneau, N., et al. (2015). Examining women's perceptions of their mother's and romantic partner's interpersonal styles for a better understanding of their eating regulation and intuitive eating. *Appetite* 92:156–66.

Carraça, E.V., Leong, S.L., and Horwath, C.C. (2018). Weight-focused physical activity is associated with poorer eating motivation quality and lower intuitive eating in women. *Journal of the Academy of Nutrition and Dietetics*. doi: 10.1016/j.jand.2018.09.011.

Christoph, M.J., et al. (2018). Nutrition facts use in relation to eating behaviors and healthy and unhealthy weight control behaviors. *Journal of Nutrition Education and Behavior* 50(3):267–274. el. doi: 10.1016/j.jneb.2017.11.001.

Cole, R., et al. (2016). Normal weight status in military service members was associated with intuitive eating characteristic. *Military Medicine* 181(6):589–595.

Cole, R., and Horace, K. (2010). Effectiveness of the "My body knows when" intuitive-eating pilot program. *American Journal of Health Behavior* 34(3):286–297.

Cole, R., et al. (2019). The "My body knows when" program increased intuitive eating characteristics in a military population. *Military Medicine.* doi: 10.1093/milmed/usy403.

Craven, M., and Fekete, E. (2019). Weight-related shame and guilt, intuitive eating, and binge eating in female college students. *Appetite.* Oi.10.1016/j.eatbeh.2019.03.002.

Da Silva, W.R., et al. (2018). A psychometric investigation of Brazilian Portuguese versions of the caregiver eating messages scale and intuitive eating scale-2. *Eating and Weight Disorders: Studies on Anorexia, Bulimia and Obesity.* doi:10.1007/s40519-018-0557-3.

Daundasekara, S.S., et al. (2017). Validation of the intuitive eating scale for pregnant women. *Appetite* 112:201–209.

Denny, K., et al. (2013). Intuitive eating in young adults: Who is doing it, and how is it related to disordered eating behaviors? *Appetite* 60:13–19.

Dockendorff, S., et al. (2012). Intuitive eating scale: An examination among early adolescents. *Journal of Counseling Psychology* 59(4):604–611.

Duarte, C., et al. (2017). What makes dietary restraint problematic? Development and validation of the inflexible eating questionnaire. *Appetite* 114:146–154.

Eneli, I., Tylka, T., and Lumeng, J. (2015). Maternal and child roles in the feeding relationship: What are mothers doing? *Clinical Pediatrics* 54(2):179–182.

Ellis, J., et al. (2016). Recollections of pressure to eat during childhood, but not picky eating, predict young adult eating behavior. *Appetite.* 97:58-63. doi: 10.1016/j.appet.2015.11.020.

Galloway A., Farrow, C., and Martz, D. (2010). Retrospective reports of child feeding practices, current eating behaviors, and BMI in college students. *Obesity, 18,* 1330–1335.

Gan, W.Y., and Yeoh, W.C. (2017). Associations between body weight status, psychological well-being and disordered eating with Intuitive Eating among Malaysian undergraduate university students. *Int J Adolesc Med Health.* Sept 13.

Gast, J., Madanat, H., and Nielson, A. (2011). Are Men More Intuitive When It Comes to Eating and Physical Activity? *American Journal of Men's Health.* doi: 10.1177/1557988311428090.

Gast, J., et al. (2015). Intuitive eating: Associations with physical activity motivation and BMI. *American Journal of Public Health.* 29(3):e91-9. doi: 10.4278/ajhp.130305-QUAN-97.

Gravel, K., et al. (2014). Sensory-based nutrition pilot intervention for women. *Journal of the Academy of Nutrition and Dietetics* 114 :99–06.

Gravel, K., et al. (2014). Effect of sensory-based intervention on the increased use of food-related descriptive terms among restrained eaters. *Food Quality and Preference.* 32:271–276.

Hahn, K., et al. (2012). Intuitive Eating and College Female Athletes. *Psychology of Women Quarterly.* doi: 10.1177/0361684311433282.

Hawks, S., et al. (2005). The relationship between intuitive eating and health indicators among college women. *American Journal of Health Education* 36, 331–336.

Hawks, S., Merrill, R., and Madanat, H. (2004). The intuitive eating validation scale: Preliminary validation. *American Journal of Health Education, 35,* 90–98.

Hawks, S., et al. (2004). Intuitive eating and the nutrition transition in Asia. *Asia Pacific Journal of Clinical Nutrition, 13, 194–203.*

Heileson, J., and Cole, R. (2011). Assessing motivation for eating and intuitive eating in military service members. *Journal of the American Dietetic Association,* 111 (9S): Page A26.

Herbert, B., et al. (2013). Intuitive eating is associated with interoceptive sensitivity. Effects on body mass index. *Appetite* 70:22–30.

Homan, K.J., and Tylka, T.L. (2018). Development and exploration of the gratitude model of body appreciation in women. *Body Image.* 2018 Feb 8;25:14-22. doi: 10.1016/j. bodyim.2018.01.008.

Horwath, C., Hagmann, D., and Hartmann, C. (2019). Intuitive eating and food intake in men and women: Results from the Swiss food panel study. *Appetite.* 1(135):61–71. doi:10.1016/ *Journal of Appetite.* 2018.12.036.

Humphrey, L., Clifford, D., and Neyman Morris, M. (2015). Health at Every Size college course reduces dieting behaviors and improves intuitive eating, body esteem, and anti-fat attitudes. *Journal of Nutrition Education.* 47(4):354–360.

Iannantuono, A., and Tylka, T. (2012). Interpersonal and intrapersonal links to body appreciation in college women: An exploratory model. *Body Image* 9(2):227–235.

Jarvela-Reijonen, E., et al. (2016). High perceived stress is associated with unfavorable eating behavior in overweight and obese Finns of working age. *Appetite* 103:249–258.

Jarvela-Reijonen, E., et al. (2018). The effects of acceptance and commitment therapy on eating behavior and diet delivered through face-to-face contact and a mobile app: a randomized controlled trial. *International Journal of Nutrition and Physical Activity.* 2018 Feb 27;15(1):22. doi: 10.1186/s12966-018-0654-8.

Katzer, L., et al. (2008). Evaluation of a "nondieting" stress reduction program for overweight women: a randomized trial. *American Journal of Health Promotion* 22(4):267–274.

Kelly, A., and Stephen, E. (2016). A daily diary study of self-compassion, body image, and eating behavior in female college students. *Body Image.* 17:152-160. doi: 10.1016/j.bodyim.2016.03.006.

Kelly, A.C., Miller, K.E., and Stephen, E. (2016). The benefits of being self-compassionate on days when interactions with body-focused others are frequent. *Body Image.* Dec;19:195-203. doi: 10.1016/j.bodyim.2016.10.005.

Kerin, J.L., Webb, H.J., and Zimmer-Gembeck, M.J. (2019). Intuitive, mindful, emotional, external and regulatory eating behaviours and beliefs: An investigation of the core components. *Appetite.* Jan 1;132:139-146. doi: 10.1016/j.appet.2018.10.011.

Keirns, N.G., and Hawkins, M.A.W. (2019). The relationship between intuitive eating and body image is moderated by measured body mass index. *Eating Behaviors.* 23(33):91–96.

Khalsa, A.S., et al. (2019). Parental intuitive eating behaviors and their association with infant feeding styles among low-income families. *Eating Behaviors, 32, 78–84.* doi:10.1016/j.eatbeh.2019.01.001

Koller, et al.

Kroon Van Diest, A., and Tylka, T. (2010). The Caregiver Eating Messages Scale: Development and psychometric investigation. *Body Image* 7:317–326.

Leahy, K., et al. (2017). The relationship between Intuitive Eating and postpartum weight loss. *Maternal Child Health.* 21(3):1591–1597.

Lee, M., et al. (2019). Striving for the thin ideal post-pregnancy: cross-sectional study of intuitive eating in postpartum women. *Journal of Reproductive Infant Psychology.* Apr 30:1–12.

Leong, S., et al. (2016). Weight-control methods, 3-year weight change, and eating behaviors: A prospective nationwide study of middle-aged New Zealand women. *The Journal of the Academy of Nutrition and Dietetics* doi: 10.1016/j.jand.2016.02.021.

Linardon, J., and Mitchell, S. (2017). Rigid dietary control, flexible dietary control, and intuitive eating: Evidence for their differential relationship to disordered eating and body image concerns. *Eating Behavior.* 26:16–22.

MacDougall, E. (2010). An examination of a culturally relevant model of intuitive eating with African American college women. University of Akron, 2010. Dissertation 218 pp.

Madanat, H., and Hawks, S. (2004). Validation of the Arabic version of the Intuitive Eating Scale. *Global Health Promotion* (Formerly *Promotion and Education*) 11:152–157.

Madden, C., et al. (2012). Eating in response to hunger and satiety signals is related to BMI in a nationwide sample of 1,601 mid-age New Zealand women. *Public Health Nutrition,* Mar:1–8.

Mensinger, J., Calogero, R., and Tylka, T. (2016). Internalized weight stigma moderates eating behavior outcomes in women with high BMI participating in a healthy living program. *Appetite.* 102:32–43.

Mensinger, J.L., et al. (2016). A weight-neutral versus weight-loss approach for health promotion in women with high BMI: A randomized-controlled trial. *Appetite* Oct 1;105:364-74. doi: 10.1016/j.appet.2016.06.006.

Miller, K., Kelly, A., and Stephen, E. (2019). Exposure to body focused and non-body focused others over a week: A preliminary investigation of their unique contributions to college women's eating and body image. *Body Image.* doi: 10.1016/j.bodyim.2018.12.003.

Moy, J., et al. (2013). Dieting, exercise, and intuitive eating among early adolescents. *Eating Behaviors.* 14: 529–532.

Nielsen, T., and Powell, R. (2015). Dreams of the *Rarebit Fiend*: food and diet as instigators of bizarre and disturbing dreams. *Frontiers in Psychology* 6:47.

Oswald, A., Chapman, J., and Wilson, C. (2017). Do interoceptive awareness and interoceptive responsiveness mediate the relationship between body appreciation and intuitive eating in young women? *Appetite* 109:66–72. PMID:27866989.

Outland, L., Madanat, H., and Rust, F. (2013). Intuitive eating for a healthy weight. *Primary Health Care* 23:9, 22–28.

Paterson, H., et al. (2018). Validation of the Intuitive Eating Scale in pregnancy. *Journal of Health Psychology* 23(5):701–709. doi: 10.1177/1359105316671186.

Peschel, S.K.V., et al. (2018). Is intuitive eating related to resting state vagal activity? *Autonomic Neuroscience.* Mar; 210:72–75. doi: 10.1016/j.autneu.2017.11.005.

Plante, A., et al. (2019). Trimester-specific intuitive eating in association with gestational weight gain and diet quality. *Journal of Nutrition Education and Behavior.* (10):20025-9. doi: 10.1016/j.jneb.2019.01.011

Plateau, C.R., Petrie, T.A., and Papathomas, A. (2017). Learning to eat again: Intuitive eating practices among retired female collegiate athletes. *Eating Disorders* 25(1):92–98.

Reel, J.J., et al. (2016). Development and validation of the intuitive exercise scale. *Eating Behaviors.* 22:129–132.

Reichenberger, J. (2019). "I will fast . . . tomorrow": Intentions to restrict eating and actual restriction in daily life and their person-level predictors. *Appetite* Sep 1;140: 10–18.

Ricciardelli, B.L. (2016). A systematic review of the psychosocial correlates of intuitive eating among adult women. *Appetite* 96:454–472.

Richards, P.S., et al. (2017). Can patients with eating disorders learn to eat intuitively? A 2-year pilot study. *Eating Disorders*. 2:1-15. doi: 10.1080/10640266.2017.1279907.

Romano, K.A., et al. (2018). Helpful or harmful? The comparative value of self-weighing and calorie counting versus intuitive eating on the eating disorder symptomatology of college students. *Eating and Weight Disorders—Studies on Anorexia, Bulimia and Obesity*. doi:10.1007/s40519-018-0562-6.

Ruzanska, U.A., and Warschburger, P. (2017). Psychometric evaluation of the German version of the Intuitive Eating Scale-2 in a community sample. *Appetite* 117: 126–134.

Ruzanska, U.A., and Warschburger, P. (2019). Intuitive eating mediates the relationship between self-regulation and BMI: Results from a cross-sectional study in a community sample. *Eating Behaviors*. 18;33:23–29. doi: 10.1016/j.eatbeh.2019.02.004.

Sairanen, E., et al. (2015). Psychological flexibility and mindfulness explain intuitive eating in overweight adults. *Behavior Modification*. 39(4):554–579.

Sairanen, E., et al. (2017). Psychological flexibility mediates change in Intuitive Eating regulation in acceptance and commitment therapy interventions. *Public Health Nutrition*. 20(9):1681–1691.

Saunders, J.F., Nichols-Lopez, K.A., and Frazier, L.D. (2018). Psychometric properties of the intuitive eating scale-2 (IES-2) in a culturally diverse Hispanic American sample. *Eating Behaviors*. Jan;28:1-7. doi: 10.1016/j.eatbeh.2017.11.003.

Schaefer, J., and Zullo, M. (2016). Validation of an instrument to measure registered dietitians'/nutritionists' knowledge, attitudes and practices of an intuitive eating approach. *Public Health Nutrition* 1:1–19.

Schaefer, J., and Magnuson, A. (2014). A review of interventions that promote eating by internal cues. *Journal of the Academy of Nutrition and Dietetics* 114,734e760.

Schaefer, J., and Zullo, M. (2017). U.S. registered dietitian nutritionist's knowledge and attitudes of Intuitive Eating and use of various weight management practices. *Journal of the Academy of Nutrition and Dietetics* 117(9):1419–1428.

Schoenefeld, S., and Webb, J. (2013). Self-compassion and intuitive eating in college women: Examining the contributions of distress tolerance and body image acceptance and action. *Eating Behaviors* 14(4):493–6.

Shouse, S., and Nilsson, J. (2011). Self-silencing, emotional awareness, and eating behaviors in college women. *Psychology of Women Quarterly* 35:451–457.

Smith, T., and Hawks, S. (2006). Intuitive eating, diet composition, and the meaning of food in healthy weight promotion. *American Journal of Health Education* 37:130–136.

Smitham, L. (2008). Evaluating an Intuitive Eating Program for Binge Eating Disorder: A Benchmarking Study. University of Notre Dame, Dissertation. 26 November 2008.

Spoor, K., and Madanat, H. (2016). Relationship Between Body Image Discrepancy and Intuitive Eating. *International Quarterly of Community Health Education* 36: 189–197.

Tylka, T. (2006). Development and psychometric evaluation of a measure of intuitive eating. *Journal of Counseling Psychology 53*:226–240.

Tylka, T., and Homan, K. (2015). Exercise motives and positive body image in physically active college women and men: Exploring an expanded acceptance model of intuitive eating. *Body Image*. 15:90–97.

Tylka, T., and Kroon Van Diest, A. (2013). The Intuitive Eating Scale–2: Item refinement and psychometric evaluation with college women and men. *Journal of Counseling Psychology* 60(1):137–153.

Tylka, T., and Wilcox, J. (2006). Are intuitive eating and eating disorder symptomatology opposite poles of the same construct? *Journal of Counseling Psychology, 53*, 474–485.

Tylka, T., Calogero, R., and Daníelsdóttira, S. (2015). Is intuitive eating the same as flexible dietary control? Their links to each other and well-being could provide an answer. *Appetite* 95: 166–175.

Tylka, T., Calogero, R., and Daníelsdóttira, S. (2019). Intuitive eating is connected to self-reported weight stability in community women and men. *Eating Disorders*. 1:1–9. doi: 10.1080/10640266.2019.1580126.

Tylka, T., Lumeng, J., and Eneli, I. (2015). Maternal intuitive eating as a moderator of the association between concern about child weight and restrictive child feeding. *Appetite*. Dec 1;95:158–65.

Tylka, T., et al. (2013). Which adaptive maternal eating behaviors predict child feeding practices? An examination with mothers of 2- to 5-year-old children. *Eating Behaviors* 14(1):57–63.

Van Dyke, N., and Drinkwater, E. (2014). Relationships between intuitive eating and health indicators: literature review. *Public Health Nutrition* 17(8):1757–66.

Van Dyck, A., et al. (2016). German version of the intuitive eating scale: Psychometric evaluation and application to an eating disordered population. *Appetite* 105:798–807.

Warren, J.M., Smith, N., and Ashwell, M. (2017). A structured literature review on the role of mindfulness, mindful eating and intuitive eating in changing eating behaviours: effectiveness and associated potential mechanisms. *Nutrition Research Reviews.* Dec;30(2):272–283. doi: 10.1017/S0954422417000154.

Webb, J., and Hardin, A. (2016). An integrative affect regulation process model of internalized weight bias and Intuitive Eating in college women. *Appetite.* 102:60–69. doi: 10.1016/j.appet.2016.02.024.

Wheeler, B., et al. (2016). Intuitive eating is associated with glycaemic control in adolescents with type I diabetes mellitus. *Appetite* 96:160–165.

Willig, A.L., et al. (2014). Intuitive eating practices among African-American women living with type 2 diabetes: A qualitative study. *Journal of the Academy of Nutrition and Dietetics* 114(6):889–96.

Wirtz, A., and Madanat, H. (2012). Westernization, intuitive eating, and BMI: an exploration of Jordanian adolescents. *International Quarterly of Community Health Education* 33(3):275–28.

Notes

Foreword and Introduction

Bacon, L., and Aphramor, L. (2011). Weight Science: Evaluating the evidence for a paradigm shift. *Nutrition Journal,* January 10:9. [http://bit.ly/f4CKOK].

The Center for Mindful Eating's website: [https://www.thecenterformindfuleating.org /Principles-Mindful-Eating accessed May 20, 2019].

Heraldkeeper. (2019). Weight loss and weight management market 2018 global analysis, opportunities and forecast to 2023 (Press Release). *MarketWatch.* [https:// www.marketwatch.com/press-release/weight-loss-and-weight-management-market-2018 -global-analysis-opportunities-and-forecast-to-2023-2018-09-27 accessed 5-20-19].

Kristeller, J.L., and Hallett, B. (1999). Effects of a meditation-based intervention in the treatment of binge eating. *Journal of Health Psychology* 4(3): 357–363.

Levine, P.A. *Waking the Tiger—Healing Trauma.* North Atlantic Press, 1997.

Siegel, D. (2010). *Mindsight: The New Science of Personal Transformation.* New York, NY: Bantam.

Chapter 1. The Science Behind Intuitive Eating

Craig, A.D. (2014). *How Do You Feel: An Interoceptive Moment with Your Neurobiological Self.* Princeton, NJ: Princeton University Press.

Mehling, W., et al. (2018). The multidimensional assessment of interoceptive awareness, version 2 (MAIA-2). PLOS One. [https://doi.org/10.1371/journal.pone.0208034].

Quadt, L., et al. (2018). The neurobiology of interoception in health and disease. *Annals of the New York Academy of Science* 1428:112–128.

Also see, Intuitive Eating studies listed in p. 331 under references.

Chapter 2. Hitting Diet Bottom

Bellini, et al. (2017). A journey through liposuction and lipoculture: Review. *Annals of Medicine and Surgery.* 24:53–60.

Department of Health and Aging. (2013). National and Medical Research Council. Clinical practice guidelines for the management of overweight and obesity in adults, adolescents and children in Australia, Melbourne, p. 161.

Field, A.E., et al. (2003). Relation between dieting and weight change among preadolescents and adolescents. *Pediatrics* 112:900–906.

Fothergill, E., et al. (2016). Persistent metabolic adaptation 6 years after "The Biggest Loser" competition. *Obesity.* doi.10.10020oby.21538.

Harrison, C. (August 10, 2018). What is diet culture? [https://christyharrison.com/blog/what-is-diet-culture accessed May 20, 2019].

Keys, A., et al. (1950). *The Biology of Human Starvation*, vol II. p. 834. University of Minnesota: St. Paul.

Lissner et al.

Mann, T. (2007). Medicare's search for effective obesity treatments: Diets are not the answer. *American Psychologist* 62(3): 220–233.

Mundel, E.J. (October 19, 2018). Almost half of Americans are trying to lose weight: CDC. *Health Day.* [https://consumer.healthday.com/vitamins-and-nutrition-information-27/dieting-to-lose-weight-health-news-195/almost-half-of-americans-are-trying-to-lose-weight-cdc-738808.html accessed 5-20-19].

Neumark-Sztainer, D., et al. (2006). Obesity, disordered eating, and eating disorders in a longitudinal study of adolescents: how do dieters fare five years later? *Journal of the Academy of Nutrition and Dietetics* 106(4):559–568.

O'Hara, L., and Taylor, J. (2018). What's wrong with the "War on Obesity?" A narrative review of the weight-centered health paradigm and development of the 3C framework to build critical competency for a paradigm shift. *Sage OPEN*, page 8.

Pietilainen, K., et al. (2011). Does dieting make you fat? A twin study. *International Journal of Obesity* 1–9.

Pittman, D. (June 17, 2013). Obesity not a disease, AMA Council says. *Medpage Today.* [https://www.medpagetoday.com/MeetingCoverage/AMA/39918 accessed 5-20-19].

Shisslak, C.M., Crago, M, Estes E. (1995). The spectrum of eating disorders. *International Journal of Eating Disorders* 19(3):214.

Taylor, S.R. (2018). *The Body Is Not an Apology: The Power of Radical Self-Love.* Berrett-Koehler Publishers: Oakland, CA.

"Bush declares war on fat America." *The Guardian,* June 23, 2002. [https://www .theguardian.com/world/2002/jun/23/usa.georgebush1 accessed May 20, 2019].

". . . the representations of women's bodies across all media have shrunk dramatically in the last 30 years" in https://beautyredefined.org/newsroom/faqs/.

Chapter 3. What Kind of Eater Are You?

Berg, F. *The Health Risks of Weight Loss.* (1993). Hettinger, ND: Healthy Living Institute.

Bever. L. (April 5, 2019). Bad diets kill more people around the world than smoking, study says. *Washington Post.* [https://www.washingtonpost.com/health/2019/04 /05/bad-diets-kill-more-people-around-world-than-smoking-study-says/?noredirect =on&utm_term=.ba3c434e8b41 accessed May 20, 2019].

Birch, L.L. (1987). The role of experience in children's food acceptance patterns. *Journal of the American Dietetic Association* 87(9 supplement):S-36.

Birch, L.L. (1993). Children's eating: Are manners enough? *Journal of Gastronomy* 7(1):19–25.

Birch, L.L., et al. (1991). The variability of young children's energy intake. *New England Journal of Medicine* 324:232.

Eating guilt. (1992). *Obesity and Health* 6(2):43.

Eneli, I., et al. (2008). The trust model: A different feeding paradigm for the management of childhood obesity. *Obesity* 16(10):2197–2204.

Forbes, G.B. (1991). Children and food—order amid chaos. *New England Journal of Medicine* 324:262.

Gallup Organization. (January 1990). Gallup Survey of Public Opinion Regarding Diet and Health. Prepared for American Dietetic Association/International Food Information Council. Princeton, NJ: Gallup Organization, Inc.

Livermore, S. (June 5, 2015). 16 foods you didn't know could kill you. *Cosmopolitan.* [https://www.cosmopolitan.com/food-cocktails/news/a41525/foods-you-didnt-know -could-kill-you/ accessed 5-20-19].

Press Association (January 19, 2013). Women own up to guilt over eating habits. *The Guardian.* [https://www.theguardian.com/lifeandstyle/2013/jan/20/binge-eating-food -women accessed 5-20-19].

Satter, E. (1987). Comments from a practioner on Leann Birch's research. *Journal of the American Dietetic Association* 87(9 supplement):S-41.

Satter, E. (1987). *How to Get Your Child to Eat . . . but Not Too Much*. Palo Alto, CA: Bull Pub, page 6.

Smit, H.L. (May 21, 2015). New poll reveals that 80 percent of women suffer from food guilt. [https://www.huffpost.com/entry/new-poll-reveals-that-80_n_7348024 accessed 5-20-19].

Smith, B. (TK). 12 foods that can kill you. *Men's Journal*. [https://www.mensjournal.com/food-drink/12-foods-can-kill-you/ accessed 5-20-19].

Tufts University Diet & Nutrition Letter. (1993). Warning: Keep dieting out of reach of children. 11(10):3.

Tylka, T. (2006). Development and psychometric evaluation of a measure of intuitive eating. *Journal of Counseling Psychology* 53(2):226–240.

Chapter 6. Principle 1: Reject the Diet Mentality

Associated Press (Washington). (1994). Vitamin retailer to pay fine. *AP Online,* April 29, 1994.

Berdanier, C.D., and McIntosh, M.K. (1991). Weight loss–weight regain: A vicious cycle. *Nutrition Today* 26(5):6.

Berg, F.M. (1993). *The Health Risks of Weight Loss*. Hettinger, ND: Healthy Living Institute.

Blackburn, G.L., et al. (1993). Why and how to stop weight cycling in overweight adults. *Eating Disorders Review* 4(1):1.

Blackburn, G.L., et al. (1989). Weight cycling: The experience of human dieters. *American Journal of Clinical Nutrition* 49:1105.

Ciliska, D. (1990). *Beyond Dieting*. New York: Brunner/Mazel.

Dehnart A. (May 13, 2019). The Biggest Loser is coming back—but should it? [https://www.realityblurred.com/realitytv/2019/05/biggest-loser-returning/ accessed 5-22-19].

Foreyt, J.P., and Goodrick, G.K. (1993). Weight management without dieting. *Nutrition Today*. March/April:4.

Foreyt, J., and Goodrick, G.K. (1992). *Living Without Dieting*. Houston, TX: Harrison Publ.

Gallup Organization. (June 1993). Women's knowledge and behavior regarding health and fitness. Conducted for American Dietetic Association and Weight Watchers.

Garrow, J.S. (1992). Treatment of obesity. *The Lancet* 340:409–413.

Goodrick, G.K., and Foreyt, J.P. (1991). Why treatments for obesity don't last. *Journal of the American Dietetic Association* 91(10):1243.

Grodner, M. (1992). Forever dieting: Chronic dieting syndrome. *Journal of Nutrition Education* 24(4):207–210.

Hartmann, E. (1991). *Boundaries in the Mind. A New Psychology of Personality*. New York: Basic Books.

Hill, A.J., and Robinson, A. (1991). Dieting concerns have a functional effect on the behaviour of nine-year-old girl. *British Journal of Clinical Psychology* 30:265–267.

Hunger J. Smith, and Tomiyama, A. (2020). An Evidence-Based Rationale for Adopting Weight-Inclusive Health Policy. *Social Issues and Policy Review* 14(1): 73–107.

Katherine, A. (1991). *Boundaries: Where You End and I Begin*. Park Ridge, IL: Parkside Publishing Company.

Kern, P.A., et al. (1990). The effects of weight loss on the activity and expression of adipose-tissue lipoprotein lipase in very obese human. *New England Journal of Medicine* 322(15):1053–1059.

Lee, I., and Paffenbarger, J. (1992). Change in Body Weight and Longevity. *Journal of the American Medical Association* 268:2045–2049.

Lelwica, M. (2009). *The Religion of Thinness: Satisfying the Spiritual Hungers Behind Women's Obsession with Food and Weight*. Carlsbad, CA: Gurze Books.

Polivy, J., and Herman, C.P. (1992). Undieting: A program to help people stop dieting. *International Journal of Eating Disorders* 11(3):261–268.

Rodin, J., et al. (1990). Weight cycling and fat distribution. *International Journal of Obesity* 14:303–310.

Stice, E., et al. (2013). Caloric deprivation increases responsivity of attention and reward brain regions to intake, anticipated intake, and images of palatable foods. *NeuroImage* 67:322–330.

Wilson, G.T. (1992). Short-term psychological benefits and adverse effects of weight loss. *NIH Technology Assessment Conference: Methods for Voluntary Weight Loss and Control*, March 30-April.

Wooley, S.C., and Garner, D.M. (1991). Obesity treatment: The high cost of false hope. *Journal of the American Dietetic Association* 91(10):1248.

Yanovski, S.Z. (1993). Are anorectic agents the magic bullet for obesity? (Editorial). *Archives of Family Medicine* 2(Oct):1025–1027.

Chapter 7. Principle 2: Honor Your Hunger

Becker C.B. et al (2017). Food insecurity and eating disorder pathology. *International Journal of Eating Disorders* 50:1031–1040.

Birch, L.L., et al. (1991). The variability of young children's energy intake. *New England Journal of Medicine* 324(Jan. 24):232.

Boyle, M.A., and Zyla, G. (1992). *Personal Nutrition,* 2nd edition. St. Paul, MN: West Publ, pages 77, 217.

Cameron, J., et al. (2014). Fasting for 24 hours heightens reward from food and food-related cues. *PLOS One* 9(1): e85970.

Ciampolini, M., and Bianchi, R. (2006). Training to estimate blood glucose and to form associations with initial hunger. *Nutrition and Metabolism*, vol. 3, article 42, 2006. [http://bit.ly/bXRdkD].

Ciampolini, M., et al. (2010). Sustained self-regulation of energy intake: Initial hunger improves insulin sensitivity. *Journal of Nutrition and Metabolism*, vol. 2010, article ID 286952, 7 pages. doi:10.1155/2010/286952 [http://bit.ly/9OYSsw].

Ciampolini, M., Lovell-Smith, D., and Sifone, M. (2010). Sustained self-regulation of energy intake: Loss of weight in overweight subjects: Maintenance of weight in normal-weight subjects. *Nutrition and Metabolism*, vol. 7, article 4.

De Koning, L., et al. (2011). Low-carbohydrate diet scores and risk of type 2 diabetes in men. *American Journal Clinical Nutrition* 93:844–850.

Drott, C., and Lundholm, K. (1992). Cardiac effects of caloric restriction-mechanisms and potential hazards. *International Journal Obesity* 16:481–486.

Favaro, A., Rodella, F. C., & Santonastaso, P. (2000). Binge eating and eating attitudes among Nazi concentration camp survivors. *Psychological Medicine*, 30(2), 463–466.

Franchina, J.J., and Slank, K.L. (1988). Effects of deprivation on salivary flow in the apparent absence of food stimuli. *Appetite* 10:143–147.

Garner, D.M., and Garfinkel, P.E. (eds). (1985). *Handbook of Psychotherapy for Anorexia and Bulimia*. New York: Guilford, chapter 21.

Judge, B. S., & Eisenga, B. H. (2005). Disorders of Fuel Metabolism: Medical Complications Associated with Starvation, Eating Disorders, Dietary Fads, and Supplements. *Emergency Medicine Clinics of North America,* 23(3), 789–813. doi:10.1016/j.emc.2005.03.011

Kosinski, C., and Jornayvaz, F. (2017). Effects of ketogenic diets on cardiovascular risk factors: Evidence from animal and human studies. *Nutrients* 9:517.

Leibowitz, S. (1991). Brain neuropeptide Y: An integrator of endocrine, metabolic and behavioral processes. *Brain Research Bulletin* Sept–Oct:27 (3-4)33–7.

Lydecker, J.A. & C.M. Grilo, (2019). Food insecurity and bulimia nervosa in the United States. *International Journal of Eating Disorders.* 52(6):735–739

Marano, H. (1993). Chemistry and craving. *Psychology Today* Jan–Feb:31.

Nicolaidis, S., and Even, P. (1992). The metabolic signal of hunger and satiety, and its pharmacological manipulation. *International Journal of Obesity* Dec (16 suppl 3): S31-41.

Polivy, J., and Herman, C.P. (1985). Dieting and binging: A causal analysis. *American Psychologist* Feb:193–201.

Polivy, J., and Herman, C.P. (1987). Diagnosis and treatment of normal eating. *Journal of Consulting and Clinical Psychology* 55(5):635–644.

Scrimshaw, N.S. (1987). The phenomenon of famine. *Annual Review of Nutrition* 7:1–21.

Seaton, C., et al. (2018). A case study of breastfeeding ketoacidosis: A rare but important diagnosis for emergency physicians to recognize. *American Journal of Emergency Medicine.* doi.10.1016/j.aje,.2018.10.014.

Wolf, N. (1991). *The Beauty Myth.* New York: Anchor Books, pages 179–217.

Wroble, K. et al. (2019). Low-carbohydrate, ketogenic diet impairs anaerobic exercise performance in exercise-trained women and men: A randomized crossover trial. *The Journal of Sports Medicine and Physical Fitness* 59(4):600–7.

Chapter 8. Principle 3: Make Peace with Food

Baldwin, A.L. (1980). *Theories of Child Development,* 2nd edition. New York: John Wiley and Sons.

Berk, L.E. (1994). *Child Development,* 3rd edition. Boston: Allyn and Bacon.

Benton, D. (2010). The plausibility of sugar addiction and its role in obesity and eating disorders. *Clinical Nutrition* 29:288–303.

Berridge, K.C., and Kringelbach, M.L. (2008). Affective neuroscience of pleasure: Reward in humans and animals. *Psychopharmacology* (Berl) 199(3): 457–480.

Carr, K. (2011). Food scarcity, neuroadaptations, and the pathogenic potential of dieting in an unnatural ecology: Binge eating and drug abuse. *Physiology & Behavior* 104:162–167.

Epstein, L.H. (2009). Habituation as a determinant of human food intake. *Psychological Review*. 116(2): 384–407.

Epstein, L.H. (2011). Long-term habituation to food in obese and nonobese women. *American Journal of Clinical Nutrition*. doi: 10.3945/ajcn.110.009035.

Erikson, E.H. (1982). *The Life Cycle Completed. A Review*. New York: W.W. Norton and Company.

Ernst, M.M. (2002). Habituation of responding for food in humans. *Appetite* 38:224–234. doi:10.1006/appe.2001.0484.

Gearhardt, A., et al. (2009). Preliminary validation of the Yale Food Addiction Scale. *Appetite* (52):430–436.

Gilbert, D. (2006). *Stumbling on Happiness*. New York: Knopf, page 130.

Herman, C.P., and Polivy, J. (1980). Restrained eating. In A. Stunkard, *Obesity*. Philadelphia: WB Saunders, pages 208–225.

Jansen, E., et al. (2007). Do not eat the red food! Prohibition of snacks leads to their relatively higher consumption in children. *Appetite* 49:572–577.

Keeler, C., et al. (2015). Anticipatory and reactive responses to chocolate restriction in frequent chocolate consumers. *Obesity* 23:1130–1135.

Kristeller, J.L., and Wolever, R.Q. (2011). Mindfulness-based eating awareness training for treating binge eating disorder: The conceptual foundation. *Eating Disorders* 19(1):49-61 PMID: 21181579.

Larson, E., MS, RD. Personal Communication. Research dietitian for NIH, Phoenix, AZ.

Long, C., et al. (2015). A systematic review of the application and correlates of YFAS-diagnosed "food addiction" in humans: Are eating-related "addictions" a cause for concern or empty concepts? *Obesity Facts* 8:386–401.

Loro, A.D., and Orleans, C.S. (1981). Binge eating in obesity: Preliminary findings and guidelines for behavioral analysis and treatment. *Addictive Behaviours* 6(2): 155–166.

Markus, C., et al. (2017). Eating dependence and weight gain: No human evidence for a "sugar addiction." *Appetite* 114:64–72.

Miller, P.H. (1993). *Theories of Developmental Psychology*. New York: W.H. Freeman and Company.

Mydans, S. (1993). 8 bid farewell to the future: Musty air, roaches and ants. *New York Times*, Sept 27, page A1.

Ogden, J., and Wardle, J. (1991). Cognitive and emotional responses to food. *International Journal of Eating Disorders* 10(3):297–311.

Penzenstadler, L., et al. (2018). Systematic review of food addiction as measured with the Yale Food Addiction Scale: Implications for the food addiction construct. *Current Neuropharmacology* 16:1–13.

Ruddock, H., and Hardman, C. (2017). Food addiction beliefs amongst the lay public: What are the consequences for eating behaviour? *Current Addiction Reports* 4:110–115.

Salimpoor, V.N. (2011). Anatomically distinct dopamine release during anticipation and experience of peak emotion to music. *Nature NEUROSCIENCE* 14(2): 257–262.

Satter, E. (1987). *How to Get Your Kid to Eat . . . but Not Too Much.* Palo Alto, CA: Bull Publishing Company.

Seamon, J.G., and Kenrick, D.T. (1994). *Psychology,* 2nd edition. Englewood Cliffs, NJ: Prentice Hall.

Smitham, L. (2008). Evaluating an intuitive eating program for binge eating disorder: A benchmarking study. University of Notre Dame, November 26.

Snoek, H.M., et al. (2004). Obese and normal-weight women. *American Journal of Clinical Nutrition* 80(4):823–831.

Westwater, M.L., Fletcher, P.C., and Ziauddeen, H. (2016). Sugar addiction: The state of the science. *European Journal of Nutrition* 55(Suppl 2):S55–S69.

Chapter 9. Principle 4: Challenge the Food Police

As the Chicken Turns. (1994). *Tufts University Diet and Nutrition Letter* 11(11):1.

Berne, E. (1964). *Games People Play.* New York: Grove Press.

Ellis, A., and Harper, R.A. (1975). *A New Guide to Rational Living.* North Hollywood, CA: Melvin Powers, Wilshire Book Company.

Food guilt. (1993). *Utne Reader* Nov–Dec:53.

Hiser, E. (1993). Butter paroled, margarine charged. *Eating Well* Nov–Dec:104.

King, G.A., Herman, C.P., and Polivy, J. (1987). Food perception in dieters and nondieters. *Appetite* 8:147–158.

Seid, R.P. (1989). *Never Too Thin.* New York: Prentice Hall Press.

Chapter 10. Principle 5: Discover the Satisfaction Factor

Anderson, S.L. (1990). A look at the Japanese dietary guidelines. *Journal of the American Dietetic Association* 90(11):1527–1528.

Epstein, L.H. (2009). Habituation as a determinant of human food intake. *Psychological Review.* 116(2):384–407.

Oldham-Cooper, R.E., et al. (2011). Playing a computer game during lunch affects fullness, memory for lunch, and later snack intake. *American Journal of Clinical Nutrition.* 93(Feb):308–313.

Visser, M. (1993). On having cake and eating it. *Journal of Gastronomy* 7(1):5–17.

Wisniewski, L., Epstein, L.H., and Caggiula, A.R. (1992). Effect of food change on consumption, hedonics, and salivation. *Physiology and Behavior* 92(52):21–26.

Chapter 11. Principle 6: Feel Your Fullness

Bray, G.A. (1993). The nutrient balance approach to obesity. *Nutrition Today* 28(3): 13–18.

De Castro, J.M. (1988). Physiological, environmental, and subjective determinants of food intake in humans: A meal pattern analysis. *Physiology & Behavior* 44:651–659.

De Castro, J.M. (1991). Weekly rhythms of spontaneous nutrient intake and meal patterns of humans. *Physiology & Behavior* 50:729–738.

Chapter 12. Principle 7: Cope with Your Emotions with Kindness

Arnow, B., Kenardy, J., and Agras, W.S. (1992). Binge eating among the obese: A descriptive study. *Journal of Behavioral Medicine* 15(2):155–170.

Barnett, R. (1993). Appetite and the meal. *Journal of Gastronomy* 7(1):59–72.

De Castro, J.M. (1990). Social facilitation of duration and size but not rate of the spontaneous meal intake of humans. *Physiology and Behavior* 47:1129–1135.

De Castro, J.M. (1991). Weekly rhythms of spontaneous nutrient intake and meal pattern of humans. *Physiology and Behavior* 50:729–738.

De Castro, J.M., and Brewer, E.M. (1991). The amount eaten in meals by humans is a power function of the number of people present. *Physiology and Behavior* 51:121–125.

Goldman, S.J., Herman, C.P., and Polivy, J. (1991). Is the effect of a social model on eating attenuated by hunger? *Appetite* 17:129–140.

Heatherton, T.F., Herman, C.P., and Polivy, J. (1992). Effects of distress on eating:

The importance of ego-involvement. *Journal of Personality and Social Psychology* 62(5):801–803.

Herman, C.P., and Polivy, J. (1991). Fat is a psychological issue. *New Scientist* Nov:41–45.

Herman, C.P., and Polivy, J. (1988). Psychological factors in the control of appetite. *Current Concepts in Nutrition* 16:41–51.

Herman, C.P., et al. (1987). Anxiety, hunger, and eating behavior. *Journal of Abnormal Psychology* 96(3):264–269.

Hill, A.J., Weaver, C.F.L., and Blundell, J.E. (1991). Food craving, dietary restraint and mood. *Appetite* 17:187–197.

Morton, C.J. (1988). Weight loss maintenance and relapse prevention. In R.T. Frankle and M.-U. Yang, *Obesity and Weight Control*. Rockville, MD: Aspen Publishers.

Ogden, J., and Wardle, J. (1991). Cognitive and emotional responses to food. *International Journal of Eating Disorders* 10(3):297–311.

Polivy, J., et al. (1986). The effects of self-attention and public attention on eating in restrained and unrestrained subjects. *Journal of Personality and Social Psychology* 50(6):1253–1260.

Weissenburger, J., et al. (1986). Weight change in depression. *Psychiatry Research* 17:275–283.

Chapter 13. Principle 8: Respect Your Body

2011 Succeed Foundation Body Image Survey [http://www.responsesource.com /releases/rel_display.php?relid=63713&hilite=BOdy%20image *accessed June 6, 2011*].

Bacon, L., and Aphramor, L. (2011). Weight science: Evaluating the evidence for a paradigm shift. *Nutrition Journal* January 10:9. [http://bit.ly/f4CKOK].

Brownell, K. (2006). The debate to nowhere. Posted August 23. [http://bit.ly/je8eFU accessed June 12, 2011].

Daníelsdóttira, S. et al. (2010). Anti-fat prejudice reduction: A review of published studies. *Obes Facts* 3:47–58.

Diet winners and sinners of the year. *People Weekly,* January 10, 1994.

Dietary Guideline Advisory Committee. (1990). *Report of the Dietary Guidelines Advisory Committee on the Dietary Guidelines for Americans 1990*. USDA.

Dietary Guidelines For Americans 2015-2020 Eighth Edition Hhs Publication #: HHS-ODPHP-2015-2020-01-DGA-A USDA Publication #: Home and Garden Bulletin No. 232

Lavie, C. (2014). *The Obesity Paradox: When Thinner Means Sicker and Heavier Means Healthier.* New York: Hudson Street Press.

Mensigner, J., Tylka, T., and Calamari, M. (2018). Mechanisms underlying weight status and healthcare avoidance in women: A study of weight stigma, body-related shame and guilt, and healthcare stress. *Body Image.* Jun;25:139-147.139–147.

O'Hara, L., and Taylor, J. (2018). What's wrong with the war on obesity? SAGE Open, April-June. https://doi.org/10.1177/2158244018772888.

Puhl, R.M. (2009). The stigma of obesity: A review and update. *Obesity.* doi:10.1038/oby.2008.636.

Puhl, R., and Suh, Y. (2015). Health consequences of weight stigma: Implications for obesity prevention and treatement. *Current Obesity Reports.* doi 10.1007/s13679-015-0153-z.

Rodin, J. (1992). *Body Traps.* New York: William Morrow.

Rudd Report. (2009). Weight Bias: A Social Justice Issue Policy Brief. Yale University.

Stice E. et al. (2009). An effectiveness trial of a dissonance-based eating disorder prevention program for high-risk adolescent girls. *Journal of Consulting and Clinical Psychology* 77(5):825–834. [http://bit.ly/bw6gLV].

Tomiyama, A.J., et al. (2016). Misclassification of cardiometabolic health when using body mass index categories in NHANES 2005–2012. *International Journal of Obesity* doi:10.1038/ijo.2016.17.

Tomiyama, A.J., et al. (2018). How and why weight stigma drives the obesity "epidemic" and harms health. BioMed Central *(BMC) Medicine* 16:123.

Tylka, TL and Piran, Niva (editors), Handbook of Positive Body Image and Embodiment, *Constructs, Protective Factors, and Interventions*, Chapter 7: Intuitive Eating by Elyse Resch and Tracy Tylka, pp. 68–79.

Wildman, R.P., et al. (2008). The obese without cardiometabolic risk factor clustering and the normal weight with cardiometabolic risk factor clustering prevalence and correlates of 2 phenotypes among the US population. *Archives of Internal Medicine* 168(15):1617–24. doi: 10.1001/archinte.168.15.1617.

Wiseman, C., et al. (1992). Cultural expectations of thinness in women: An update. *International Journal of Eating Disorders* 11(1):85–89.

Wu, Y., and Berry, D. (2017). Impact of weight stigma on physiological and psychological health outcomes for overweight and obese adults: A systematic review. *Journal of Advanced Nursing.* doi: 10.1111/jan.13511.

Chapter 14. Principle 9: Movement—Feel the Difference

American College of Sports Medicine, Academy of Nutrition and Dietetics, Dietitians of Canada (2016). Nutrition and Athletic Performance. *Medicine & Science in Sports & Exercise*, 48(3): 543–568.

American College of Sports Medicine. (1990). Position stand: The recommended quantity and quality of exercise for developing and maintaining cardiorespiratory and muscular fitness in healthy adults. *Medicine & Science in Sports & Exercise* 22:265–274.

American College of Sports Medicine. (1998). Position stand: The recommended quantity and quality of exercise for developing and maintaining cardiorespiratory and muscular fitness, and flexibility in healthy adults. *Medicine & Science in Sports & Exercise* 30(6):975–991.

American College of Sports Medicine. (1993). (Press Release). Experts release new recommendations to fight America's epidemic of physical inactivity, July 29.

American College of Sports Medicine. (2011). Two minutes of exercise a day can keep the pain away, June 3. [http://bit.ly/mdFUog accessed June 10, 2011].

Calogero, R., and Pedrotty, K. (2007). Daily practices for mindful exercise. In L. L'Abate, D. Embry, and M. Baggett (eds.), *Handbook of Low-Cost Preventive Interventions for Physical and Mental Health: Theory, Research, and Practice,* pages 141–160). New York: Springer-Verlag.

Chaput, J.C. (2011). Physical activity plays an important role in body weight regulation. *Journal of Obesity*, article ID 360257, 11 pages. doi:10.1155/2011/360257.

Costill, D.L. (1988). Carbohydrates for exercise: Dietary demands for optimal performance. *International Journal of Sports Medicine* 9:5.

Evans, B., and Rosenberg, I. (1991). *Biomarkers: The 10 Determinants of Aging You Can Control*. New York: Simon and Schuster.

Foreyt, J., et al. (1993). Response of free-living adults to beavioral treament of obesity: Attrition and compliance to exercise. *Behavior Therapy* 24:659–669.

Gandey, A. (2011). Exercise reduces silent brain infarcts. *Medscape News,* June 10.

Garber et. al. (2011). Position Stand. Quantity and Quality of Exercise for Developing and Maintaining Cardiorespiratory, Musculoskeletal, and Neuromotor Fitness in Apparently Healthy Adults: Guidance for Prescribing Exercise. *Medicine & Science in Sports & Exercise*: 43(7): 1334–1359.

Gavin, J. (1992). *The Exercise Habit*. Champaign, IL: Human Kinetics.

Lemon, P.W.R., and Mullin, J.P. (1980). Effect of initial muscle glycogen levels on protein catabolism during exercise. *Journal of Applied Physiology: Respiratory, Environmental and Exercise Physiology.* 48(4):624–629.

McGuire, K., and Ross, R. (2011). Incidental physical activity is positively associated with cardiorespiratory fitness. *Medicine & Science in Sports & Exercise.* doi: 10.1249/MSS.0b013e31821e4ff2.

Miller, W.C. (1994). Exercise: Americans don't think it's worth it. *Obesity & Health* Mar–Apr:29.

Pollock, M.L., et al. (1987). Effect of age and training on aerobic capacity and body composition of master athletes. *Journal of Applied Physiology* 62:725–731.

Tryon, W.W., Goldberg, J.L., and Morrison, D.F. (1992). Activity decreases as percentage overweight increases. *International Journal of Obesity* 16:591–595.

Chapter 15. Principle 10: Honor Your Health with Gentle Nutrition

2010 Dietary Guidelines. [http://www.cnpp.usda.gov/dietaryguidelines.htm accessed May 30, 2011.

Basdevant, A. (1995). Prevalence of binge eating disorder in different populations of French women. *International Journal of Eating Disorders* 18(4):309–315.

Beardsley, E. (2009). In Paris, culinary education starts in day care. NPR, February 16.

Calder, P. (2010). The American Heart Association advisory on n-6 fatty acids: Evidence based or biased evidence? *British Journal of Nutrition* 104(11):1575–1576.

Callaway, W. (1992). The marriage of taste and health: A union whose time has come. *Nutrition Today* 27(3):37–42.

CDC. Social Determinants of Health: Frequently Asked Questions [https://www.cdc.gov/nchhstp/socialdeterminants/faq.html accessed 11/27/19]

CDC. Adverse Childhood Experiences (ACEs). #Vitalsigns November 2019. [https://www.cdc.gov/vitalsigns/aces/index.html accessed 11/27/19]

Egolf, B., et al. (1992). The Roseto Effect: A 50-year comparison of mortality rates. *American Journal of Public Health* 82:1089–1092.

Evans, H.M., et al. (1928). A new dietary deficiency with highly purified diets: The beneficial effect of fat in the diet. *Proceedings of the Society for Experimental Biology and Medicine* 25:390–397.

Felitti V.J. et. al. (1998). Relationship of childhood abuse and household dysfunction to many of the leading causes of death in adults: the adverse childhood experiences (ACE) study external icon. *American Journal of Preventive Medicine.* 1998;14:245–258.

Getz, L. (2009). Orthorexia: When eating healthy becomes an unhealthy obsession. *Today's Dietitian,* June, page 40.

Glore, S.R., et al. (1994). Soluble fiber and serum lipids: A literature review. *Journal of the American Dietetic Association* 94:425–436.

Guyenet, S. (2008). Butter, margarine and heart disease. *Whole Health Source,* December 27.

Holt-Lundstad J, Robles, T., Sbarra D. (2017). Advancing Social Connection as a Public Health Priority in the United States. *American Psychologist* 72(6):517–530.

Ledoux, S. (1991). Eating disorders among adolescents in an unselected French population. *International Journal of Eating Disorder* 10(1):81–89.

Mazidi, M., et al. (2019). Lower carbohydrate diets and all-cause and cause-specific mortality: A population-based cohort study and pooling of prospective studies. *European Heart Journal* 40(34):2870–2879.

McCargar, L.J., et al. (1993). Physiological effects of weight cycling in female lightweight rowers. *Canadian Journal of Applied Physiology* 18(3):291–303.

McEwen, B. (2008). Central effects of stress hormones in health and disease: Understanding the protective and damaging effects of stress and stress mediators. *European Journal of Pharmacology* 583(2–3):174–185.

National Research Council. (1989). *Recommended Dietary Allowances.* National Academy of Sciences: Washington, D.C., pages 46–49.

The Nobel Prize in Physiology or Medicine 2005 was awarded jointly to Barry J. Marshall and J. Robin Warren "for their discovery of the bacterium *Helicobacter pylori* and its role in gastritis and peptic ulcer disease." The Nobel Prize in Physiology or Medicine 2005. NobelPrize.org. Nobel Media AB 2019. [Accessed Tue. 26 Nov 2019 .https://www.nobelprize.org/prizes/medicine/2005/summary/]

OECD. (2010). *OECD Factbook 2010: Economic, Environmental and Social Statistics.* OECD Publishing.

Ramsden, C.E., et al. (2010). Omega 6 fatty acid-specific and mixed polyunsaturate dietary interventions have different effects on CHD risk: A meta-analysis of randomized controlled trials. *British Journal of Nutrition* 104:1586-1600.

Rozin, P. (1993). Food and cuisine: Education, risk and pleasure. *Journal of Gastronomy* 7(1):111–120.

Rozin, P. (1999). Food is fundamental, fun, frightening, and far-reaching. *Social Research* 66:9–30.

Rozin, P., et al. (1999). Attitudes to food and the role of food in the life in the USA,

Japan, Flemish Belgium and France: Possible implications for the diet-health debate. *Appetite* (33):163–180.

Rozin, P., et al. (2003). The ecology of eating: Smaller portion sizes in France than in the United States help explain the French paradox. *Psychological Science* 14(5):450–454.

Schardt, D. (1994). Phytochemicals: Plants against cancer. *Nutrition Action Health Letter* 21(3):1.

Schneeman, B., et al. (2006). The regulatory process to revise nutrient labeling relative to the dietary reference intakes. *American Journal Clinical Nutrition* 83(5):1228S–1230S.

Scrinis, G. (2008). On the ideology of nutritionism. *Gastronomica: The Journal of Food and Culture* 8(1):39–48.

Stacey, M. (1994). *Consumed: Why Americans Love, Hate, and Fear Food*. New York: Simon and Schuster.

Stout, C., et al. (1964). Unusually low incidence of death from myocardial infarction: Study of an Italian American community in Pennsylvania. *Journal of the American Medical Association* 188(10):845–849.

Thompson, J.L., et al. (1996). Effects of diet and diet-plus-exercise programs on resting metabolic rate: A meta-analysis. *International Journal of Sport Nutrition* (6):41–61.

Urban, N., et al. (1992). Correlates of maintenance of a low-fat diet among women in the women's health trial. *Preventive Medicine* 21:279–291.

USDA. (1992). Human Nutrition Service. *USDA's Food Guide Pyramid*. Home and Garden bulletin, no. 249, April.

USDHH. (1990). Healthy People 2000. *Nutrition Today*. 25(6):29–39.

WebMD. (2008). The Olympic diet of Michael Phelps. [http://www.webmd.com/diet /news/20080813/the-olympic-diet-of-michael-phelps accessed May 23, 2011].

Wolf, S., et al. (1974). Roseto revisited: Further data on the incidence of myocardial infarction in Roseto and neighboring Pennsylvania communities. *Transactions of the American Clinical Climatological Association* 85:100–108.

Chapter 16. Raising an Intuitive Eater: What Works with Kids and Teens

American Academy of Pediatrics. (2016). [https://www.aap.org/en-us/aap-voices/Pages /Minding-Childrens-Media-Use.aspx].

Bacon, L. *Body Respect: What Conventional Health Books Get Wrong, Leave out, and Just Plain Fail to Understand About Weight*. Dallas: BenBella Books, page 30.

Birch, L.L., Fisher, J.O., and Davison, K.K. (2003). Learning to overeat: Maternal use of restrictive feeding practices promotes girls' eating in the absence of hunger. *American Journal of Clinical Nutrition* 78: 215–220.

Carper, J.L., Fisher, J.O., and Birch, L.L. Young girls' emerging dietary restraint and disinhibition are related to parental control in child feeding. *Appetite* 35:121–129.

Eneli, I.U., Crum, L.P.A., and Tylka, T.R. (2008). The trust model: A different feeding paradigm. *Obesity* 16:2197–2204.

Field, A.E., et al. (2003). Relation between dieting and weight change among preadolescents and adolescents. *Pediatrics* 112:900–906.

Neumark-Sztainer, D., et al. (2007). Why does dieting predict weight gain in adolescents? Findings from Project EAT-II: A 5-year longitudinal study. *Journal of the American Dietetic Association* 107:448–455.

Rapley, G., and Murkett, T. (2010). *Baby-Led Weaning: The Essential Guide to Introducing Solid Foods and Helping Your Baby to Grow up a Happy and Confident Eater.* New York: The Experiment Publishing Company.

Resch, E. (2019). *The Intuitive Eating Workbook for Teens.* Oakland, CA: New Harbinger.

Satter, E.M. (2000). *Child of Mine, Feeding with Love and Common Sense.* Boulder, CO: Bull Publishing Company.

Satter, E.M. (2005). *Your Child's Weight: Helping Without Harming.* Madison, WI: Kelcy Press.

Schilling, L., and Peterson, W.J. (2017). *Born to Eat: Whole, Healthy Foods from Baby's First Bite.* New York: Skyhorse Publishing.

Chapter 17. The Ultimate Path Toward Healing from Eating Disorders

American Psychiatric Association (APA). (2006). *Practice Guideline for the Treatment of Patients with Eating Disorders,* 3rd edition. Washington, D.C.: American Psychiatric Association (APA).

Galmiche M. et al (2019). Prevalence of eating disorders over the 2000-2018 period: a systematic literature review. *American Journal of Clinical Nutrition* 19:1402–1413.

Tribole, E. (2006). Intuitive Eating in the treatment of disordered eating. *SCAN's Pulse,* Summer.

Tribole, E. (2009). Intuitive Eating: Can you be healthy and eat anything? *Eating Disorders Recovery Today,* Winter.

Tribole, E. (2010). Intuitive Eating in the treatment of eating disorders: The journey of attunement. *Perspectives* Winter: 11–14.

Intuitive Eating Official Website
www.IntuitiveEating.org
Get the latest news from our blog and calendar of events. You will also find articles, research, interviews, and general information about Intuitive Eating.

Intuitive Eating audio CD, Sounds True, 2009
This is a set of four CDs and is an excellent companion to our book. It focuses on the practical "how-to" aspects of Intuitive Eating. This is a discussion format with guided practices, not a verbatim reading of the book.

***The Intuitive Eating Workbook*, New Harbinger, 2017**
As a complement to *Intuitive Eating,* this workbook offers a multitude of exercises and practices to help hone your skills as an Intuitive Eater. This workbook has been validated by studies that show increases in body appreciation, overall intuitive eating, and satisfaction with life!

***The Intuitive Eating Workbook for Teens*, New Harbinger, 2019**
A nondiet, body-positive approach written for teens and the teen within each of us. Drawing on the same evidence-based practices introduced in *Intuitive Eating,* the activities within the workbook will help you learn to listen to your body's wisdom, break out of diet mentality, and learn to fully enjoy your food.

Social Media
Facebook: www.facebook.com/IntuitiveEating/
Instagram: @evelyntribole @elyseresch #IntuitiveEatingOfficial

Counseling and Support

Certified Intuitive Eating Counselor Directory
https://www.intuitiveeating.org/certified-counselors/
www.IntuitiveEatingCounselorDirectory.org
This is a listing of allied health professionals who are trained and certified in the Intuitive Eating process. We receive numerous requests for local Intuitive Eating health professionals. To help fill this gap, we offer certification for allied health professionals. These health professionals include dietitians, psychotherapists, physicians, physical therapists, nurses, chiropractors, dentists, occupational therapists, licensed massage therapists, licensed physical trainers, certified health education specialists, licensed health and life coaches, and others in the health profession who espouse the Intuitive Eating principles in their work.

Intuitive Eating Online Community
www.IntuitiveEatingCommunity.org
Get inspired, share your story, and partake of the many tools to empower your Intuitive Eating journey. This is your community—it's free, but you will need to sign up.

Professional Resources

How to Become a Certified Intuitive Eating Counselor
We are eager to spread the message of Intuitive Eating through allied health professionals who qualify to be certified and listed on our Intuitive Eating Counselor Directory. There are three key steps to becoming a certified Intuitive Eating Counselor:

1. Complete a self-study program administered by Helm Publishing that is based on the *Intuitive Eating* book and *The Intuitive Eating Workbook*. This is an independent study on your own schedule. For more information, see: http://bit.ly /IEPROSelf-Study.
2. Participate in an Intuitive Eating Pro Skills training with Evelyn and supervision with either Elyse or Evelyn.

For more details and information, see these websites:

www.intuitiveeating.org
www.EvelynTribole.com

www.ElyseResch.com
www.IntuitiveEatingProTraining.com

3. Upon completion of the self-study program, the teleseminar, supervision, and passing an exam, you qualify as a Certified Intuitive Eating Counselor.

Intuitive Eating Client Worksheets

www.Intuitive-Eating-Worksheets.com

Help your clients through the Intuitive Eating process by using this easy-to-use, reproducible set of twenty-one worksheets.

Index

About the Authors

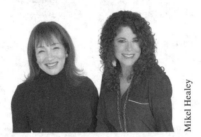

Mikel Healey

EVELYN TRIBOLE, MS, RDN, CEDRD-S (Certified Eating Disorder Registered Dietitian-Supervisor) is the author of nine books, with a private practice in Newport Beach, California. She enjoys training health professionals from around the world on how to help their clients cultivate a healthy relationship with food, mind, and body through the process of Intuitive Eating. As an international speaker and workshop leader, Evelyn is passionate and has been called, "Wonderfully wise and funny." Previously, she was the nutrition expert for *Good Morning America,* a national spokesperson for the Academy of Nutrition and Dietetics, and a contributing editor for *Shape* magazine, where her monthly column appeared for eleven years. The media often seeks Evelyn for her expertise, appearing in hundreds of interviews, including CNN, NBC's *Today Show,* MSNBC, *Fox News, USA Today, The Wall Street Journal, The Atlantic, Ten Percent Happier,* and *People.* Evelyn qualified for the Olympic Trials in the first ever women's marathon in 1984. Although she no longer competes, she is a wicked ping-pong player and avid hiker. Her favorite food is chocolate—when it can be savored slowly.

ELYSE RESCH, MS, RDN, CEDRD-S, FIAEDP, FADA, FAND, is a nutrition therapist in private practice in Beverly Hills, California, with thirty-eight years of experience, specializing in eating disorders, Intuitive Eating, and Health at Every Size. She is the author of *The Intuitive Eating Workbook for Teens,* the co-author of *Intuitive Eating* and *The Intuitive Eating Workbook,* a chapter contributor to the *Handbook of Positive Body Image and Embodiment,* and has published journal articles, print articles, and blog posts. She also does regular speaking engagements, podcasts, and extensive media interviews. Her work has been profiled on NPR, CNN, KABC, NBC, KTTV, *Los Angeles Times,* Associated Press, KFI Radio, *USA Today,* and *HuffPost,* among others. Resch is nationally known for her work in helping patients break free from diet culture through the Intuitive Eating process. Her philosophy embraces the goal of developing body positivity, with the belief that all bodies deserve dignity, and reconnecting with one's internal wisdom about eating. She supervises and trains health professionals, and is a Certified Eating Disorder Registered Dietitian-Supervisor, a fellow of the International Association of Eating Disorders Professionals, and a fellow of the Academy of Nutrition and Dietetics.

BASED ON THE WISDOM OF *INTUITIVE EATING*

Learn how to reject diet culture and raise our next generation to have a healthy relationship with food and their bodies.

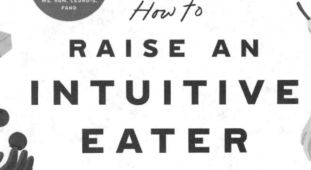

WITH A FOREWORD BY **ELYSE RESCH,** MS, RDN, CEDRD-S, FAND

How to

RAISE AN INTUITIVE EATER

Raising the Next Generation with

FOOD AND BODY CONFIDENCE

SUMNER BROOKS, *and* **AMEE SEVERSON,**
MPH, RDN · MPP-D, RDN

AVAILABLE WHEREVER BOOKS ARE SOLD

ST. MARTIN'S ESSENTIALS